The Spiral of Love

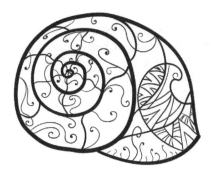

Robert W.H. Wilkins, "Woody"

Cover and Interior Design by Woven Red Author Services, www.wovenred.ca

The Spiral of Love/Robert W.H. Wilkins—1st edition
ISBN hardback large print: 978-0-9966575-5-6
ISBN paperback: 978-0-9966575-3-2
ISBN ebook: 978-0-9966575-4-9

Library of Congress Control Number: 2020910205

Printed in the United States of America

Published by Woody's Wooden Wonders Publishing
A division of Woody's Wooden Wonders, LLC
80 Olde Orchard Road, Clinton, CT 06413
Email: woodyswwpublishing@gmail.com

The information provided in this book is based on the personal experience of the author and is not intended as a medical manual. The information should not be used as a substitute for professional medical care.

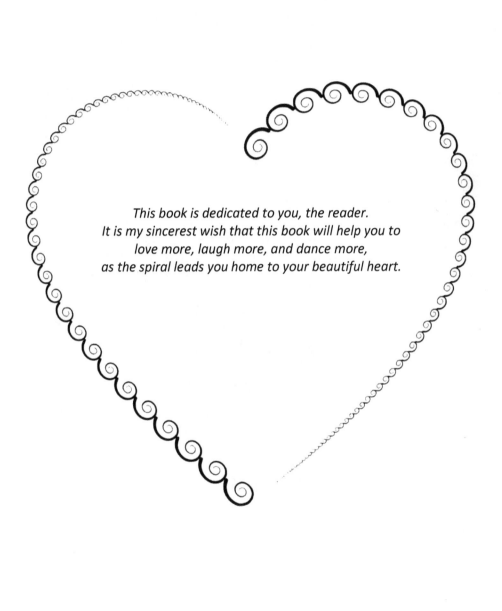

This book is dedicated to you, the reader.
It is my sincerest wish that this book will help you to
love more, laugh more, and dance more,
as the spiral leads you home to your beautiful heart.

Table of Contents

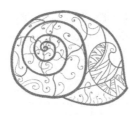

Chapter 1

Tears at Daybreak

I woke up crying at 5:00 a.m. on a rainy Monday morning. The first thing I did was clench my fist and punch the pillow next to me where my husband's head once lay. Thirty-six days ago, I told my husband to get the hell out of my bed. He went, and he has not come back. Thirty-six days ago, I thought we were in love. I thought our love would last forever. Thirty-six days ago, that love left with him. Thirty-six days ago, I was diagnosed with breast cancer. Now, my heart feels like a derelict building on the outskirts of the abandoned city I once called my marriage. There are three fears inside of me. I fear that I will never find love again. I fear that I am not worthy of love. And the biggest fear of all is that I do not know what love is.

My cancer diagnosis was like a bomb going off. My life just fell apart after it. I had been like a little girl in love with a beautiful balloon called my marriage. Then one day, a needle came along in the form of a cancer diagnosis, and pop! It was gone. Twenty-four years of marriage zapped, gone, vanished from sight. Love, what is it? Even the thought of it makes me nauseous now. I was raised believing that love was the answer. I was programmed to find someone to love. Like a heat-seeking missile, I was launched into adult life. *Mission accomplished*, I thought. How wrong I was. Whatever that thing that I called *love* was, it had only brought pain. I gave what I thought was my heart to a man who I thought loved me. Then the bastard deserted me.

I remember the moment it happened. It was at 2:38 p.m., thirty-six days earlier. My husband and I were sitting in two sterile chairs across from the paper-laden desk of my doctor. She was a bespectacled, chubby woman whose complexion matched her clinical white coat. She was sitting on the other side of her desk, flipping through my chart. She closed the file and slowly brought her eyes up to meet mine.

Her eyes were blank. She was looking at me, but it did not seem as if she was seeing me. She lacked balls. I knew she was struggling to find the right words. I also knew the words were bad. She coughed into the palm of her hand and then began talking. "Mrs. Harris...Jane, I regret to inform you that you have advanced breast cancer. Stage two." She kept talking, but I did not register the words. The words *breast cancer* echoed savagely in my head. Then I thought, *This is a dream, right? Any minute now, the alarm will go off and rescue me.* But there was no alarm. This was no dream.

When my doctor said I had breast cancer, my reaction was numbness and disbelief—a sort of "this is not really happening to me, right?" reaction.

When the words *breast cancer* left my doctor's mouth, I felt an immediate chill from my husband next to me. I waited for him to extend his warm hand to take mine, but it never came. I waited for him to wrap his arm around my shoulders to comfort me, but it never came. I waited for some warm, whispered words of comfort, but they never came. We both sat like statues frozen in an icy block of fear-filled emotion. We drove home in silence.

The evening was strange as we pretended to watch TV. We were remote with each other. At bedtime, I thought we would find a way to connect. I longed for his touch, his comfort, his warmth. He would rescue me from my icy prison, right? Wrong. Our usual bedtime ritual was well established. I went to bed around nine, leaving my husband to watch some news and sports on TV. I would have a little time to myself to read a romance novel. Around nine thirty, my husband would come to bed. Then we shared the part of our togetherness that I loved the best. He would climb into bed and roll his long, strong body toward me, and I would curl in his arms, where I felt like a child in the womb, a bear in a cave, like a piece of dark chocolate held between moist lips. It was like going to church.

I loved weekends the most. He would place his big warm hands gently on my body, and I could feel a pulsing of energy before he slowly began moving them. They would be seeking a point of entry into the magic kingdom of my pajamas. On weekends, I always left a couple of buttons undone, and it made me feel sexy. He had a soft, sensuous touch, and he knew how to tease and induce my arousal. I loved the way he made me feel. First would come the fleeting, teasing winds of passion deep in my groin, and from there they would spread throughout my body.

I loved his slowness. He would touch with a gentle pulsing, pressure, and wait. He knew the faint stir my body made. Then his hands would move again, ever so gently, like a pilgrim en route to the promised land, pausing at intervals to pray. The energy of his touch communicated the stir of his own growing arousal.

Our Friday and Saturday nights were glorious. He became a beautiful ocean, breaking on the beach of my naked body. His waves pulsed over and into me. I crested with him. Mornings would bring another surging, relentless tide. I loved lying with him in our tossed sheets with the scent of our love juices filling the air. Then the aroma of Italian roast would drift into our bedroom. He loved his tech toys, and I remember his beaming smile when he brought home a coffee pot with a timer. He was an artist of the sensual.

On the evening of my cancer diagnosis, I headed up to bed at my usual hour and waited. I hoped and prayed that soon his caring touch and loving embrace would engulf me. I lay in bed, waiting for the sound of his footsteps on the stairs. At 9:45 p.m., there was still no sound of footsteps. I felt the cold embrace of rejection as I lay alone, feeling sad, feeling abandoned.

At ten came the long-awaited footsteps on the stairs. I felt my longing for him stir. My rescue was close, or so I thought. The usual sounds emanated from our bathroom. His touch, his embrace, his warmth, all closer now. I lowered the two bedside lamps to a soft glow. I readied my body; I awaited his arms.

With my eyes half closed, I heard his soft footsteps come to the far side of the bed. I felt the weight of his body lower onto the mattress. I waited for the roll of his body toward me, but it never came. I waited for his long, caring arms to wrap themselves around me. But they never came. He just lay there. We just lay there. Like two corpses with a great frozen divide between us.

I felt a burning at the back of my eyes as tears gathered like an angry crowd. The silent seconds of loneliness became minutes. We lay apart in coffins of emotional ice. Then, I could wait no longer. I whispered softly, "Honey, you okay?"

Silence. I knew he was not sleeping. In a slightly louder whisper, I tried again. "David, you okay?"

Not even a stir. Then something sharp inside my heart prodded me, and I sat up and turned the lights up. He was lying flat on his back, staring up at the ceiling. A bolt of fear struck deep inside my heart. Then came anger. "Look at me!" I demanded in a loud, shrill voice.

He couldn't. I could feel anger surging in me. "Touch me!" I demanded.

He rolled his head from side to side.

Then my fear became rage. "Then get the hell out of my bed!" I screamed. The venom in my voice scared me. His distance scared me more.

Slowly, he rose, directing his eyes away from me. I remember the pain of disbelief I felt. He could not even look at me. He made his way slowly to the closet. With clothes draped over his arm, he walked to the bathroom. Ten minutes later, I heard his car start and pull out of the driveway.

I felt sucked into an abyss of darkness and fear. Would he come back? How could I face cancer alone? More than a month later, I still woke up crying each morning. And the first thing I did was curl my hand into a fist and hit his pillow. At first, I felt I was hitting him. Then he turned into my breast cancer. Then I was punching love for how it had betrayed me.

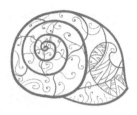

Chapter 2

A Traffic Delay

As the darkness slowly gave way to the light of day, the rain felt kind and comforting and somehow parallel to my life. As my thoughts about the day ahead began to form into some coherent order, I remembered that this was my chemo day, and I had an appointment at the clinic. A big, dark lump of anxiety and dread formed in my stomach.

Beep, beep went the alarm, and as I reached out to turn it off, I hit the radio button instead. I was shocked to hear the words of my husband's favorite country song, "We Ain't Never Coming Back." He loved that song. I hated it. I think my husband had some deep romantic notion of wanting to be a cowboy. He would often talk about buying cowboy boots but never did. Now I hated the song more than ever. The sound of it stirred anger in me, and I gave the off button a sharp thump. I slowly dragged my body to the edge of the bed and put my feet on the floor. The silence of the house seemed to echo my sense of desperate loneliness. Love had lived here once. Now love was gone, and I was left with a hurting heart.

Even though my husband had proved himself to be a miserable, cowardly asshole, I still missed his presence in the morning. The loneliness seemed more painful on chemo days. I think it was because I knew that at the end of the day, I would return to an empty house. The only good thing about clinic days was that I could dress casually. I was simply one cancer patient among many. Gray, oversized sweats was the dress of choice. But not for me; I couldn't do the gray-sweats-in-public thing and always opted for a stylish sweater and jeans.

When I was not busy being a cancer patient, I spent my days working for a grant-writing agency. I took the position for a year, twenty-four years ago. My husband said we needed steady income for the first year as he got his financial-services company up and running. It was supposed to be temporary until I found a way to launch my creative writing career. I had a master's degree in English lit and had always loved writing short stories. In my wildest dreams, I saw myself being headhunted by a Hollywood film studio to write award-winning scripts. I had given myself twelve months as a grant writer before the fast track of writing success would carry me away. It was my fantasy life to have agents and book publishers camping out at my door to get my signature on lucrative book contracts.

And here I was, twenty-four miserable, frickin' years later. My love for writing had rotted like compost inside of me. I had become a churner of grants for non-profit organizations. I had become a hired gun, only my gun was a pen.

I was well and truly trapped in my life. What I thought was love had ensnared me. I had been the sacrificial lamb, giving up my own dreams in the name of our marriage and the love I thought we shared. I had been blind to how one-sided it had been. I was a chained dog living in a compound.

One of the chains was the large mortgage for the ridiculously big house in which we lived. This was David's doing. He was now a wealth-management consultant and he needed the image of a big house in an expensive neighborhood. David never talked about his work. He gave me the sense that he thought it was a little beyond my reach. He was the expert, and who the hell was I? Just a little old wordsmith? On reflection, I realize that this was just one of the many ways he controlled me and kept me small.

I spent my days grinding out soulless grant requests for a regular paycheck and the medical benefits he kept saying we needed. As for David, he was living the good life. Once a month, he would take off for a week on an all-expenses-paid trip to some exotic place to discuss wealth with one of his clients. Never an invitation for me to join him. I had to keep my nose to the wheel to keep up with the mortgage payments. How lost and blind I had been.

His income was commission-based, and he kept a separate bank account where his commission was deposited. He would transfer a certain amount into our shared bank account to keep us in the black. He kept saying this gave us a tax advantage, but he never explained it to me. Because I loved him, or thought I loved him, I gave him blind trust. I thought that by keeping him happy, it would keep us happy. Geesh, big mistake, that one. I had joined the headless-chicken club of disempowered wives.

I glanced at the clock and saw that it was time to stir my still-weary body into action. First stop, the shower. There was something comforting about standing under warm, running water. In the absence of human touch, this helped me to feel my body again. After my shower came the donning of clothes. I picked a brightly colored sweater and a stylish pair of old, worn jeans. Then came some light makeup, and it was time for Henry—that's what I called my wig. I had lost my hair after the first two chemo treatments, and Henry had become essential to getting through each day. It was a love/hate relationship. I hated Henry for all it represented and for how it symbolized my cancer. I loved it for allowing me to hide from the world. Henry and I had forged an amicable, negotiated, working relationship.

Although I had been bald for three weeks, I still got a dark, sinking feeling deep inside my stomach every time I saw my head in the mirror. I would narrow my eyes and squint a little to blur the sight of my baldness. I kept Henry in the bathroom cupboard behind doors. Keeping him locked away seemed to give me some sense of control. It was, I admit, a pretty futile form of control.

So here I was, washed and made up. I opened the cupboard door, eased Henry out, and positioned him on my head. Now it was time for the fixing gel. All it needed was a few small dabs around the edges, and I was good for the windiest of days. I kept the gel in the top drawer of my sink unit. I pulled open the drawer and reached inside. As I picked up the tube, I immediately realized that it was hard. *Oh crap!* I thought, as I remembered being in a rush the previous day. I had tossed the tube into the drawer without putting the cap back on. Now it was rock solid. Then I remembered that it was a chemo day, and the clinic would have a new tube for me. All I had to do was pray there was no wind and make my way very carefully from the parking lot to the clinic.

Next was a cup of herb tea. I really wanted strong, dark, Italian roast, but my doctor said the tea would help me detox. Then I had one slice of gluten-free toast, which felt like porous cardboard. I lavished it with peanut butter as I said a plaintive prayer for strength to get through the day. I glanced at my watch and noted that time was on my side. It was 8:30 a.m., and my appointment was for nine with a fifteen-minute drive. Pulling out of my driveway, I put a talk show on the radio to distract me from the heaviness I was feeling inside. Chemo days sucked.

I had just pulled onto the highway when I saw it, a long winding line of red lights ahead of me. The highway was a parking lot. *Unbelievable*, I thought, giving the steering wheel a thump of frustration. I reached for my phone to call the clinic to let them know and change my appointment. The clinic's receptionist Deborah was rude and cold. She had a miserable attitude, and my interactions with her were always strained. Deborah answered with a curt "hello." Caller ID told her who was calling, and in a smug way, she said that she knew I would be late and had already shifted my appointment to 10:45. She did not say, but I knew, that one of the doctors lived in my neighborhood, which is how she knew about the traffic. Geesh, she was a bitch.

With a dull sense of resignation, I sank back in my seat and took a piece of sugar-free gum from my bag. A few minutes passed, and the cars in front of me started to move very slowly. They were being ushered off an emergency exit to a B road. This was going to be a very, very slow journey.

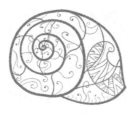

Chapter 3

The Coffee Shop

Stop, crawl, stop crawl, on and on the traffic went. I had been off the highway for about a mile when I saw a funny-looking building with a large sign advertising, "Good Coffee." I was feeling really down and thought that a cup of kick-ass coffee would brighten my mood. A flip of the steering wheel, and I pulled into the parking lot. The building was an old house that had been converted into a sort of quirky coffee place. I parked near the door and checked Henry in the mirror to make sure he was on straight.

The rain had become a drizzle, and I held Henry in place for the few short paces to the door. As I pushed against it, it jammed on the bottom and jerked me backward, making Henry slip down to one side. Oh crap! I stood in the doorway, and the people in the coffee shop seemed frozen in shock. *Oh no, this is not happening*, I thought. Seated patrons were looking at me. Do I turn and run? Or give the game away by pulling Henry back into position? Or should I just pretend it's a new hairstyle? I felt vulnerable and embarrassed. The backs of my eyes began to burn, and I knew tears were close. It had been a simple plan: walk in slowly, get a coffee, and walk gently back to my car. Suddenly, cancer had ambushed me. The instant exposure made me want to run and hide. Instead, I took a deep breath and locked my eyes on the back of the head of the person at the end of the queue.

Even though I was on the verge of tears, I decided to push through and move forward. I could feel my throat beginning to close. I wasn't sure I could get the word *latte* out. I visualized a plan. When it was my turn at the counter, I would keep my head down to avoid eye contact and pretend to fumble through my purse as I said the word *latte*. That was it. I could do that, right? There were two people in front of me, and when I glanced over their shoulders to the cashier, I got a real shock. The young woman behind the counter wore alarming makeup. Thick, dark circles of black eyeliner and dark, blood-red lipstick stood out against her whiter-than-white complexion, and her black hair was streaked with red. She also wore a large, rather disconcerting silver ring through her nose. *This*, I thought, *is one scary-looking woman*. The best I could figure out was that she must be what they call a Goth. I had seen photographs in magazines of similar women with bizarre-looking makeup. I had read in a self-help book that naming something you fear will minimize that fear. I never discovered if this actually worked, but in this pressured, fragile moment, I decided to give her the name *Goth Girl*.

She was, one scary-ass looking lady. And she was going to serve me coffee? The line moved slowly forward; there was no backing out now.

I furtively stole another glance of her over the shoulder of the person in front of me. Though she looked scary and intense, I could also see a real sense of precision in how she had made herself up. It must have taken hours. And her hair, jet black with bright-red streaks, was beautifully groomed and cared for. I had to admit that there was a strange sort of beauty about her. I also sensed a rebellious freedom in her that some deep, lost part of me yearned for.

As the line moved forward, I rehearsed keeping my head down and saying *latte* without making eye contact with Goth Girl. I would swipe my credit card, pick up my latte, and then lopsided Henry and I could beat a speedy retreat. The plan was good. Or so I thought. I was still on the verge of tears. I could feel Henry slanted down over one eye and thought how odd I must look. Would people guess it was a wig? Could they guess I had breast cancer? I suddenly felt very conspicuous—as if my cancer was on display—which added to my fragility.

The woman in front of me moved away with her drink. "Next," Goth Girl said.

As per my plan, I pulled out my purse and pretended to look through it as I order a latte with my head down. Goth Girl did not move. There was silence. She must not have heard me. I could feel tears forming in my eyes. *She needs a latte size*, I thought. I summoned all my remaining emotional energy and made the effort to say, "Large latte." Still, Goth Girl did not move. More silence. Then, very slowly, I looked up to find Goth Girl's piercing eyes locked onto me. A tear rolled down my cheek, and I tightened my lips. I was cornered with no way out. Goth Girl turned to a colleague prepping a coffee pot and said, "Hey, Mare. Cover me for five, will ya?"

A tall, thin girl in blue jeans and a white shirt said, "Got it, Dar," and moved toward the counter. Goth Girl did not say anything. With her penetrating eyes upon me, she pointed to the right, toward a quiet corner of the coffee shop. Then she tipped her head sideways as if to say, "Follow me." Meekly, I followed her to the end of the counter, where she met me on the other side of a big Coke machine. Goth Girl did not say a word. She walked out from behind the counter, opened her arms, and wrapped them around me. It was then that my fragile emotional control broke, and I crumpled into her protective, caring arms, sobbing uncontrollably.

I was out of control now and lost in the white water of my emotional brokenness.

She kept whispering, "Just breathe, honey. I've got you. I've got you. I've got you." For a few minutes that seemed like an eternity, my tears poured out onto her shoulder, and my body convulsed with overflowing sadness and despair.

Slowly, I regained my sense of control and pulled away from her. Through my tears, I looked questioningly into her eyes, wanting to know what had just happened. Her piercing eyes locked onto mine, and she whispered, "Please don't move, honey." Then she lifted her hands and with great tenderness caught hold of the right and left sides of Henry and centered it on my head. I was stunned, shocked, embarrassed, speechless. And what she did next completely hit me into left field. From her pocket, she pulled a tube of wig gel and squeezed small, clear globs onto three of her fingers. Gently lifting one corner of Henry at a time, she dabbed gel on my hairline and then softly pressed Henry in place. She did it just as they had taught me in the clinic.

After pressing Henry down, she stood back and said, "There you go, girl. Now you are ready for the ball." I was absolutely stunned and silent. Then Goth girl asked, "You got fifteen?"

I looked at my watch and nodded yes.

Goth Girl led me over to a corner table and pulled out a chair that faced the window, and I sat down with my back to the counter. She pulled a couple of napkins from the container on the table and handed them to me. I looked up at her and said, "You need to explain what just happened!"

She nodded and smiled. "Large latte, right?" She walked toward the counter and called, "Barney."

I turned to see a short, bearded guy come out of the back room. He was wearing an apron, so I guess he was a roaster. "Going on break. Need fifteen," she said to him.

"Sure thing, Dar," he said.

I turned my head to look out the window at the trees. Soon, I heard footsteps behind me, and a very large, steaming latte was placed in front of me. I looked up to thank her and was blown away by what I saw. She was completely bald! As she sat down, I burst into tears. We both reached across the table and grabbed each other's forearms. We lowered our heads until our foreheads touched. We were both lost in tears. We had become a human pyramid of sobbing.

"Ya get it now?" she asked, pulling her head away. I nodded in silence. She looked so beautiful with tears in her eyes. The thick, black lines of makeup around her eyes seemed to showcase a sparkle in her tears. They caught a glint from the lights in the shop and reminded me of diamonds.

For the first time since my diagnosis, I felt a true human connection. And to a Goth-girl stranger of all people! But she was not the stranger. It was I who was the stranger—to myself. There was something magnetic about Goth Girl that drew me to her. Some form of freedom, some aliveness in her that I craved for myself. She seemed wild. I felt tame. I did not like tame. It felt as though I was trapped inside a cold metal container that I called my life. Inside this empty container, I could barely breathe, and I was slowly dying.

Goth Girl pushed the latte closer to me, encouraging me to take some sips.

As I held the cup close to my lips, I watched her beautifully lipsticked lips form gorgeous shapes as she began to talk. She explained that she had begun chemo nine months ago and how the first week had been a living hell. "Gotta tell you my New York wig-and-taxi story, so you have to come back, right?" she said holding me in her gaze.

"Got that right, Goth Girl," I said.

She repeated "Goth Girl" and laughed aloud. I laughed aloud too. I had a comrade in arms now. I was no longer isolated and alone. There were two of us.

I was struck by her energy, her warmth, her confidence, and her ability to reach out to a stranger. She had just rescued me. I wanted just a small amount of whatever it was she had.

Goth Girl was studying me and could see I had a question. She leaned toward me and raised one of her beautifully crafted, black Goth eyebrows at me. "So, Wig Girl, you have a question?"

I laughed at the name Wig Girl and felt an immediate closeness and kinship to her. It was as if she had reached into me and lovingly touched my heart. I felt safe and protected by her. I just wanted to crawl up in her arms and never come out.

"Breathe, honey. It's all good. It's all way cool," she whispered to me. "But I gotta pee. Hold the question. I'll be back in two." She stood and headed to the restroom.

I sat there quietly breathing and started to feel a flicker of warmth deep in my cold and abandoned heart. It kind of shocked me. Since David left, my heart had been so full of pain that it felt cold all the time. I had felt betrayed by love. And now, in the most bizarre of occurrences, this Goth Girl woman had stirred it to life again. What was this flicker in my heart? It was hope. But hope for what?

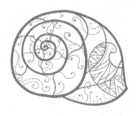

Chapter 4

More about Goth Girl

It was good to have a few quiet moments to gather my thoughts. The trees outside the window seemed to soothe me. Goth Girl soon returned to the table and as she took her seat, I could sense her eyes scanning me in a caring way.

She beamed me a big smile and said, "And the question is?"

"Gee," I said, "I have so many questions."

Goth Girl waited for me to collect my thoughts.

"Well, to start with," I said, "how were you able to do what you just did for me?"

"Good question," she said. She took a deep breath. "Ya see, when I was a little girl, I had this sense about people. I could sort of see inside their thoughts. I could see angels, as well. I was living in this beautiful world inside of myself. Then I told my mom about seeing angels, and being real religious, she thought I was delusional. They called in a priest and did various healing ceremonies to try to rid me of this ability.

"That made me very distrustful of the gift of seeing, and I learned how to suppress it. I did this right up to the time I was diagnosed with cancer. The diagnosis really broke me open, and I crashed. Or, I should say, the life I had created crashed. All the learned beliefs and pretenses that I was living with just crumbled around my feet. It was pretty scary initially. But as I have learned, if ya wanna build a new building, ya gotta take the old one down. And boy, did my old life crash and burn. Had some really crap days, I can tell you. Anyway, then came this sort of *birth* thing, when the real me, who had been locked away inside, began to appear. The little girl I had abandoned when I was a child was actually still alive and wanting to live. Up to the point when I was diagnosed with cancer, I was a little corporate bunny of sorts, hopping through my days with all the other bunnies. Looking back, I realize that I was quietly dying inside. I tell people that the cancer diagnosis broke me open like an egg, and I started to claim who I really was under all the conditioning.

"This is when my Goth Girl look emerged, and I really came home to the psychic gifts I had been given. Friends began to call me for advice and direction. I would ask them why they were asking me, and they would say that there was just something about me that was kind of medium-or-mystic-like. When you walked into the coffee shop, I could sense your pain and emptiness. Even before you got to the head of the line, I could feel your energy. The more I use these psychic gifts, the more I have come to understand what my soul wants from this life. We all got 'em, honey—you too. Just some people have them a bit more than others do."

I asked another question. "So, is working in the coffee shop now your career in life?"

Goth Girl laughed aloud. "Oh, no!" She pulled a business card out of her pocket. "This is who I am."

I took the card and read it. On the front, it said, "World-Famous Psychic" above a telephone number. On the back was a drawing of three rings, one inside the next, like a target.

I was a little confused and gave her a puzzled look.

"You see, Wig Girl, this is the law of attraction at work. I am in the process of manifesting this career in my life. An important part of the manifestation process is to live and feel as if I'm already a world-famous psychic. I am co-creating this with the Universe, God, the divine creator, Mother Nature, or whatever you want to call it. It's what I call IPB—intention, patience, and belief.

"I set the intention with the business card and live as if I am already a world-famous psychic. Then I need to have patience to allow the Universe, the higher power, or whatever you want to call it transform my life into the intention that I am sending out. Then I hold true to my belief and never let it falter. It's not a magic wand, but you can create whatever you want. Your intention has to be in accord with your soul's purpose, and each soul has within it the necessary gifts and inclinations that will be activated once you align with it. You just gotta tune into your deeper wisdom and not let the world push you off course with pressure to live to in some predetermined, socially accepted, but empty norm.

"Once I set my intention, I activated all the beautiful and invisible creative forces in the Universe to live the life I came here to live and experience. The key is to allow time for this to happen and to never stop believing in the process. Nature offers a good example of how it manifests. An intention is like a seed planted in the garden of your soul. I love the acorn. So sweet and innocent, but who could guess the beautiful oak tree that it contains within? Both you and I, honey, have great oak trees inside us. Only thing is, they aren't made of wood, just something beautiful. Trust me. I see it in your eyes and feel it in your soul.

"The acorn, like my ambition, needs to be watered and protected. For me, protection means that I am very discerning with whom I share my deep intention with. Many of my family and friends think I am nuts wanting to be a famous psychic. They would rather I had stayed in a secure corporate job. I respect that, but that is their path, and I have my own path, so I follow IPB with power, passion, and discretion. In the meantime, I like working in the coffee shop because of the many people who come in, and I also feel that I am developing my psychic gifts here. And, of course, then you came in, and *ta-da*, we get to share this beautiful process together."

I asked Goth Girl about the symbol of the rings on the back of the card.

She laughed. "After my cancer diagnosis, what really changed my life was 'the way of the three loves.' I know I was led to this coffee shop and the way of the three loves. It has completely changed, empowered, and inspired me."

I mulled over those words. The way of the three loves? I couldn't get one love right, so how the hell would I ever get three loves right?

"The way of the three loves saved and transformed my life. But it is not for me to say more about them. You really need to meet a dude called Brock and let him explain," Goth Girl said. "All I can say is that up to my cancer diagnosis, the word 'love' had only brought heartache and suffering into my life. I tried so hard to find love, to be loving, and to love someone, and I met with failure after failure. I had decided that the word *love* was far more trouble than it was worth. I kind of gave up on it, and in the process, gave up on ever loving myself. Then cancer and Brock came along. He is one cool-ass kind of a guy. You gotta meet him, right?"

I nodded enthusiastically.

"Only Brock can share with you the way of the three loves, but I can tell you a little bit about him. Like me, he was screwed by love. He had trained as a cabinetmaker and woodcarver but went into the corporate world in search of a higher salary to support the rather lavish spending habits of his very materialistic wife. He became a successful sales-account manager for an engineering company, and he had the ideal life, or so everyone thought. Within the span of three months, he was diagnosed with colon cancer and prostate cancer. Bad deal, eh? Anyway, he lost his job, and without the big income, his wife went off with his best friend."

I sipped my coffee, completely entranced by this young woman and her stories.

"He went through a very dark period, which led him to a path of spiritual searching. Although he lost everything in the outside world, his spiritualty began to open and grow," she said. "For a short period, he went to live with an order of Benedictine monks to explore monastic life. This only partially satisfied him, and he ended up going to Asia in search of his true spiritual path. In a small fishing village on the coast of Myanmar, he used his cabinetmaking skills doing some boat-repair work. It was there that he learned about a small group of Shaolin monks who lived on an island five miles from the mainland.

"The Shaolin monks followed a spiritual practice that dates back some three thousand years and is only communicated verbally, from generation to generation. Brock is a crazy-ass skilled woodcarver, and the villagers told the monks about him because one of their old temples needed restoration. The Shaolin monks invited Brock to live with them for three months to restore their temple. The three months turned into nine years, and the monks took him into their community and taught him their spiritual practices. As Brock will tell you, he found the answer his heart had been seeking, and he wanted to spend the rest of his days with the monks.

"The Shaolin monks were known for their loving and kind ways. Often, villagers from nearby islands would go to the monks for help with problems of relationships and love. To help the villagers, the monks developed a process or philosophy called the way of the three loves. It is a transformational way of living and loving that comes out of their most ancient and wise spiritual teachings and practices. The island the monks lived on was surrounded by three oceans, and the way of the three loves came from living in harmony with the three oceans. The monks said that to live a fulfilled life, there are three loves in every life. The first love has to do with our lives in the world—loving our families, friends, a special partner, animals, and all of nature. The second love has to do with loving ourselves. The third love has to do with loving the Divine Presence, or whatever word we use to describe the higher power. It could be God, Mother Nature, the beloved, or any one of many others that have been used.

"Brock grew very close to the abbot and became his personal student. When the abbot was ninety-eight, he asked Brock to return to the West to share the way of the way of the three loves with people here. Shortly thereafter, the abbot passed away, and to honor him, Brock returned to the West to teach," she said. "And this cool-ass three-loves thing is what makes me who I am today."

Goth Girl paused and took a sip of her latte. I was quick with questions. "So, what is it? Please tell me about it."

"Can't do. You gotta talk to Brock about it. He does not share it with everyone. He has this way of looking into people that he learned from the monks. It's as if he sees into your heart. He says he's looking for 'pure intent.' If he sees it in someone, then he will share the way of the three loves.

"Only he can decide, Wig Girl, which is why you gotta meet him. When you came to the counter with tears in your eyes, I could sense that you had this pure intent. Just my guess, of course. But you just gotta meet him. Then, what is meant to be, will be." Goth Girl looked at her watch and said, "Gotta go, honey, but I want to tell you about how I met Brock. Now that's a fun story. You're coming back, right?"

I nodded an enthusiastic yes.

She stood and opened her arms for a hug. I was quick to my feet and fell into her embrace. For the first time, I noticed that she was wearing a beautiful scent. I took in a long inhale as she held me. Then she pulled back and gave me a quick kiss on the forehead. "My number's on the card. You can call me anytime, right? Just know that you ain't ever gonna be alone again, got it?" With that, she went back to the counter.

I sat down and cradled my latte as I gazed out of the window to savor all that had just happened. Her final words struck me. She must have sensed how alone and abandoned by life I had been feeling. I glanced at the time and saw that I should head to the clinic. I slid her business card into my pocket. When I paused to drop my empty latte container into the trash, I looked up to see

Goth Girl behind the counter beaming a big smile at me. I smiled back and headed to my car.

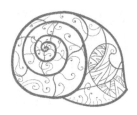

Chapter 5

A Day in the Clinic

Traffic was moving quickly, and in minutes, I was back on the highway. I looked at the clock on the dash and calculated that I had been in the coffee shop for about forty-five minutes. It had felt like a beautiful eternity. I wanted it to last forever. When I turned into the hospital parking lot, I felt as though a dark cloud was forming in my chest. My breath became heavy, and the old familiar feeling of dread returned.

The elderly security guard gave me his usual friendly wave and a nod. He could easily have kept his head down in his newspaper, but he took the time to look up and smile. Even though we had never spoken, I could tell he was a warm man with a kind heart. I wonder if he knew how important his one friendly smile was to me. A simple nod from a stranger that seemed to say, *I see you, I welcome you.*

My first task was to register at reception. And this was where the dreaded receptionist Deborah hung out. Cold and grumpy, she was my first hurdle of the day. Of the many things that pissed me off and hurt me about her greeting style was that she always had her eyes on her computer screen, even though I knew that she could see me coming when I walked toward her desk.

It felt as if she wanted to keep me waiting for a few moments until she had finished her all-important computer work. Then she would move her eyes toward me before her head followed, which made me feel of little importance to her.

I was always annoyed with myself for getting ensnarled in her little games.

Then I would think it was just me, being a depressed neurotic. After her acknowledgment that I had had arrived, she would ask my name. I would say my last name aloud, feeling like a naughty schoolgirl in front of a teacher. Sometimes she would flash her eyes at me without seeing me, and sometimes she kept her eyes on the computer screen. I hate to use this word, but she really was a bitch. She never said hello or good-bye; just "Name?" and "You are all set." I gave her the name *Ice Bitch*. I am not sure why, but giving her a secret, snide nickname seemed to give me some small, pathetic way of claiming back the power she had stolen from me. Then I would feel sorry for myself because I had been brought so low. And this is how my miserable day in clinic would always begin.

After Ice Bitch gave me the okay, I headed to the clinic. Another wave of dread would wash over me whenever I walked into the clinic area with its line of sterile chairs, some with the limp bodies in them and glassy eyes staring at nothing or at their little TV screens. Two nurses ran the clinic. One was reasonably friendly, and the other was another grump. I had a name for her, too. It was "Grumpy Nurse."

I always hoped that I would get the happier nurse, but inevitably, I got Grumpy Nurse. When I arrived in the clinic, I had to wait by the nurses' station until I was assigned a chair. I hated standing there. Some of the other patients would steal glances at me, and I knew they were wondering what cancer I had and what my prognosis was. This is something I had begun to do as well. I stopped seeing people in the clinic; all I saw were their illnesses, and I would try to guess whether I was better or worse off than they were.

After I had been at the nurses' station for about five minutes, Grumpy Nurse looked over at me and pointed toward a chair she had selected for me to sit in.

No words, no greeting, no, *So. how are you feeling today?* Just the pointing finger. A direction and a destination. By this time, I was always feeling miserably depressed, and my chemo treatment hadn't even begun. The treatment would last between four and five hours, which again brought a new wave of dread. I once asked Grumpy Nurse if she could give me a sleeping pill, so I could sleep for the four hours. The look she gave me was classic. No words. She just narrowed her eyes and slowly shook her head from side to side. I knew she was thinking that I was a real wimp. The look said more than her words ever could have.

As I took my seat and waited for Grumpy Nurse to hook me up to the chemo pump, my thoughts went to Goth Girl. Was she just a dream? Did our conversation really happen? How could I travel from heaven to hell in under one hour? I pulled out her card and pictured her in my mind sitting across from me in the coffee shop. Then I pondered the way of the three loves and tried to imagine what it meant.

My daydream ended suddenly when the stony cold voice of Grumpy Nurse barked my last name. "Harris!"

I opened my eyes. There she was, standing over me holding my medical file and a bag of chemo.

"Hi. You okay?" she asked in a disinterested tone. Although it was sort of a question, it was also her form of distanced ritual for getting my attention.

I wanted to shout, *Say my first name, bitch!* But I figured that she was already grumpy enough; no need to piss her off even more. Then I wondered how Goth Girl would deal with Grumpy Nurse. Goth Girl would not take this shit.

Grumpy Nurse brought over a small tray with the needle resting innocently on a light-blue cloth. Without any eye contact or small talk, she swabbed my arm with a cotton ball and searched for a vein. I turned my head away and clenched my other fist to brace myself. My veins were sunken and not easily found. Nurses usually struggled to find a vein in my arm with their first stick. As Grumpy Nurse readied the needle, I cast my eyes upward and away and said a quick, silent prayer. *Please get it the first time.*

Then came the stick, a sharp pain, and I heard Grumpy Nurse curse quietly. She had missed my vein. *Bitch!* I wanted to shout.

"Sorry," she said curtly as she swabbed another area on my arm.

Just my day, I thought. I clenched my fist and turned my head away again. In it went with a sharp pain that made my whole body wince.

"Shit," she said in a muffled whisper. "This is not my day." She missed again.

Okay. Now I wanted to punch her out. I pulled my bottom lip between my teeth to stop myself from saying something I would regret. Then I turned to her and asked, "Why don't you use the warming pad the other nurse uses to raise my veins first?"

In an impatient tone, she said that she really didn't have time.

I felt blood rush to my face. I turned to her, narrowed my eyes, and gave her a menacing look of hell about to break loose. In a cold and angry tone of voice, I said, "I want the frickin' heating pad."

She stopped in her tracks and stared at me with her eyes wide open. I had gotten her attention. She gazed in shocked silence at me, deciding how to react. I could sense that a part of her wanted to tell me to go screw myself. She lowered her eyes from my gaze compliantly and nodded her assent. "On its way," she whispered as she headed for the warming cabinet. With warming pad in hand, she eyed me as she returned. I could tell that her thoughts about me were not favorable. I didn't give a shit anymore.

Without any verbal communication, she placed the heating pad on my arm and went off to attend to a pump that was beeping. I was seething and was close to losing control. Under the anger was a deep and desperate sadness. Then there was the fear, then the depression, and I felt so utterly alone. I was being sucked into a pit of sadness and self-pity. Then a voice in my mind screamed, *Hold it together! Lock it down. Get through this. Get through this.*

I am not sure where this voice came from. It was a strong and rescuing part of me that seemed to show up in moments like this. I locked my emotions down and froze my jaw to get through the treatment. All but one of the eleven other chemo chairs were now occupied, and I stared at each person one by one. They all seemed so desperately alone in their individual plights. There was a woman on the end I had seen before and felt drawn to chat with. She had been staring at the same magazine page for five minutes.

I hated the hospital. I hated the medical system, I hated cancer, I hated chemotherapy, and I hated Grumpy Nurse for treating me so badly. Then I decided to hate love, which I thought was behind all my unhappiness. Goth Girl's words echoed in my head. *The way of the three loves.* I couldn't get one love right; how on Earth could I ever succeed with three loves? But Goth Girl had. And she was glorious. Who was this Brock guy, and would he let me in on this Shaolin wisdom and the three loves? I wanted to know more, and the thought of returning to the coffee shop the following morning seemed to bring some relief from the misery of the clinic.

I pulled one of the TVs in front of me and searched for some distraction. There were nine stations, and all had ads playing at the same time. The hospital headphones were tight on my head, adding to my irritation. I just wanted to go home and have a good cry.

Then Grumpy Nurse returned with her needle again. I turned my head away in silence. She removed the warming pad and swabbed down a small area of skin. I braced myself for the needle stick. "Got it," she said, more to herself than to me, and soon I was hooked up to my chemo. I could tell that she was pissed at me. I could tell that she knew I was pissed at her. And here we were, thrust together in this cauldron of human suffering called a chemo clinic.

Eye contact with other patients was always tricky. A part of me wanted to be social, but a part of me was feeling depressed, and another part of me was frightened to get too close to anyone in case he or she died. The wide spacing of the chairs made it hard to have a private conversation. Even though people did not look at me, I knew they were all listening. This made me even more intimidated and afraid to start a conversation.

One chair was still empty. After a quick scan, I realized that a youngish man with a friendly face was missing. Last week, he'd looked really pale and threw up twice during his treatment. He looked bad. I feared the worst but didn't dare to ask about him. An empty chair was like a bad smell that nobody wanted to acknowledge. It hung in the air and pushed people further down inside themselves. About bad air, there was an elderly guy who was always put at the end of the line of chairs. My guess was that he had some form of stomach complaint that resulted in the occasional loud fart. I figured we could expect him to let one rip every fifteen to twenty minutes.

I hate to admit this, but I did begin to award him points—one to ten, like in ice skating. In one fantasy moment, I imagined giving everyone in the group a scorecard so that we could hold them up every time he farted. A short whimper of a fart would get a one or a two. A loud, rasping fart would get an eight or a nine. For a ten, he would receive a standing ovation. And this is what my life had become during these interminable chemo sessions. I hated the feeling of disempowerment I had whenever I spent time in the clinic. As for the woman I felt drawn to chat with, I kept wanting to ask if I could sit next to her. But again, I just felt disempowered and never quite got up the courage to ask.

Then there was the clear chemo fluid going into a vein in my arm. I would stare at the full bag hanging over me like a dark rain cloud and wish somehow the flow would speed up. The fluid moved so slowly I could never see the level go down. I wished that it was out of sight. It was a constant irritation. Our eyes are so powerful in how they perceive images to feed our minds. Couldn't somebody come up with a way to make medical equipment look less intimidating? Everything seemed so very ugly. The bags of chemo, the little blue pumps that hung near our heads, the clear thin pipes you prayed would not block so they had to be flushed.

I fantasized about taking the chemo pumps to a local school and having schoolchildren paint flowers on them and then sign them.

And so, this was how my day of chemo treatment unfolded. It reminded me of when I took my car in for service. I would hand over my keys, surrendering my car. Only in this case, I was surrendering my body.

At last, after four-and-a-half hours that seemed like an eternity, my chemo bag was empty. I waited impatiently for a nurse to set me free. The cranky nurse was slowly making her way to me as she checked other patients.

After five minutes of waiting, I coughed aloud and said in her direction, "Ready when you are." Her back was toward me, and she looked over her shoulder with narrow eyes and just nodded in my direction. I knew I had just pissed her off again. Another five minutes passed, and I sat upright on the edge of my chair.

Finally, Grumpy Nurse came to me. No eye contact. She just pulled the line from my arm, stuck a Band-Aid over it, and said, "See ya," as she headed over to another patient. I gave the back of her head a long, nasty look. I felt sorry that that was all I could muster. Really pathetic. My exit from the clinic was always the same: I put my head down and walked as fast as I could to the parking lot. I got in my car and had a quick cry. The chemo I was on took about twenty-four hours to become fully active, and that meant some lethargy and often nausea. The good news was that I could always drive myself home.

Usually when I arrived home, I would park the car in the driveway and have another cry. Sometimes the day in the clinic made me cry; sometimes the loneliness in the empty house awaiting me made me cry. Sometimes the feeling that there was no love in my life made me cry. I had so many tears and so many reasons to cry.

The evenings of my days in the clinic were the same. A frozen dinner I pecked at but never fully ate as I slumped in a recliner, flipping stations on the TV, watching anything to distract my mind from biting holes in me.

I had some meds to take before bed, and I always added a couple of melatonin tablets to suck me into a deep sleep. As my weary head hit the pillow, I lay in darkness, reviewing the day. Chemo hell, coffee house heaven. These two worlds felt far apart and so far away. The awareness of my empty bed shot an arrow of loneliness that hit me right in the heart.

To redirect my mind, I thought about getting up early and making another visit to the coffee shop. I wanted to see Goth Girl. I needed to know that she was real. I wanted to feel again what she made me feel. I wanted to be seen again in the way she had seen me. I wanted to be held in her arms and comforted again. I set the alarm and burrowed down into my cold, lonely sheets.

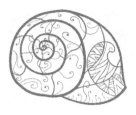

Chapter 6

Filing for Divorce

I did not sleep well and woke up in the middle of the night. The empty pillow next to me once again prompted anger at my husband, and I punched it several times. Our Saturday mornings together had always been so special. The memory was painful to me, and I curled up in a ball and cried. Then I dozed and napped and dozed and napped. When I rolled over on my back and glanced at the clock, it was 8:00 a.m.! Then a word came out of nowhere and flashed like a blinking neon light: DIVORCE!

Screw my husband, I thought. *I am going to divorce the bastard. Gotta get him out of my life and out of my head.* Then my big brother, Bob, flashed into my thoughts. He was a hotshot attorney in Los Angeles. He had moved there some twenty years ago to marry his college sweetheart. Bob had always been protective of me, and he had invited me out to LA to visit since I kicked David out. My respect for Bob was enormous. My father had served in the army in World War II, and Bob followed in his footsteps and went to Vietnam. After being there for eighteen months, he stepped on a land mine, which took his leg off from the knee down. He came back angry and crippled. He took to drinking heavily, and I thought he was a lost cause. Then, some program for disabled vets took him under its wing and completely turned his life around. The army paid for his college education, and he became an attorney. He always said that what he lost in flesh and bone, he gained in character.

He's always raising funds for the vets in his area and is committed to giving back.

I decided to ask Bob to file divorce papers to get this moving. I wanted my life back. It was five o'clock on the West Coast. Bob was an early bird, and I knew he would be sitting with his morning cup of joe reading the paper. I dialed his number and waited. Bob was one of the few people in my life who I could be honest with. He was now the only male in my life I could trust. As a brother, he was always like a big, warm, soft-hearted bear. But as an attorney, as I heard on the phone one day, he was cold and ruthless. Just what I needed in an attorney. He would kick my husband's ass!

After three rings, he picked up, and his warm, deep voice greeted me. "Hi, Sis. This is a nice surprise. How you doing?"

"So-so," I replied. "Listen, Bob, I need to ask a favor."

"Sure thing."

"Can you file divorce papers against my shithead husband?"

There was silence. Then he said, "Let me go into my study so we can talk about this." I heard him tell his wife, Mary, what he was doing, and in a few moments, I heard the door of his study close. Then came his voice again. "Now, Sis, you know I will do anything for you. Have you thought this through? Is it really over?"

The question annoyed me. "The night he walked out of the bedroom, he walked out of my life. *He is gone!* History! I want out!"

"Got it," he said. "What reason do you want to use?"

"Well, I guess him being a dickhead, ball-less jerk is not so good a reason?" I said. "How about desertion?" Sure, I had told him to get out. But that was my fear talking. I'd wanted him to react, and he had—by leaving. He had not stopped by since that night. He had not called. He had lost interest in trying to make our marriage work.

There was silence at the other end. Then Bob said, "That works. Do you want a straightforward process with this, Sis, or would you like me to terrorize him a little?"

"Oh, could you?"

He was quick to reply. "Oh, I will make his life hell. In hurting you, he hurt me; and to that, I just don't take kindly. What is your timetable for this, Sis?"

"Like, now!" I said.

He went quiet for a moment. "Actually, I have two interns I can put on it first thing on Monday. We need to gather financial data and testimony from you, and they can begin the process, okay? Later this morning, I will fax you some of the financial questions you'll need to answer."

"Oh, Bob, you're just the best!" I said.

"Cool," he said. "Let's pluck this turkey!"

"Go for the throat!" I said. "I want to make his sorry ass bleed."

"To spook him, I will send him a notice of filing first thing on Monday. This is a shot across the bow. It will take a couple of weeks before we are ready to officially file, but he will be unsettled by what I will be asking of him—mostly detailed financial information, which will include personal information about his clients. Technically, a good attorney will know how to block this, but it will take David time and a boatload of money to hire one. In the meantime, I'll hit him with some penetrating questions. A bit like what picadors do to a bull to weaken and anger it before it gets killed. This will break the emotional skin, and he will start bleeding. I will ask for names and addresses, and he'll fear that I will contact them directly. Thus, he will be afraid of losing all credibility and respect. Again, this is sort of a terrorist approach. I should be able to fax him the primary document of intention to file in the next couple of days. Sound okay?"

I was quick to respond. "You betcha! Thanks, Bob. You are my rock, and I love you a bunch."

"Anything for you, Sis. Just want to see you happy again. I understand your need to move beyond this. This asshole is going down for what he has done to my little sister."

I started to cry, and he went silent.

After a few moments, I gathered myself again and thanked him for all he was doing. After putting the phone down, I lay in bed, staring at the ceiling. For the most part, it felt really good to be getting my shithead husband out of my life. But there was a part of me that was uncertain about being alone in the world again. I did not like the word *divorced*. It had a certain connotation of failure. Like a tattoo I would wear on my forehead. Would I ever find love again? Could anyone ever love me again? Nagging thoughts that I had failed at love and, perhaps, I was in some way broken inside began to dance around in my head.

I clicked on the bedside radio to some mindless morning music and talk show to numb my turbulent thoughts. Then that awful country song came on. "We Ain't Never Coming Back." I hit the stop button so hard I knocked the radio to the floor. I cursed aloud, then curled into a ball again and cried. And cried and cried.

After lying in a pit of gloom, I glanced at my watch, which told me it was 8:30 a.m. and time to start my day. Then a small ray of sunshine appeared when I remembered that I was going to see Goth Girl again.

I decided on a pair of dark-blue jeans and a light-blue blouse. Just before I left the house, I glanced at myself in the full-length mirror in the hallway. I had a sinking feeling in my stomach. It was the word *divorce*. I was feeling unsettled—as if a big wave was headed my way, and I could not get out of its way. There was also a strong sense of aliveness stirring inside me, though, and I had Goth Girl to thank for it.

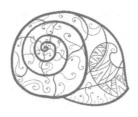

Chapter 7

How Goth Girl Met Brock

As I pulled into the coffee shop parking lot, I tried to see if Goth Girl was there, but the reflection on the glass prevented it. When I reached the door, I knowingly gave the bottom of it a little kick with my foot as I pushed the handle.

With great ease, I sailed into the coffee shop and was relieved to see Goth Girl behind the counter, organizing the pastry shelves. When she saw me, she shouted, "Hey, Wig Girl, glad you dragged your sorry ass out of bed to come visit!"

I liked her familiar, cheeky greeting. It communicated her fondness for and comfort with me. I was also aware that her greeting conveyed the fact that I wore a wig. I was surprised that this did not bother me. There was strength in knowing she wore a wig as well, and somehow this seemed to make me immune from embarrassment. Also, I had a sense that she called this out deliberately to minimize the drama I could so easily create around my wig.

Goth Girl pointed to the empty corner table, and I headed toward it. In a few minutes, she arrived with two large lattes. She put them down and then held her arms out for a hug. I stood and dove into her waiting embrace. Once again, I felt her big energy field engulf me. That immediate sense of being loved and accepted washed all over and through me. It made me feel safe and loved. As we sat down, she asked, "So tell me, how are you doin', girl?"

Gee, where to begin? I told her about how I punched the pillow each morning and waited to see if she thought I was nuts.

"You go, girl! You punch that sorry-assed bastard of a pillow. Get the anger out; it will only turn to poison."

I was struck by her words. I had felt embarrassed and sorry for myself for punching a pillow at the start of each day. She had just shifted my whole perspective, helping me to see that the punching had an inherent emotional release.

"Anger gotta keep movin' out," she said. "Don't let it fester; that's when it becomes poison."

"Got it," I said, nodding in agreement.

It felt good to have her fiercely beautiful eyes upon me again. I felt the same feeling of being looked at, but she was looking into me. It was as if she was reading my emotions in some way. Her gaze held both curiosity and care.

She reached out and gave my hand a warm squeeze as she said, "And you want to hear the story of how I met Brock, right?"

"Got that right."

Nodding and smiling, she took a sip of her latte. "When I went for my first chemo treatment three months ago, I was just one big emotional mess. I felt as if my life had been smashed into a thousand pieces. Whatever control I thought I had over my life had been stolen from me. I was the world's biggest victim and loser. *Why me?* I asked myself repeatedly. Why had life done this to me? Anyway, I was driving home after my first chemo treatment completely distraught and broken apart. I felt a deep, deep sadness and could not stop crying. It was actually hard to see where I was going, so I pulled into a grocery store parking lot to take a time-out. As I was parking the car, my tears made it hard to focus, and I rear-ended a pickup truck.

"I had a complete emotional meltdown, right then and there behind the wheel of my car. My first reaction was to lock all the doors in case the other driver tried to attack me. I saw the driver's door open, and a tall guy made his way to my door. I was a basket case. I was hunched forward over the steering wheel with my head in between my arms. I was sobbing uncontrollably.

"Out the corner of my eye, I could sense this guy standing outside my door, looking at me having this meltdown. Then he walked back to his truck and went to the passenger-side door to get something. I got really scared at that point. I thought it was maybe a baseball bat to smash my window. Worse scenario, it could be a gun. I saw the guy reach down and get something and then make his way back to my car. I was expecting the worst. I kept my head down between my arms while discreetly stealing glances to monitor the stranger. If he so much as tried to smash in my window, I was going to hit the horn.

"Then he tapped on the window. I ignored him at first, then he tapped again. I slowly turned my head, and much to my surprise, instead of seeing a very angry man, I saw a bar of dark chocolate pressed up against my car window. I rubbed my eyes to make sure I was not seeing things. Then I lifted my eyes to the man. He had a smile on his face and spoke to me through the window. 'Thought you may need a first-aid kit,' he said. Then he gestured for me to roll down my window just an inch or two. I was still in disbelief, but I lowered it a crack. In came the chocolate.

"'Please,' he said, 'eat some chocolate.'

"I felt like saying, 'Excuse me, I am having a complete emotional breakdown here. What the hell has chocolate got to do with it?' But I peeled back the paper, snapped off three blocks of dark chocolate, and promptly placed them in my mouth. Gee, it was the most glorious dark chocolate, and the transformation was instant. The burst of flavor in my mouth completely distracted me from my freak out. I slowly chewed as the chocolate melted in my mouth.

"'Eat more,' the guy said through the window. I broke off three more pieces and popped them in my mouth. What happened next completely blew me away. I started laughing. He started laughing as well. It was hard to keep my mouth closed, and soon a little dribble of chocolate rolled down my chin, which made me laugh even harder. Then I rolled down my window a couple of inches and looked right at him. 'Are you frickin' real?' I asked him.

"In a very gentle, deep voice, he said, 'When life sucks, I have found it helps to have something to suck on, and chocolate seems to really help.'

"I knew I must have looked a complete mess with teary, bloodshot eyes and chocolate dribbling out of my mouth. But somehow, I was also feeling kind of good. It was as if the sun just came out inside me. I snapped off three more pieces and pushed the remaining chocolate back out through the window.

"'Give this to your pickup truck with my apologies,' I said. Then we both burst into laughter again.

"What a sight we must have looked. We laughed together for a while, and then he said, 'May I buy you a cup of coffee?' and pointed to this coffee shop.

"Needless to say, I went with him for coffee. The driver of the pickup truck was—you guessed it—Brock. This is the guy who introduced me to the way of the three loves, which completely changed my life."

I was sitting there spellbound. After a silent moment, I said, "So when can I meet this guy, Brock?"

Goth Girl was smiling at me. "Sometime soon. He has some big things going on now, but he should be available soon. Lemme track him down and see how I can hook you two up." She looked toward the counter, where a line of people stood. "Gotta go, honey," she said, standing up. I stood too, and we opened our arms for a parting hug.

As we eased apart, she gave me a mischievous wink. I turned to look at the trees outside the window and thought about the story she had just shared with me. I took the last few sips of my latte and headed out to buy some groceries.

Later that day, Bob called to tell me that he had faxed me some questions about my financial setup, and he sent a preliminary notice of intent to file for divorce to my husband. "That'll unsettle him," he said. "How are you doing?"

"Kind of numb."

"Not unusual," he said. "Divorce is a fierce process regardless of who initiates it and what the reason is. You are going to get through this and move beyond it real soon, Sis. Trust me." His words were comforting and seemed to fill the hole I was feeling inside. For the moment, at any rate.

After I put down the phone, I sat back in my chair to tune into myself. As I thought about being a single woman again, a cold shiver went through me. Then I thought about love and how it had betrayed me, and I could feel myself slipping into a depressed state. Negativity was circling me like a pack of hungry dogs.

Although Goth Girl had given my day a magical start, I really had to talk myself into doing housework and the laundry, which was stacked a mile high. At four o'clock I decided a trip to the liquor store was in order. I wanted a soothing bottle of white wine for company that evening.

On the drive back from the liquor store, I tried to shift my heavy mood by focusing on something creative. If I was going to write my autobiography, what would I call it? I wondered. Then it came to me: *Shitfaced in Wonderland.*

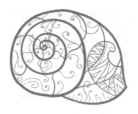

Chapter 8

His Car in My Driveway

Listening to classical music was helping me unwind as I drove home. But as I turned left onto my street, what I saw thrust a cold dagger into my heart: my husband's car in my driveway. My whole body stiffened.

I gripped the steering wheel and drove right past my house to the end of the street. Turning left, I pulled over where I'd be out of sight from the house and turned off the engine. He had really caught me off guard. I had to quiet myself. Quiet my heartbeat. Breathe, breathe, I kept telling myself.

Then it dawned on me. Of course. He received my notice to file for divorce, and he's not a happy camper. But what did he want? Why was he here? Why the hell hadn't I changed the locks?

Breathe, breathe, I told myself, fighting the tears that welled up. Then I thought of Goth Girl and her words, *You can call me anytime, okay?* I pulled her business card out of my wallet and entered her number. The phone rang three times before she picked up, but her warm voice brought immediate comfort.

"Breathe, breathe, breathe," she said over and over like a mantra. I breathed in silence, and slowly my emotions began to gather themselves.

"Wassup, girl?" she asked softly.

I took a long, deep breath and said, "His car is in my driveway. What do I do?"

"Keep breathing, girl. Jusssss breathe and listen within. Let your emotions be free. Just feel what you need to feel."

And so I did, and anger, fear, confusion, hurt, and rage all flooded through me. All the peace and empowerment of the past couple of weeks suddenly disappeared. I felt hurt, torn open, confused, vulnerable, and angry. And yet, I also felt sad. My emotions churned like a washing machine on steroids.

As I calmed down, my mind slowly began to take control. My husband's sudden leaving had hurt me more than I realized. The pain around his rejection was still very much alive and raw. Seeing his car in my car driveway was like a knife stabbing at the pain I had buried within myself.

"He ain't nuttin'," Goth Girl said. "Remember who you are, girl."

Her words felt like one of her warm hugs. I could feel my strength and confidence—my power—slowly returning.

"Remember; I got your back," she said. "You are not alone. He is in your home, but it is also his home. This is part of your healing process. You gotta face this shit and begin to move through and beyond it. I am guessing you're ready, or else the Universe would not have brought him back into your life like this."

Her words brought a sudden vibrational resonance to me. This was not something for me to run from. It was time for me to turn and face him so I could begin to move forward. I could feel my sense of centeredness return and thanked Goth Girl for being there for me.

"Want me to come over?" she asked.

"No, I'm good," I replied.

"Don't forget; you can call me anytime, right?"

I was now sitting upright behind the steering wheel. It was as if somebody had just given me a clean pair of glasses. Everything seemed new and fresh. I pulled out my cosmetic bag and touched up my makeup, choosing some bright-red lipstick. I sucked in a couple of deep breaths, looked at myself in the rear-view mirror, and said, "Hey girl, you got this. Go kick some ass."

I started my car, drove slowly to my house, parking in the street so my car would not block his exit.

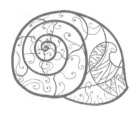

Chapter 9

The First Meeting with David

As I walked up the path to my house clutching my bottle of wine, I felt a core of strength in me. I turned the key in the front door and pushed it boldly open. I followed my usual routine. Car keys on the hallway table, coat into hallway closet. I kicked off my shoes and walked into the kitchen without hearing a sound. The house was silent. Then to the cupboard for a wineglass and drawer for a corkscrew. I pulled the cork and slowly poured the wine. Then I stood motionless gazing out the kitchen window at the bird feeder and my little feathered friends.

I waited in silence. After a few minutes, I heard some footsteps come from the living room and a voice behind me. "Hi, Jane."

I turned slowly and deliberately to find my husband standing in the doorway to the living room. He was holding what looked like a fax, which I guessed was the notice to file divorce papers. I gave him a half glance and took a sip of wine. "Oh, it's you. I thought the car in the driveway looked familiar." I was feeling good, and an image of Goth Girl flashed across the screen of my mind. I think she would have liked that response. I stayed facing the window, giving him my back, and waited in silence as I eased my glass of wine to my lips.

Still with my back to him, I said. "If you are looking for the rest of your clothes, then look no further. I burned them along with your frickin' golf clubs." I liked the way those words poured out of me. I had actually taken them to Goodwill, but I figured Goth Girl would have encouraged my creative license.

For one moment, I felt the urge to throw my glass of wine at him. Then I thought, *Waste good white wine on this shithead? I don't think so.* I waited silently with my back to him.

His voice lacked his usual confidence as he said, "Jane, can we talk?"

"What do you think we are doing? Baking a cake?" I imagined Goth Girl laughing at that one.

"Please, can we sit and talk, Jane? This fax from your brother, you know, just really hurt because it was so sudden."

"May I fix you a drink?" I asked without turning.

He responded quickly, sounding appreciative and a little surprised. "Sure, yes. Ah, thank you."

Quick as a flash, I bent down and opened the cabinet under the kitchen sink and pulled out a bottle of bleach. "With or without ice?" I asked. I felt a sudden pang of guilt for enjoying this smart-ass remark.

"Okay, okay," he said rather pathetically. "Please, this fax. So sudden. Can't we just sit and talk about this?" His question hit a raw nerve. Even though it sounded like a rehearsed line, it caught me off guard. After all, we had spent twenty-four years together. His leaving had ripped those years away from me, and I was still emotionally bleeding. Then I felt a surge of anger, and I spun around flashing venom from my eyes.

"What the hell do you want?"

As I waited for his response, I noticed that he was looking very unkempt. Three days of beard growth and the beginning of a pot belly. Mr. Spic and Span was looking a little shabby. He also looked tired. I wondered what he had been up to.

"Jane, please, can we sit and talk?" he asked, lifting the fax.

"Standing is better for the blood flow in my legs," I said with a little twinge of attitude. "What do you want?"

"I know what I did was not good. I just don't know what happened. Something inside of me seemed to snap. The cancer thing was just too much for me. Something in me froze. I was and am lost."

His voice sounded a little shaky. I felt a little tweak in my heart. I wanted to go at him again. But he was not his usual self. He seemed unusually vulnerable. This was not something I had witnessed in him before. I was confused, not sure how to respond.

He reached into his pocket, pulled out a business card, and dropped it on the kitchen table. "I will leave you alone, but I want you to know I am trying," he said, as he started to move toward the front door.

Annoyance that he had just waltzed into my home without invitation stirred again, and I barked at him. "And never just show up again. Please respect my privacy. Future visits by appointment only. Got it?"

He stopped by the front door and turned. "I know. I was wrong to just show up. But I wanted you to know that I am looking at what in me failed you that night." As he lifted the fax up to eye level, he added, "All I am asking is that we pause this divorce process. Can we find a way to move forward without animosity?"

It took every ounce of control I had to stop myself from screaming at him. He turned quietly and left. I stood there dazed, clutching the bottle of bleach and staring at the front door.

I was full of mixed emotions that confused me. I was really angry at him, yet somehow, I felt almost sorry for him. He seemed a little broken. I reached for the card he left on the table. It was for a relationship specialist. On the back, he had scribbled, "Sorry, Jane. I am trying."

My husband's sudden appearance had unnerved me, and suddenly I felt uncertain. I needed to hear my brother's reassuring voice. I called his cell. He picked up quickly. His voice was urgent. "Hey, Sis. You okay?"

"Sure, sure," I said. "Only David just turned up at my home, and it really threw me."

"Yeah, this process is very unpredictable. You gotta remember to lock and load on this one. Be ready for anything at any time. Okay? While I have you on, let me get some financial background so I know our footing. So, tell me, how are your finances set up?"

I was a little confused as to what he meant. "Sorry, Bob. This is a bit new to me. What exactly do you mean?"

"Well, for example, whose name is on the house mortgage? How are your bank accounts set up? What debts do you have and in whose name are they? Where are all your financial records? I will also need full statements of income for you both with details about how you spend your money."

I felt a churning in my stomach. I responded rather meekly, "Well, Bob, we have an unusual situation here."

"What does that mean?"

"Well, as he is the financial expert, he kind of set things up in accordance with what he felt was best."

"Be specific," Bob said.

I could feel his frustration, and he started to shift into his stern attorney mode. I took a sip of wine and a deep breath and started to explain. "Well, we have two main bank accounts. One is in both our names, and my salary goes into it. We run the household and miscellaneous spending on that. The second account in his name is where his income goes, and he transfers monies into our joint account when needed."

"Do you have access to the account that is in his name?" Bob asked.

I felt a bit stupid in answering, "Well, no. He said because his income is mostly commission and fee based, it was better to set it up that way."

I heard him murmur, "*Balls.* Go on."

"He put his BMW and the loan for it in my name for tax purposes."

I heard a long sigh on that one. I continued, "He just said that it would be better if he ran our finances, which I realize was also a message that he was smart and I was dumb."

"So, tell me about your savings, Sis."

The question made me feel like a little schoolgirl who had just failed an exam. "Well, I don't actually know how much we have saved or where he keeps it."

This time I heard a loud, "Oh, shit." Then in his stern attorney voice, he said, "You gotta hack the bastard. We need to get all, and I mean all, his financial data, okay?"

This was really upsetting me, and Bob picked up on it right away and switched into his loving, brotherly voice. "Listen, Sis, we just gotta get some info to help you with the divorce. Ask around and see if you can find someone to help. This is the timeframe for us: you have sixty days from when we actually file the papers. This gives him time to find an attorney and get his ducks in a row. After that, the legal wheels start to turn, and this is when we need the financials, okay?"

"Yeah," I responded meekly.

"I know this is hard for you, so let's talk again in a few days."

"Sounds good," I said, and we hung up.

The conversation had really thrown me a curve ball. I felt nauseated, fragile, and vulnerable. Thoughts were bouncing around in my head like wild, demonic cats. Then I remembered my date for the night. The bottle of wine.

I reached for my glass. "Just you and me," I whispered. "It's time for us to get this on."

With the opened wine bottle and a monster bag of chips, I headed into the living room. As I eased myself onto the sofa, I picked up the remote and flipped on the evening news. I needed something to take my mind away from what just happened. I was ruffled, uncertain, and hurting. I drained my first glass of wine in three gulps and filled it again. I needed relief. I needed to escape. I needed to be numb for a while.

Soon the wine bottle was empty, and so was my glass. A woozy feeling took over. My head began to spin, and the sofa seemed to suck me down into it. Next came a deep, drunken sleep.

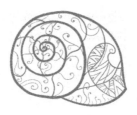

Chapter 10

Meeting Mare

The phone startled me awake at 7:00 a.m. I sprang to my feet, dashed to the kitchen, and grabbed the phone. I thought it was one of those telemarketers and was ready to give someone hell.

I was shocked to hear my doctor's voice on the other end of the phone. It was always her secretary I spoke with; she never called me directly. I looked at the caller ID and did not recognize the number because she was using her cell phone. I could feel my heart beginning to race. Then a cold fear seemed to fill me. My head was pounding from the wine the night before. I tried to pull myself together.

She spoke in a quiet and professional voice. "Hi, Jane. Sorry to call you so early. I need to review your last blood work with you and wondered if you could come into the office tomorrow morning at nine."

This really scared me. "What is it?" I asked urgently.

"Just something I need to look at deeper with you, Jane. We need to discuss this in person. Can you be here at nine?"

In the calmest voice I could muster, I said, "Sure, sure, I can be there." I put the phone down, feeling a dark sense of dread. Then my negative thoughts took over. Has she found new cancer? Has my current cancer started to grow? Am I going to die? Then it dawned on me that this was Sunday, and a sharp piercing fear ran through me from head to toe.

I felt frightened and in a really bad way. It was now 7:15 a.m. I needed coffee and a visit with Goth Girl. She would know how to help me deal with this.

I showered and dressed quickly. I left through the kitchen door, and when I did not see my car parked in the garage, I felt a wave of panic, thinking it had been stolen. Then I remembered that it was parked in the road outside my house. I drove eagerly to the coffee shop for a healing hug from Goth Girl. I left a voice mail for my boss saying that I would be in late on Monday.

As I drove to the coffee shop, I could feel my emotions beginning to fragment and disintegrate. Screw my doctor for doing this to me. Couldn't she have done this another way? It helped to be angry at my doctor. It distracted my thoughts from what I would find out the following morning.

As I swung open the door to the coffee shop, my eyes went straight to the counter. No sign of Goth Girl. Just the tall Asian-looking young woman I had seen there before. I glanced urgently into the storeroom, thinking she may be there. No sign. Shit! Where is my friend, Goth Girl? I suddenly felt deserted and alone. I moved slowly to the counter. The Asian woman was studying me with her big hazel eyes.

"Large latte," I said, handing her my credit card while searching for Goth Girl.

The woman leaned forward and whispered, "She's off today."

I gulped a deep breath and without making eye contact, I collected my latte and headed to the corner table. I sat with my back to the counter. Then, something inside of me seemed to crack in half, and from the dark abyss came a torrent of tears.

I huddled over my latte, hoping no one would see me as sob after sob poured out of me. I was completely losing it and felt powerless. Then it happened. I felt a very gentle touch on my shoulder. Then a second touch in the middle of my back. Then came the softest of voices whispering in my ear. "Hey sweetie, you are going to be okay."

An incredible wave of love seemed to pour into me from the hand on my back. It flooded my whole being. "Take some big breaths," the voice said again.

In a few moments, the sobbing stopped, and I turned to see the tall slender, Asian woman standing behind me with a pure light of love pouring out of her eyes at me and into me.

She released her hands and came around to sit opposite me. Through my teary eyes, I could see an aura of light all around her. She was like an angel.

Her beautiful almond eyes were locked onto me, sort of holding me. She had long, beautiful hair, I noticed. She was drop-dead gorgeous.

She reached into her apron, pulled out some tissues, and placed them in front of me. I blew my nose and slowly began to regroup. After some moments of silence, she said in a quiet, warm voice, "Hi, Jane. My name is Mare."

As my tears cleared, I met Mare's eyes. Then more tears came, but these were not tears of sadness or brokenness. These tears felt full of love. Mare had tears in her eyes too, and for a glorious moment, we both seemed to inhabit an ethereal world of teary light. Then I took a big breath and asked, "What the hell did you just do?"

She smiled and replied, "Welcome to the spiral of love."

I shivered all over remembering Goth Girl's reference to the three loves. It felt like some magical potion. "Thank you, thank you, thank you, Mare."

Mare reached out and grasped my hands gently. "Thank you," she said. "We are now sisters, right? Dar, you, and I. And this is what sisters do, right?"

I nodded a slow, heartfelt yes. Then I asked, "What was it you just did? How did you know? Why me?" I seemed full of questions.

She paused for a few seconds then said, "It's the spiral of love."

Those words again. "What do you mean by that?"

"The three loves is an ancient healing tradition that empowers the heart to love fully and unconditionally. Brock is the guy you need to talk to. All I can say is that it completely transformed my broken and lost life. It has made me who I am today. It's what makes me able to support you in this way."

"Your life was broken and lost?" I asked.

"Like, big time," she replied. "Brock will tell you about the spiral of love, and I am happy to share the journey of woundedness and abuse that brought me here."

"Would you?" I asked.

She glanced at the counter and then back at me. "Let me get someone to cover me. I'll be back in a few."

It was good to have some moments to settle and reflect. I had just traveled from the realm of brokenness into the realm of unconditional love. They seemed so close, as if the thinnest of veils separated the two. How could this be? I pondered this question as I sat quietly, gazing out at the trees swaying in the breeze.

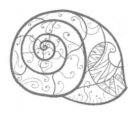

Chapter 11

Mare Tells Her Story

Mare soon returned and slid her drink onto the table near mine. She eased herself into the chair, took a big breath, and began. "I was born in the Philippines, and my parents were both killed in a car crash when I was nine. I was adopted by a young married couple who could not have children of their own. For the first three years, everything was fine. Then my adopted father lost his job and began to drink heavily. At night when his wife slept, he would sneak into my room and fondle me. He was physically very powerful, and I was frightened he was going to kill me.

"This went on for several months before I plucked up the courage to run away to stay with my aunt on the far side of the city. I did not know it before I went there, but my aunt was a prostitute. She was my only refuge. In the Philippines, we did not have things like social services that protected children. There were many homeless children on the streets, and children having to beg to eat was commonplace. Even though my aunt was a prostitute, she did, in her own way, care for me. She allowed me to stay with her.

"It wasn't long before I ended up selling sex, and by the time I was fourteen, I was a full-time prostitute. It was a terrible, terrible time. I was trapped and did not know how to escape. The men who came to us were often drunk and violent. My aunt taught me how to hurt men if they became threatening. A kick between the legs, fingers to eyes, and even how to use underwear to choke a man almost to the point of death. Several men did become violent, so my attack skills became well practiced, I am sorry to say. The house where I lived was essentially a brothel, and one day, it was raided by the police. I was taken from the brothel to a convent, of all places, to be rehabilitated and educated. It was out in the country.

"It was a surreal time. It was as if I'd gone from hell to heaven. The sisters were so very loving and helped me to believe in myself again. They discovered that I had artistic talent and encouraged it. They had a sister house in America and arranged for me to come here and study art.

"To start with, I stayed at the convent and eventually moved into an apartment with two other girls and started taking college courses. I did well for about a year, then I mixed with the wrong people. They introduced me to drugs and drinking, which led to addiction. The emotional pain inside of me from all the years of abuse was eating me alive. I was assigned a social worker, who arranged for me to attend a three-month rehabilitation program. This was a very dark period for me. The searing inner pain was more than I could handle. After a month in rehab, I ran away in the middle of the night. I found my way back into prostitution and back to the streets. All those old destructive patterns just kicked right in again. Everything crashed for me, and I spiraled down into a dark and depressed state. I had no self-confidence and ended up living in homeless shelters.

"I was in a shelter one night, waiting in line for a meal. Ahead of me was a single mother and a young child. A man under the influence of drink came in and pushed his way in front of the mother. I couldn't be bothered to react until he pushed the little girl to the ground. When I saw that, something flipped inside of me. It was as if I became the little girl. I jumped on his back and with his own dirty shirt began to choke him to death.

"Years of rage just poured out in that one searing, violent moment. The man collapsed on the floor, and I kept my choking lock on his neck. I really wanted to kill the bastard. But in some way, I was wanting to kill myself to end the pain.

"Even though I could hear the police sirens in the distance, I continued to choke him. He was lying facedown, and I was straddling him, twisting his shirt tightly, squeezing his neck. I remember his body convulsing as he desperately tried to gulp in air. Then I felt a warm hand on the middle of my back and heard the words, 'You have a right to be angry. You have vanquished him. You can set him free when you are ready.'

"I felt an immediate shift in energy. Had anyone tried to use force to make me let him go, it would only have strengthened my grip. Looking back, I would say that this was a moment of divine intervention. All my pent-up rage seemed to flow out through the warm hand on my back. The softly spoken words poured into me like a soothing balm.

"As soon as I released the man, he scrambled to his feet and ran out the door. I turned to see this guy called Brock standing behind me. When the police arrived, Brock stepped in and directed them away from me, saying the situation was in hand. He had just saved me from arrest and a possible prison sentence for aggravated assault.

"Brock took me to a quiet corner of the shelter, and we chatted. I told him my story, and for the first time in my life, I saw tears of compassion in the eyes of a man. Up to that point in my life, men had been lousy, sex-driven, violent animals. I hated them. Now, just one man, through his own caring and compassion, had suddenly turned my world upside down. Brock saw something in me that I did not see in myself. It was Brock who introduced me to the way of the three loves. And that is what gave me back my life. That night, Brock took me from the shelter to the person who would become my spiritual sister. She is the person you call Goth Girl.

"She let me camp out on her sofa and gave me a sense of security that I had never had before. She became a big sister to me, and I am devoted to her. Brock got me some house-painting gigs so I could generate income, and Goth Girl let me borrow space in her art studio to start painting. That's when I started to learn about the way of the three loves." Mare paused, took a sip of her latte, and then glanced out the window as if gathering her thoughts. Then she turned her beautiful eyes back and gazed at me in silence.

I was struck by the violence and abuse in her life. How had she become such a loving and kind person?

"As strange as this may seem," she said, "all the violence and abuse I have experienced has now been transformed into who I am today, thanks to the spiral of love. I went from being the world's biggest hater to being the biggest lover!" She broke into a big smile. "No, I am only kidding. I'm just one of the world's biggest lovers." She gave me a wink.

"With your art and healing hands, what are you doing now?" I asked.

"Good question," she said. "Well, there are three parts to my working life. For a third of my work week, I offer people healing body work. I actually trained as a massage therapist and have studied many energy healing modalities. I also paint and sell my work. And then there is the coffee shop. I love serving the public and meeting new people, like you." She smiled.

"Wow," I said. "What a fabulous work schedule you have."

"It's there for you too," she said. "We gotta get you connected to Brock and the way of the three loves. Lemme check in with Goth Girl, and we will set it up, okay?"

"Can't wait," I said. I was mesmerized, in awe of, and enchanted by Mare. Here was another healing angel who emerged at the worst of moments to transform agony into ecstasy.

Then Mare glanced at her watch and said, "Time for me to go, sweetie." She reached across the table and gently grasped both of my hands. "Just know that with this cancer thing, Dar and I have your back. Come back soon. I want to get the lowdown on your life and what's cooking for you."

I nodded a yes.

We both stood, and we hugged. Then she reached into her back pocket, pulled out her business card, and placed it on the table.

As she headed back to the counter I glanced down at the card. In light-blue ink were the words *Healing Angel Hands*. Her name and phone number were printed below. Soft fuchsia butterflies decorated the edges. Even the card was beautiful and full of presence.

I picked up my latte and headed for the door, turning to glance at Mare, who was busy serving customers. She was aware of me and looked up to give me a wink and a smile. All I could think about for the twenty-minute drive to the office was how full of pain and abuse her life had been and how it had all been transformed. She was an angel with almond eyes. And this spiral of love...perhaps there was a glimmer of hope for me in it. I drove home slowly and spent the rest of the day watching old movies doing all I could to not think about why my doctor wanted to see me. I went to bed at nine and set my alarm for 7:00 a.m.

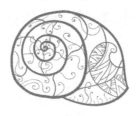

Chapter 12

Mistaken Tests

I kept waking up in the night, and all I could think about was my doctor's concerned voice and her need to review my bloodwork. At 7:00 a.m. the alarm went off, and I hit the snooze button with a sharp, angry motion of my right hand. I needed a long hot shower to wash away all the fear and stress.

I had been in the shower around five minutes when I heard the phone ring. I felt panic; nobody ever called me this early. I had a sense it was urgent. In a flash, I grabbed the towel, ran dripping into my bedroom, and grabbed the phone. "This is Jane." I said urgently. I felt another bolt of fear when I recognized the voice as that of my doctor's secretary.

"Hi, Mrs. Harris. It is Julie from your doctor's office. Dr. Hughes has asked me to call you to let you know that we do not need you to come in this morning. Seems the lab mixed up your blood tests, and now that we have the correct ones, there is no urgent reason for her to meet with you. She offers her sincere apologies for any undue stress this may have caused."

As I put the phone down, I felt a surge of annoyance. I felt the urge to say, *What the hell are you doing down there? Can't you even write a name on a bottle of blood?* Then came the sense of deep relief that all was okay. I headed back to the shower and decided to head into work early to get the jump on a grant request I was working on.

At 10:00 a.m. the phone rang. It was Goth Girl. "Hey, Wig Girl. Got some frickin' good news for you. Spoke with Brock today, and he said he would love to meet you. Any chance you can drag your sweet ass out of bed early tomorrow and meet him at 6:30 a.m. in the coffee shop?"

I felt a burst of excitement. "You betcha," I said.

Goth Girl shot back, "See ya then. I am on the run. Catch you tomorrow, Wig Girl. 'Bye!"

I put the phone down in something of a daze. I sat back in my chair and savored the delicious feeling the prospect of meeting Brock had created in me. For the rest of the afternoon, I tried to focus on my work, but I kept daydreaming about this Brock guy.

I came up with all sorts of visuals for him. Handsome or not so handsome? Young? Old? Tall? Short? Pot-bellied? Friendly? Distant and aloof? Married? Kids? Gee, my mind was having a field day.

My thoughts about Brock shifted into what I would wear. No boring business suit, for sure. I settled on a pair of faded and rather tight-fitting blue jeans that had rhinestones down the sides. I added a slim-fitting blouse, and I was set. Then there was my wig, Henry. He was due for a wash and blow dry. I flipped off my computer and headed home for the night. My evening date with a bottle of shampoo was set.

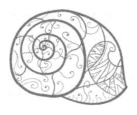

Chapter 13

Meeting Brock

I woke before the alarm, and my first thoughts were of my meeting with Brock.

I think it was the sense of mystery about the guy and this way of the three loves that was really intriguing me. Then another voice inside snapped me out of it with the thought of my husband and my recently filed divorce papers. It was the love thing again. I had given it everything, and it had given me only heartache in return.

After showering, I had fun putting on my tight jeans with rhinestones. The thought of seeing Goth Girl made me feel happy, and I decided to be a little daring and chose a black lace bra that would show ever so slightly through my white blouse. I guessed that Goth Girl would approve.

I packed my dark-blue business suit in a bag so that I could change in the office restroom after my meeting with Brock. Henry, my wig, was looking bright and cheery as I placed him on my head and dabbed on a couple of extra spots of holding gel. No sticky coffee house door was going to ambush me today.

For the first ten minutes of my twenty-minute drive to the coffee house, I was feeling happy and quite elated. Then I started to feel a little uneasy. Something about this spiral of love. I felt my life was in a spiral down and wondered how this spiral of love could stop my descent. I was simply not good at love. Then there was meeting this mystery guy called Brock. I revised my vision of him to make him pot-bellied, elderly, and grandpa like. This reduced the charisma that I had imagined around this guy. I pulled into the parking lot at 6:25 a.m. and peeked into the coffee shop to see if I could see Brock and Goth Girl. Our corner table was empty, so I guessed Brock had not yet arrived.

I did my usual kick on the bottom of the door and strode confidently into the coffee house. I was pleased to see Goth Girl behind the counter, and she beamed me a big smile. I glanced at the empty corner table, and for a second, I feared that Brock may not show up.

I took a quick look around the coffee shop to get a sense of who was there. Two yuppie-type guys sat at separate tables, lost on their iPhones. Near them was an elderly man poring over the sports section of a newspaper. There were three gym bunnies sitting around another table chin wagging over their coffee. In the far corner was an elderly man who looked very disheveled. He could have been homeless or perhaps mentally ill. He was gazing at a newspaper laid out in front of him and had a very sad look on his face. At the table next to him was a student, pecking away on his laptop. At the end of the counter, partly hidden by the Coke machine, was a slim guy in a checked shirt and blue jeans. He was perched on a stool with his head buried in a book. And so it was. No sign of the mystery guy, Brock. Light jazz music played in the background, and all seemed at peace in the world of the coffee shop.

Goth Girl slapped me a high five over the counter and slipped a large latte in front of me. I leaned in toward her and pointed to the corner table, whispering, "So, is he still coming?"

She bellowed a big laugh and pointed toward the guy sitting on the stool. As I turned to look at him again, he got up and walked toward me.

I was immediately struck by his big blue eyes, which were locked onto to me. He was around six feet tall and had a slim, wiry build. I felt a shiver go down my back. Then Goth Girl said, "Ta-da, and this is Mr. Brock!"

My mouth fell open, and I stumbled to find appropriate words as I extended my hand to him. He moved toward me with his arms open and inviting. This felt like a scene in a movie. As we closed toward each other, his arms went past the weak offering of my handshake and wrapped themselves around me, pulling me close, and I caught the scent of pine. My arms were caught helplessly by my sides, and I was lost in his hug. In a soft voice, he whispered in my ear, "Hi, Jane. It's great to meet you."

He released me, and I stumbled back, trying to regroup. He stood silently in front of me, holding me in his beautiful gaze with a soft smile on his face.

He was doing this not-looking-at-me-but-sort-of-into-me thing with his gaze. For just a few seconds, everything else in the room seemed to disappear.

Then Goth Girl snapped us out of our little spell. "Okay, guys. How about the corner table?"

As I walked the few steps to the table, I took some deep breaths and pulled myself together. I could feel my heart beating a little faster, and a little voice in my head said, *Wow, this guy is hot!* Then another voice said, *Remember the spiral of love. Focus!*

I took my usual seat with my back to the counter, and Brock took the corner seat with his back against the wall. Goth Girl sat at the end of the table.

As Goth Girl offered some opening conversation, I did my best to keep my focus on her, but I kept stealing glances at Brock. His face was warm and gentle, and he had a strong brow. His facial features were nicely proportioned and were framed by curly, red hair that had the touch of wildness. He had a warm sort of aura. Being near him was like sitting near a log fire on a cold winter's day.

Goth Girl steered the conversation toward the three loves and asked Brock if he would share about this. He took a couple sips from his drink and started to talk. It was then that I realized he had a rather suave British accent. He briefly recounted how he met Goth Girl. As he spoke, I did my best to keep my gaze focused on his big, blue eyes. Whenever he glanced at Goth Girl, my eyes darted to the chest hair visible beneath his open shirt collar. I was feeling a little—and rather nicely—untethered by this. I could sense that Goth Girl was watching my eyes and knew exactly what I was stealing glances of.

Then I felt a wave of embarrassment, and I could feel my neck flushing red. I had no control over the blush and used every ounce of willpower to keep my eyes locked on his.

I turned to look at Goth Girl, who was looking at me with her eyes sort of half open as if to say, *Naughty, naughty. I can see your neck and know what is going on.* But I also sensed from her a form of shared conspiracy. She was really on my side and enjoying this.

When Brock finished recounting how he met Dar, he rested his eyes on mine, tilting his head slightly and raising an eyebrow, inviting me to share. She was also focused on me. I took a sip of my latte as I gathered my thoughts about what to say. First, I looked at Dar and thanked her for arranging this meeting. Then I turned to look at Brock. I was more at ease with his dazzling blue eyes now and was able to formulate an outflow of intelligible words.

"Well, Brock, it is a pleasure to meet you. Dar has told me good things about you. She mentioned the spiral of love, and this really caught my interest. I was wondering if you would be open to share more of this with me." I went quiet, waiting for a reply.

He gazed at me in silence for a few seconds, and I could sense that he was processing his thoughts. Then, in his gentle British brogue, he said, "Jane, it is a pleasure to meet you. I have heard great things about you, and I was looking forward to spending this time with you."

I felt Dar's knee suddenly touch my leg under the table and had to use all my willpower not to smile at her.

"Ah yes, the way of the spiral of love," Brock said. "This comes from an ancient form of Shaolin teaching. It is not for everybody, though."

That felt like a door closing. A voice inside my head said, *Oh crap. Maybe I am not appropriate for this teaching.* I flashed a look at Dar, who also seemed a little concerned that perhaps I was not going to get access to the way of the three loves.

For a moment, Brock looked distant and removed. Then he spoke again. "It may be good if I share something of my own journey in life first, which will lead us naturally into how the three loves came into my life and why it helped save my life."

The "saved my life" part really caught my attention. I thought, *This is not going to be a home run, after all. What on Earth will it take to gain access to the wisdom of the spiral of love?*

Then I felt a tweak in my bladder and knew I needed a pee break. "Pause just there," I said as I deliberately leaned toward Brock. I rose, guiltily knowing that my movement would allow him a peek at my bra through my loosely buttoned shirt. I glanced quickly at his eyes and noticed that they flashed first to my shirt then out through the window.

I felt a sparkle of flirtation that felt oh so good. Dar gave me a sly glance as I headed toward the restroom. She was onto everything. No place to hide with her.

After I used the toilet, I took a few seconds to gather myself. I was feeling a flow of flirty energy that I thought was completely lost to me. After my husband walked out on me, it was as if something had died in me, never to be resurrected again. But here it was, alive and kicking me. I was feeling kind of sexy again.

I splashed some cold water on my face and gave Henry the quick once over. He was looking good and with the extra fixing gel, he was not going anywhere in a hurry. Then Dar burst into the restroom and stood with her back against the closed door, looking at me with a sly smile. I turned and looked at her. She continued to stare at me in silence. "What?" I exclaimed.

Speaking through a big grin, she said, "Amazing, eh, how that bad thing you just did with your flash of the black bra can make you feel so good?"

I blurted, "So, is he single? In some form of relationship?"

"He's a free bird, honey!"

At that point, we both broke out into guffawing laugher like two naughty schoolgirls. When the laughter eased, she moved toward me and cupped my face in her hands. "Listen, girl. I know you are going through some stinky shit right now with your cancer and asshole husband and all. Just remember that roses will pop up from time to time for you to smell, so enjoy this moment, right?"

Once again, she penetrated my defenses, and tears rolled down my cheeks. She knew just the right moment and just the right thing to say. She moved away from the door to allow me out. I pulled open the door, turned to her, and said with a smile, "Amazing how some roses smell of pine, eh?" We both laughed again, and I headed back to our table.

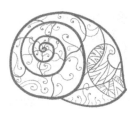

Chapter 14

Brock's Story

As I returned to the corner table, I noticed that Brock was sitting with the disheveled-looking man, listening attentively to him. After a moment, they stood up and hugged each other. When the man sat down, I could see that the sad expression on his face had become a cheerful one. I wondered what Brock had done that cheered up this sad, old guy.

I took my seat and waited. In a moment, Brock slid back into his corner seat, and Goth Girl arrived. I rested my eyes on Brock again, beamed him a smile, and said, "So, Mr. Brock, I am all ears."

I could tell he liked my casual invitation to share. He took a sip of his coffee. "I think it will be best if I share with you a snapshot about my journey in life, as I feel it is relevant to your journey. I am going to start with my college days. I trained as a cabinetmaker and woodcarver. Woodworking is my true joy in this world. I also played semipro football and mixed with a lot of driven young guys. The chairman of our football club offered me a job in his corporation with a scary good salary. It was far more than I would ever have made as a woodcarver, so I allowed myself to be pulled into the pressured, fast-moving, and very well-paid corporate world. After five years, I was pretty unhappy. Outwardly, I was successful. A flashy company car, a suit for every day of the week, and a knock-your-socks-off salary. As for how my spirit was doing on the inside? The metaphor I like to use is that of an apple pie: I was beautiful pastry on the outside, and my life looked good; but on the inside, there was no filling. I was empty.

"Then one day, I got the phone call you never want to receive. It was my mother, calling to tell me that my father had passed away unexpectedly at sixty-five. Some form of opportunistic blood infection, the hospital said. Over the years, my father and I had never really been emotionally close, but we had developed a quiet respect for each other. He had been physically present through my childhood but not at all emotionally present.

"I remember a moment, two days before we buried him," Brock said. "I was standing by his cold body, feeling really sad. The sadness came from standing by a man with whom I share the same blood, knowing that he never knew me, and I never really knew him.

"My father's sudden death was a loud wake-up call. Corporate life was fast and competitive, and I really did not fit in. My mother had been a nurse, and I had more of her tendency of wanting to care for people as opposed to competing. I knew deep inside that the corporate life was not my path. I was really lost and fell into a very dark place. The funny thing is that during my time in corporate, I had been volunteering in a home for young people with special needs. They had a variety of challenges, some physical, some mental. Some had Down syndrome, and some were without vision and/or hearing.

"Strangely, when I was with these special people, I felt like I was at home and with family. I just really liked being with them. I used to volunteer one evening a week. We would do jigsaw puzzles, drink coffee, and listen to music. I am not sure I can explain why, but I felt a deep happiness when I was with them. I was really struggling to find direction, and after burying my father, I decided that I wanted to see the world. I hoped that this would give me some perspective and a sense of direction in my life."

Brock's story made me reflect on my own direction in life—or rather my lack of direction. I was hungry to hear more.

"I resigned my corporate position, gave my business suits to Goodwill, and bought a backpack and a train ticket. To start, I headed across Russia on the Trans-Siberian Express to Japan, where I spent time studying Zen Buddhism. From Japan, I traveled around China before arriving in Hong Kong. I was staying in a youth hostel, and the guy in the bunk above me told me about a community of Shaolin monks who lived on a small island off the coast of Myanmar in Southeast Asia. I was really intrigued and traveled to the island for a short stay.

"The Shaolin monks were very hospitable and welcoming. When they learned that I was a woodcarver, they asked if I would help restore their old temple. In return, they allowed me to live and study with them. Their spiritual lives were based on the teachings of the way of the three loves. I became enamored with the way of the three loves and wanted to dedicate my life to that philosophy. I had initially agreed to stay three months, but it turned into seven years. I fell deeply in love with their traditions and teachings. I became very close to the abbot, who took me under his wing as a special student. It was the abbot who personally taught me about the way of the three loves, which totally changed and transformed my life. The abbot was very elderly, and one day he called me into his room to share with me that he was soon to leave this world. He asked me to return to the West and share his teachings."

The words "'his teachings" sparked an interest deep inside me. What were these, I wondered. Would I be able to learn more about this?

Brock continued. "Initially, I was very reluctant to return. The monastery had become my home, and the other monks were like family to me. Out of respect to my teacher, I agreed and came back about four years ago. I had made several friends at the home for the people with special needs and shortly after returning, I popped in to have tea with them. The director pulled me aside asked to see me in his office. He offered me a job as a care assistant. This was the lowest of the low jobs in terms of salary and social status. I would help wash and care for the residents, feed them, and break up fights. I would earn just a fraction of what corporate had been paying me. The position was residential, and I would live in a camper at the back of the property that had no running water or electricity. My rational mind went nuts, but I listened to my heart and took the job. It turned out to be one of the happiest periods of my life.

"A few months into my new job, the director suggested that I go for a physical. I was feeling good and did not think I needed one. To keep him happy, I went, expecting to be told that I was one healthy dude. But this physical completely changed my life. I walked out of the doctor's office with a duel diagnosis of prostate and colon cancer. My life in color had suddenly gone to black and white."

As he said that, I felt a bolt of fear go through me. I wanted to jump in and ask if he was okay now and if he still had cancer. I held back this urge, and Brock continued his story.

"My life as I knew it had suddenly come crashing down all around me," he said. "The cancer diagnosis really shook me up. I went deeply into both cancer conditions, learning all I could about them. I wanted to understand every aspect of what the diagnosis meant from a physical and spiritual perspective.

"When I emailed the news to my friends at the Shaolin temple, another life-changing event took place. Tuku, a monk who I was close to, jumped on a plane to be with me. Tuku had been trained in the ancient ways of their healing arts and came over to help me with the cancer and to teach me about their healing wisdom. This began a new journey in life with my two new teachers, Tuku and cancer.

"Two months after the initial diagnosis of colon cancer, I was sitting in the cancer specialist's office waiting for the latest test reports. The specialist came into the office carrying the test results. As he thumbed through the pages, he asked me a question. 'Mr. Williams, I am curious, do you take a vitamin C supplement?'

"'Yep, sure do,'" I said. He looked a little apologetic, then he said, 'Well, it seems that the results of the test your primary-care physician carried out on you was triggered by an excess of vitamin C in your system. He really jumped the gun in giving you the cancer diagnosis. I am happy to report that your colon is in perfect health, and no cancer is present.' I could have fallen off my chair.

"Then, fast forward another six months. I was scheduled for a final prostate biopsy, which I had kept putting off. This test was invasive and usually led to internal bleeding for several days. Real nasty!"

I felt a pang of fear in my heart at the words "internal bleeding."

Brock continued. "During the eight months since my original diagnosis, I had made some major life changes. I went to several nutritionists and completely changed my diet. I developed a yoga practice and set free many of my overly driven, stress-filled friends. I was put on prayer lists all over the country and started doing guided imagery to heal my prostate. Tuku began to teach me about the monks' ways of healing, which opened a whole new world for me regarding how to heal cancer. Tuku even suggested I start belly dancing to loosen up my rather tight pelvic region and get energy flowing again. I have to say that belly dancing was really fun. You name it, I did it!

"Another thing I was taught was to eliminate my fear of dying, strange as this may sound. But with a cancer diagnosis came a tremendous fear of dying. Tuku explained that with any life-threatening illness there comes a natural fear of dying, and the fear grows into a sort of energy body that lives in and deplete your physical body. The energy body of fear then begins to feed off and drain the good energy. This ultimately weakens the immune system, making it easier for the cancer to grow. Tuku gave me special processes to do to dissolve the fear body and claim my wholeness. This was mostly to do with focusing on what I am passionate about in life and not focusing on the fear.

"On the day of the biopsy, I woke up early and went deep within myself to ask for guidance. Tuku had taught me how to communicate with my prostate," he said.

That surprised me. "How do you talk to an organ?" I asked.

"It is a real simple process," he said. "The aim is to maintain a sense of wholeness and connection to your body as a whole. For example, I would write a question to my prostate with my dominant hand. I'd take a few deep breaths, allowing my mind to go down into my prostate. Then, using my non-dominant hand, I would write a response.

"The subtle thing that happens when you are diagnosed with cancer is that you can easily develop a negative relationship to the part of your body that has cancer. In my case, I felt as if my prostate had really let me down. I thought that it was weak and diseased. These thoughts were sending negative energy to my prostate, which only made it weaker. Tuku helped me to understand how this debilitating thought process would negatively affect not only my prostate but my health in general. The journaling process completely changed my way of relating to my prostate."

I understood. I was already feeling that way about my breasts. "Do you mean writing the questions and answers?" I asked.

Brock nodded. "I have to admit that when I started this process, I was skeptical. My first question to my prostate was, 'Why have you got cancer?' I sent my awareness down into my prostate and then wrote the response. The reply shocked me, 'Please do not ask me that question. Please tell me that you love me.' What my prostate needed was love, not judgment and abandonment."

As Brock said this, he seemed to choke up, and tears came to his eyes. I was in shock. I had never seen a man so emotionally open and vulnerable. I wasn't wearing socks, but had I been, this would really have blown them off.

Brock did not try to hide his tears. He just took in some deep breaths as the tears rolled down his face. I was almost weeping myself at this point. I flashed a glance at Goth Girl, and I knew that she was close to tears as well.

The three of us seemed held in a beautiful bubble of energy that had originated with Brock's tears. The tears had made his already beautiful blue eyes even more beautiful. He went quiet for a few moments.

"Through this process of communicating with my prostate," he continued, "I learned that instead of being a weak organ, it was, in fact, really strong and that it was time for me to marshal all of the creative forces within my body to support and strengthen my prostate. Sort of sending in the cavalry. For the first time in my life, I began to appreciate and love every part of my body, organs included. You begin the communication with journaling, and as you get used to this process, you can begin to do it in your mind, using your imagination. The negative energy I had been sending my prostate had been transformed into healing energy. As Tuku said, I had become my own primary-care physician, dispensing medicine in the form of loving thoughts from within.

"On the day of my prostate biopsy, I arrived at my doctor's office ten minutes early and took this time to tune into my body. I had the sense that I should ask my doctor to repeat the digital examination before he did the biopsy. The digital process is done with a finger, and it was this process that my primary-care doctor had used to find large nodule on my prostate.

"I knew that the specialist was a very busy man, and when I asked him to repeat the digital exam, he seemed a little impatient. He pointed to the nine needles that were all laid out and ready for the invasive biopsy and suggested we proceed as planned. But my inner sense of wanting to repeat the digital exam was really strong, and I held my ground. Eventually, he agreed and redid the digital exam with his finger. Picking up my patient file, he flipped through some of the pages with a very puzzled look on his face. Then he said, 'Mr. Williams, if you had just walked in off the street as a new patient, I would say that there is nothing abnormal about your prostate. I have no justification for doing a biopsy.' And then he said something that still reverberates in my ears today. He said. 'Mr. Williams, I don't know what you have been doing for the past eight months, but it seems that you have beaten the rap!' You could have knocked me down with a feather. I was a free—and healthy—man!"

I felt a surge of joyful emotion and held back the impulse to slap him a high five.

"It was as if cancer had come into my life to teach me how to love myself," Brock said. "He gave me the all-clear. I was really elated." Then Brock stopped and went into deep thought. Dar and I waited in silence.

With an expression of seriousness, he said, "I need to say that I am not suggesting that there is some form of easy fix for cancer and all you have to do is visualize and belly dance to heal yourself. Quite the opposite. This was just my journey. To balance my story, I need to tell you about my friend Joe who also had prostate cancer. How about we take a bathroom break, get fresh drinks, and then continue?"

I headed to the restroom for another much-needed pee.

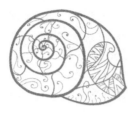

Chapter 15

Joe and His Prostate

After ten minutes, we reconvened with three hot lattes steaming away on the table. Brock picked one up and took a long sip before beginning to talk. "I would like to tell you about my buddy Joe and his journey with prostate cancer. Tuku taught him about the dialoging process with his prostate, and he ended up having the biopsy. Lucky for him he did, as they found a big tumor. He decided to have the prostate taken out surgically. One of the questions Joe asked Tuku was about the cause of his cancer. Tuku cautioned him about creating excessive stress by blaming himself for causing the cancer. The best course of action going forward was to create a healthy lifestyle—eating well, minimizing stress, exercising, finding his passion in life, and so on.

"Tuku said the key was not to blame himself, but rather to learn how to truly love himself *as is*. Tuku said that the monks believed that cancer was a form of vibrational imbalance—like energy that goes haywire. The energy then affects cells in the body, and these grow and start to kill the healthy cells. There are several ways to eradicate cancer cells. Sometimes you can do it energetically with guided imagery and other positive-thought strategies. Sometimes the cells need to be removed with surgery. Sometimes radiation or chemotherapy can eradicate them. The key is to listen to all the options and follow your deeper instincts for what is right for you.

"With the approval of his prostate and his doctors, Joe felt that it was best to remove his prostate, which would also remove the cancer. He was into battle and war movies, and he said that he imagined that his prostate was like the three-hundred Spartans who sacrificed themselves to save Sparta. We always had a good laugh about that. Joe also got creative, and he told the surgeon that he wanted his prostate to take home with him. After signing mountains of release forms and meeting with hospital attorneys, he eventually took his cancer-ridden prostate home in a special container. I know it sounds kind of bizarre, but it does get better.

"Joe wanted to create a sort of farewell and thank-you service for his prostate. By enacting this ritual of loss, he was also healing his psyche. This was a sort of grieving process for his prostate that allowed him to feel his loss emotionally and then heal. He said, 'I wanted to honor the prostate that had served me valiantly and pay my final respects.' In this way, he emerged from this process feeling more of a man, rather than less.

"Joe understood that many men who lose their prostates also lose the ability to have an erection, which means no more sex. Unfortunately, we live in a culture that puts an unhealthy and misdirected pressure on men to measure themselves by their ability to have sex. This way of seeing things is very distorted. Tuku helped Joe to understand that when something dies, there is the potential for something new to be born. He said that losing his prostate had made him more vulnerable, and he found new and deeper ways of connecting to his wife. When sexual intercourse was removed from their relationship, they found new ways to care and be with each other physically. On his fiftieth birthday, his wife bought Joe a do-it-yourself massage-training program they could do at home together. As Joe would be the first to tell you, when his prostate went, so did a part of his ego and male identity around sex. He said it was very freeing, and he now has a more loving and deeper emotional relationship with his wife.

"He also started to look at the process of when one thing ends, a new thing can begin. As a child, Joe had always wanted to play the saxophone but never had the opportunity. So, after having his prostate removed, he started taking saxophone lessons. As Joe likes to say, instead of his life being full of great sex, it is now full of great sax. Joe always laughs when he says that he is a real saxy guy!

"When Joe shared this with his male friends, it sparked a lot of interest, and he started what he calls a prostate-empowerment group. He chose not to use the words *support group* as he felt the message should be one of empowerment.

"They meet monthly and create rituals for the release and honoring of a lost prostate. It is a form of empowered bereavement, a process that helps men move on with a greater sense of self. Many of the men had already had their prostate removed, but as Joe says, you can do this work any time. Some of the wives of these men wanted to be a part of the process, and the group has grown. I attend the meeting each month, and it always opens and fills my heart. One of the wives who attended with her husband got breast cancer, and next month, they will be creating a process and ritual to support her journey. Cancer is not just about the person who has it; it also affects the family and the community. Joe has created an amazing way for men and women to come together to 'grieve each other's grief,' as he says. I have to say that this is also a real celebration of life. We do deal with some serious issues, but everybody comes away glowing with unconditional love."

I was sitting there dumbfounded by what Brock had shared. My whole world around cancer and my relationship to my body had just been flipped upside down. This had stirred something deep inside me that I needed to get in touch with.

Brock started to talk again. "The way of the three loves now guides and informs every aspect of my life. I am working with Tuku to share the way of the three loves with people who we feel are ready."

He paused and took a long sip of his latte. I was completely spellbound and felt the urge to ask him if he thought I would be a suitable student for the way of the three loves. I decided to hold back, as I felt that I was being presumptuous.

"Funny thing is," Brock said, "Tuku went back to East Asia for a few months but is returning to run a series of evening classes to teach the way of the three loves here in the coffee house. It is by invitation only."

He paused, his eyes holding me in his penetrating gaze. My eyes locked on his eyes, and I entered the silence with him. Then I felt this sort of energetic light embrace us. It was like a spark plug going off. Everything in the room vanished, and for a few seconds, it felt like the two of us became one. It was surreal, to say the least.

A big smile broke out on his face, and in a soft voice, he invited me to join the program. Then came the tears. They just started pouring out of me. They were not my usual tears of sadness and pain. These were happy tears. I felt very humbled by the fact that he thought me worthy of being a part of the program.

Goth Girl jumped in, saying, "I'm going too, so we can hang together."

This really brought me back into the moment, and a big bubble of joy seemed to explode inside of me, making its way out in the form of a beaming smile.

Brock said, "I take it you would like to join the program, right?" At that point we all started laughing.

I slapped Brock a high five and thanked him for the honor of being invited to join the program.

Brock looked at his watch and said that he had to run. The first session would be in a couple of days, and Dar would let me know the details. I nodded that this would be fine. He stood and opened his arms again for a hug. This time, I was prepared and made sure I was able to give him back the strong, embracing hug he had given to me. As he pulled me in close, I inhaled his beautiful pine scent. This made me feel light-headed in a really good way. He gave Dar a hug and then headed out. She and I sat down for a few moments and shared our excitement about me being invited to join the program.

"Tell me about Tuku," I said excitedly.

"Don't know nothing," she said. "And you don't need to know nothing. Just show up, honey. Trust and let it all flow."

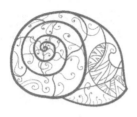

Chapter 16

The Black Ball of Sadness

As I pulled onto the highway, I started to reflect on all that Brock had shared. My attention was drawn to the dialoging process with the prostate. Then I started to ponder what this process would mean to me in connection to how I relate to my breasts. As I thought about it, I began to feel a black ball of sadness forming deep down in my groin. It was expanding and starting to move upward through my body. It was like a tidal wave of sadness that was about to engulf me. I knew that driving a car was the last thing I should be doing right now. I pulled into a small shopping center and parked at the far end of the lot where there was some privacy.

I lowered the two front windows about an inch and then lowered the back of my seat. I checked to see that all the doors were locked and eased back into the seat. I did not have a pen and paper to communicate with my body, but I remembered Brock saying that once you understood the concept, you could do it with your imagination.

The big black ball of sadness inside of me was beginning to rise, and I was beyond the point where I could stop it. I started taking deep breaths and kept saying the word *allow*. "Allow, allow, allow." The ball of sadness was getting bigger and was moving slowly up through my chest, and then it burst out of me in a torrent of anguished tears and wails. I became lost in a tidal wave of sadness. I lost all sense of where I was. Wave after wave of sadness and tears seemed to flood through me like a torrent. They felt as if they had been buried a long time ago. They were breaking free now and seeking release. I did my best to keep my breathing deep to allow whatever it was that was calling for release to be released. I lost all sense of time as the wave of tears coursed through me. It felt as if deeply held emotional energy was breaking free within me. It was as if my tears were carrying away old, stored sadness and anguish.

Eventually, the tears began to ease, and a stillness came upon me. I felt as if my mind had been hiding in a bunker to ride out the storm, and now it was emerging to assess the situation. My first awareness was the sense of deep peace I felt inside. This was in stark contrast to the emotional turmoil and pain of just a few short minutes ago.

The emotional release reminded me of a tropical rainstorm I once experienced in Florida. The skies suddenly filled with black clouds, and a tremendous deluge of rain fell. Then, within minutes, the clouds passed, and there was warm sunshine everywhere.

I had just been through my own emotional tropical storm. I started to review what happened and assess the damage. I had a sense this was about my breast cancer. It was also about my relationship with my breasts. I started to tune into them and imagined what I would say if I wrote them a letter. As I did, I felt an emotional pain around them. I had never really thought of my breasts as having any form of intelligence. But, as I was realizing very, very painfully, this was not the case. Not only did my breasts have an intelligence, but they held emotional memory as well.

Initially, I thought my letter to them would be in the form of a question, sort of. *How are you? How can I help you?* But I was sensing how poorly I had treated them. When my husband left, I remember looking at them in the bathroom mirror one morning and blaming them for getting cancer and driving him away. It was a bizarre twist of fate because my husband had always professed that he loved my breasts. Did he really love them, or did he love how they made him feel sexually? This distinction stung me. It brought another wave of deep sadness that washed through me. If he had loved them and loved me, how could he have walked out on us? It slowly dawned on me that I was really estranged from my breasts. I became aware of a sadness they were holding, as if they had been abandoned. It wasn't easy to admit, but I had abandoned them a long, long time ago.

I had needed to blame someone or something for my husband's leaving, and I'd turned this blame on my breasts. I remembered being proud of my naturally plump breasts during my dating days. I knew that they caught the attention of men. But as I was slowly and painfully realizing, I had been using them as a form of enticement—a means to an end. I turned heads, but I did not turn hearts. I also remembered how I used to compare my breasts to the breasts of other young women in the locker room at college. Mine were well developed, and looking back on it, I know it gave me a certain arrogance. The more I thought about how I had been relating to my breasts, the more the surges of sadness washed through me.

I kept my attention on my breasts and listened. It felt as if they were grieving in some way. Even though it felt emotionally painful, it was freeing at the same time. I could not remember a time when I saw them simply as two beautiful aspects of my body. They had always had some role to play in my identity as a woman who wanted to attract males.

I had the feeling that for many years, I had wronged them in some way. They had always been there when I needed them, but when cancer came along, I turned on them emotionally. As this thought sank in, another wave of sadness came. As I began to ponder what I would put in a letter to them, I could think of only one word. Sorry, sorry, sorry, sorry. More tears flowed, but instead of coming from my breasts, it now felt as if the tears were coming from my heart. I was crying for being such a selfish and cruel person. Then came a sense of shame that slashed me like a razor. I had treated them poorly and had never valued them.

Each tear seemed to hold a sting of pain. There was a sharpness in each tear that seemed to cut and tear at me. But what was being torn? Were they really tearing me or were they tearing at an old self that I created to protect a vulnerable little girl I hid away many years ago?

I felt as if something was dying inside of me while, at the same time, something was being born. I raised my arms to cradle my breasts. I held them as I would babies. I lowered my head toward them and kept saying, "Sorry, sorry, sorry." Wave after wave of tears washed through me. As hard as it was to cry, I also had a sense of some dark, long-held energy being released. My right hand held my left breast, and my left hand held my right breast. As if for the first time, I explored their shape and firmness. Only this time, it was not a fear-filled search for a lump. This time, I was exploring their beauty.

My hands were communicating to me how beautiful my breasts were. The sadness seemed to ease, and slowly my tears became full of gratitude. The words that Joe had shared about loving yourself "as is" echoed in my head. Then the letter to them began to appear in my head. "My dearest breasts, I love you. I love you. I love you. I am sorry that I abandoned you. I will always protect you. I will care for you. I will do everything in my power to heal you. I will never use you or take you for granted again."

Then I pondered the letter my breasts would write to me. "We forgive you. We want to be loved by you. We want to love you." My tears of sadness had transformed into tears of joy and union.

For the first time in my life, it felt as if I was truly falling in love with my breasts. It was like a homecoming. Like two lost and abandoned children had just returned home. We had found each other, and nothing would ever, ever come between us again. The tears were now pouring out of my heart and soul, and I imagined that they were washing over my breasts as if in some form of sacred baptism. I cradled my breasts in my arms and whispered, "You are home. You are loved. I will never leave you again."

The tears slowed to a stop, and I lay back in the car seat, reflecting on what had just happened. It felt as if a hundred-ton weight had just been lifted off me. I felt light and so wonderfully full of love and good energy. I also had a sense of my body being one big, beautiful, loving field of energy. It was the most glorious of feelings. I looked into the rear-view mirror at what I thought would be very bloodshot eyes. Instead, my eyes were clear and full of sparkles.

I glanced at the clock and noticed I had been there for fifty minutes. I punched in a text to my boss.

Sorry, delayed. Had a major meltdown. Then a major melt up. I love my breasts. Feeling fabulous. See you soon.

I pondered whether to send it and then hit the delete button. Instead, I typed,

Sorry! Delayed. Be there in ten.

With a beaming smile that reached from ear to ear, I pulled back onto the highway and headed to the office.

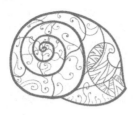

Chapter 17

The Offer

When I arrived at the office there was a message from my boss, Mark, asking me to meet with him at 11:00 a.m. in his office. *Okay,* I thought, *what's this all about?* Even though I had taken off time from my regular schedule, I had made up the time and was on track with all my projects.

Just before eleven, I made myself a cup of strong black tea and headed to his office with a notepad in hand. Mark was in his late forties, a few years older than I was. He had all the bad health habits—eating fast food, drinking gallons of Coke, and judging by his bugling belly, he had never seen the inside of a gym. But he was a kind and thoughtful man. He was meticulous with details but rather average when it came to leadership skills.

He was the original to-do list kind of guy. Always making notes on his schedule with a pencil that he kept sharp with a box cutter. He kept a master work-flow sheet for me and the other six grant writers, and he used it to control the flow of grant-writing requests. He was well liked, which helped to keep office politics to a minimum.

The door to his office was open when I arrived, and his head was buried in his computer screen. I tapped on the doorframe, and he looked up from his computer.

"Jane!" he said enthusiastically. "Come in, come in. Take a seat." He ushered me away from his desk to the couch on the other side of his office. He took a seat in a chair facing me. "So, Jane, how is everything?"

This was one of those open-ended questions I could either skim past or take an emotional dump with. Mark was a good listener and someone I trusted. He was one of the first people I had shared my diagnosis with, and he had been supportive. He never probed, but I knew he was always there if I needed an ear. "All is cool with me," I said, shooting him a friendly smile. "And you?"

"Super cool with me too," he replied returning the smile. He reached out and picked up a file from his desk and placed it on the coffee table in front of me. "New project" he said. "You were my first choice. I think this is right up your alley."

I lifted my eyebrows, trying to show some genuine interest. But quite honestly, I didn't give a monkey's ass about some new project. For the last couple of years, this grant-writing gig was really dragging. But for the fact that I needed the paycheck for the mortgage, truth is I would have split that scene a long time ago.

Mark reached forward and pulled a brochure from the file, handing it to me. "Homeless vets," he said as he studied my face for a response. "New downtown initiative by the bus depot beginning in a few months. We are heading up the fund-raising and public relations part. I know you have had some challenges of late and thought this new project would give you something to really sink your teeth into. You will have a couple of admin people under you to help with research and paperwork." He went quiet, waiting for an enthusiastic response.

All I felt was dread and heaviness in my stomach. I tried to feign some interest but knew I was failing miserably. "Why me?" I asked.

He was quick to reply. "Couple of reasons, Jane. First, you have all the skills to run a project like this. I know that you love to write, and this project is a great opportunity. For example, we want to create a book detailing the lives of local vets. This will mean interviewing them and writing up their stories. We have a publisher for it, which means you will become a published author. I remembered that during your interview, this was one of your life goals."

What he was offering me was what I had always wanted, but something inside of me was dead. There was no spark, not even a glimmer. "Sorry, Mark," I said, "I don't think I have what you need for this project."

Mark eased back in his chair and studied me. "Listen, Jane, I have this gut feeling about you and this project. I know that your dad was a vet, and I thought that having some flesh in the game would be good for you."

I sucked in a deep breath and forced a smile as I said, "I just don't have it at this time, Mark. Sorry."

"Listen," he said, "we are still finalizing the contract, so this will not start for another month or so. I am going to put this file in my drawer with your name on it. The Universe will guide us."

These last few words suddenly caught my attention. "What did you just say? 'The Universe will guide us?'"

He nodded slowly. "I keep this part of me pretty much under wraps at work, Jane, but between you and me, there is a bigger dimension to me than what I usually share. I just know my heart, and the Universe is telling me this is for you. Just don't say no for now, okay? You are working with some big stuff with your husband and cancer and all, so just know that I have your back and am cheering you on."

This gesture of kindness and support just broke me open, and I completely lost it and started gushing tears. He closed the office door and came to sit beside me, wrapping his arm around my shoulder to comfort me.

He slid a box of Kleenex in front of me. His open heart had just cracked my heart open. Between sobs and nose blowing, I started to wail. "I feel dead inside, and it scares me! I feel as if all the beautiful words I once wanted to share with the world have died inside me. They are dead, dead, dead, and they are rotting! I don't know what I am doing, where I am going, or how the hell to get out of this! I feel so utterly frickin' lost!"

The tears and snot were now flowing in abundance. Mark sat quietly, comforting me. Eventually, the tears stopped, and he moved along the couch to give me space to regroup. I turned to look at him. He seemed to have a Buddha-like gaze that was resting on me.

Then he said, "That was one cool-ass meltdown, you know!"

That was it. We both cracked up and started to laugh aloud, falling about on the couch. When we stopped laughing, I turned to him and said, "Wow, I felt like crap walking in here. Now I feel really good. I am going to have to hire you as my personal therapist for whenever I need an emotional dump!"

We both laughed again.

Then he stood up and said, "Seriously, Jane, the file is sitting in my drawer with your name on it. Do what you gotta do, and let's talk about this in a couple of weeks, okay?"

"That works for me," I said. I stood, and we hugged before I headed back to my desk very much emotionally lighter than when I had left it.

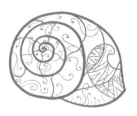

Chapter 18

The Three Loves

Midafternoon, a text arrived from Goth Girl.

Meeting tonight with Tuku. 7:00 p.m., coffee shop. Be there!

I shot a text back.

Great. See u then.

I knew nothing about this guy, Tuku, and decided to google *Shaolin monk* to give me some idea as to what to expect visually. What I found were rather thin, wiry, bald guys dressed in gray or orange outfits, who looked Asian. They were very acrobatic and seemed able to jump over tall things and kick their legs high. I guessed this was their special martial arts training. I also googled w*ay of the three loves,* but nothing came up. The prospect of seeing Goth Girl and Brock again cheered me up. I did some work for the rest of the afternoon until it was time to go.

I left time to pop home to freshen up and change my clothes. I chose a country sort of look. Faded blue jeans and a checkered shirt. As I set off for the coffee shop, I popped on a radio station. Then came that dreadful country song again, "We Ain't Never Coming Back." Ah! I hated that song and punched the off button with irritation. Why my husband liked that song was beyond me. All I knew was that I hated it. I arrived at the coffee shop a little irritated and a half hour early at 6:30.

I looked around for Goth Girl and Brock. No sign of them. Barney was behind the counter, and he nodded to me. I figured they would be bringing

Tuku and would arrive at any minute. I scanned the room and saw chairs evenly placed in a semicircle. I eyeballed the chair by the door and earmarked it for me. If this meeting turned out to be a bomb, I'd need a quick exit. I headed to the bathroom for a quick pee. As I was washing my hands, I thought about how David had taken over our finances and how I had so easily been manipulated. Angry at myself, I headed out to claim my seat. I was shocked to see a middle-aged woman in a black trouser suit had taken my chair. That really annoyed me. What was she doing here? Perhaps she did not know that we had a special event that evening. She seemed a little overweight and was obviously in the wrong place. I felt the urge to tell her this was a private meeting, but I figured Brock or Goth Girl would enlighten her when they arrived. As I eased past her, I could sense she was watching me. She said a friendly hello, and I gave a curt nod. I deliberately avoided making eye contact and took a seat three chairs away from her, turning my body slightly so as not to invite casual conversation. I still felt annoyed at her for being in my seat.

The front of the room was set up nicely with an outstandingly beautiful bunch of lilies in a striking, cut-glass vase. Someone had expensive taste, for sure. Next to the vase was a chair, and next to the chair was an empty table that matched the one the vase was on.

Soon, people started arriving, and the other chairs quickly filled. In the back room, I caught sight of Brock and Goth Girl. Seems they had been in there all along. I guessed they must be with Tuku, and I began to imagine how he would look. Dressed in orange or perhaps gray? Shiny bald head with wise, light-filled eyes? Just at seven o'clock, Goth Girl walked out of the back room and gave me a wink as she took the seat next to me. Then Brock walked out and stood in front of the room.

He was wearing a nice, crisp, white shirt that had a slim fit, showing off his broad shoulders and tapered waist. The shirt sat on top of a smart pair of dark blue jeans. He was really good on the eye. He scanned the room, and when he noticed me, he gave me a wink and a nod. I felt a little embarrassed, but I liked the extra attention. He welcomed everybody and talked briefly about how long he had known Tuku and what an esteemed teacher she was.

She? I thought. *Tuku is a* she?

Next, he invited a round of applause to welcome Tuku. At that moment, the woman in the black suit stood up and walked to the front of the room.

Oh shit! What had I just done? This woman in the black suit was Tuku! How frickin' rude of me to ignore her! She sat next to the beautiful flowers and quietly looked around the semicircle. I was feeling really embarrassed by how rude I had been and for avoiding eye contact.

Brock then took her seat. Tuku sat very quietly, looking at each of us in turn.

Then she began. "Hello and welcome to the way of the three loves. It is a pleasure and an honor to be with you this evening."

Her voice was very warm, and her whole demeanor communicated peace and gentleness. "I would like to start our series of workshops together by providing you with a background of the three loves and why it has been brought to the West. It began three thousand years ago, when a small group of holy people in the East went to live on an island off the coast of Southeast Asia. Their aim was to devote their time to prayer and to being with the divine. They developed deep meditation practices and became known for their loving and open hearts. They developed a monastic way of life that they called Shaolism.

"Across the water on the mainland was a village, and often the villagers would consult the monks for guidance about how to deal with the many challenges of their lives. The Shaolin monks were known for their loving and wise ways and helped the villagers to be more loving with one another.

"One of the recurring challenges the villagers faced was that of relationships and love. To help the villagers understand what love was and how to integrate it into their lives, the monks developed a special teaching called the way of the three loves. What I am bringing to you is this teaching. It is designed for people like you who live in the busy world and who face the many challenges of finding true and lasting love amid your challenging lifestyles.

"To help the villagers, the Shaolin monks developed special metaphors and stories to communicate their teachings. The island on which the monks lived was at the juncture of three oceans. It was the three oceans that inspired the creation of this program, which came to be known as the way of the three loves. Why three loves? The Shaolin monks said that there are three loves that exist, and it is in the full expression of these three loves that true love is found. The villagers viewed love as one single feeling that was a fit-all for all aspects of their lives. Unfortunately for the villagers, the word *love* had caused more heartache than it did joy. The Shaolin monks used the metaphor of the three oceans to explain what the three loves are and how they relate to each other.

"The first love is the love we find in our day-to-day lives and in all of our relationships. This is where our rational mind and ego live. The first love is love for a partner, our families, friends, pets, and our love of day-to-day life in general. This is represented by what we call the blue ocean. Imagine that this is a large, circular, blue ocean all around you.

"Then we have the second love. This is the love that lives within you. I would like to call it your soul. Each of you has a soul, and this is a pure form of love. Your soul existed before your life on Earth began and will continue when your journey in this life ends. The soul came to this world to learn and grow. Your body, intellect, and rational mind allow your soul to live in and experience this life on Earth.

"The soul is represented by the white ocean that is also circular. It is found within the blue ocean. Imagine a large, circular, blue ocean all around you and a smaller white, circular ocean within the blue ocean. This represents the life of your soul, which lives within your regular everyday life, the blue ocean. I will explain later why the metaphor provides a working model of how to create a beautiful and fulfilled life.

"The third love has to do with the Divine Presence that lives within your soul. There are many different names for this. The more common ones are God, the divine, Mother Nature, the Universe, the beloved, or any other name you may choose to use. The third love is the deepest and most beautiful love of all. It is the origin of all love. The third love is called the golden ocean, and it is a circular ocean within the white ocean. Imagine a target. The outer circle is the blue ocean. The white ocean is within this, and the golden ocean is in the middle and is called the bull's-eye. The golden ocean represents the divine love that loves you," Tuku said.

"The key to living a successful, love-filled life is being able to cultivate all three oceans or three loves and then knowing how to navigate between them. The villagers only lived in the blue ocean. This meant that their only source of love was their relationships to others. For this reason, love was something they bartered for and with—if you love me, I will love you back. Their relationships were based on dependency, and this led to many conflicts. Sometimes they would withhold love to punish people, which often led to conflict and wars.

"They looked for love outside of themselves and did not realize that the source of love was within. They always felt empty and searched for love in others to fill their emptiness. To help the villagers live more love-filled lives, the Shaolin monks developed a series of spiritual practices and metaphors from their own spiritual practices. The core of this work is what we call the way of the three oceans.

"The most common questions I am asked are: What does it mean to live the way of the three loves? How does it function in the world? What is a person like who has mastered the path of the three loves? To answer these questions, I would like to tell you a true story that took place some three thousand years ago.

"The Shaolin monks were living peaceful lives, devoting their days to meditation and spiritual practices. The villagers were great farmers and fishermen. From the north came a large horde of Mongol savages that were raping and pillaging every village they fell upon. The leader of the Mongols was a very cruel man called Hagza Khan. When word came to the villagers that Hagza Khan was headed toward their village, they decided to flee south. They told the Shaolin monks, and the abbot of the monastery instructed his monks to flee with the villagers. The abbot chose to stay and meditate on the way of the three loves.

When Hagza Khan and his savages arrived in the deserted village, he was angered to hear from his scouts that the abbot had not fled in fear. Hagza Khan took twenty of his cruelest mercenaries to the island to torture and kill the abbot. When Hagza Khan reached the monastery, he broke down the door of the temple where the abbot was quietly meditating. He marched up to the abbot, brandishing his blood-encrusted sword about his head.

"Spitting with rage and anger, he screamed at the abbot, 'Don't you know who I am? I am a man who can run you through without blinking an eye!'

"Hagza Khan was in his blue ocean, where anger and rage live. The abbot, who was in his golden ocean, slowly stood and looked Hagza Khan in the eye and asked him a question. 'Don't you know who I am? I am a man who can be run through without blinking an eye!'

Legend has it that Hagza Khan was so overcome with the abbot's love that he fell at his feet and asked to become his student. The abbot took Hagza Khan as a student and, after five years, instructed Hagza Khan to go out into the world to spread the way of the three loves. The abbot was in the golden ocean and came from a place of divine love. Hagza Kahn was living only in the blue ocean of rational mind and ego. It had become poisoned and distorted, which is why his behavior was so evil. Please note that I said his *behavior* was evil. I did not say that *he* was evil. When he faced the abbot, he met a man who was living in and from his golden ocean. The golden ocean in the abbot touched and woke up the golden ocean in Hagza Kahn, and it was the divine love that transformed the Mongol savage from the inside out. This is an example of what it means to live in the way of the three oceans," Tuku said.

"Each ocean represents a sort of lens through which we see life. The blue ocean provides a lens that is clouded or distorted by the ego and the rational mind.

"The white ocean, representing the soul, is a beautiful, pure lens that is not tainted by the ego, the rational mind, or self-need. The golden ocean represents a golden lens when you see with the eyes of the divine. The golden lens shone from the abbot, and this awoke the golden ocean in Hagza Kahn."

Tuku then fell silent. I was spellbound by the story. I glanced around the room and saw that everybody else was transfixed. Tuku then suggested that we take a short break. Goth Girl nodded in the direction of the door, and we headed out for some fresh air.

"Cool stuff, eh?" Goth Girl said when we got outside.

I was in a reflective mood, thinking about the concept of three loves. In many ways, it made so much sense to see life and love that way. I, for one, had always been jerked around by the one-dimensional love of the blue ocean that I had been living in. Where was my inner soul? Could I really develop a relationship to a Divine Presence? I felt my heart flood with hope just at the thought that I may be able to achieve that.

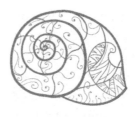

Chapter 19

Seeing the Layers

Tuku began the second half of the evening with five minutes of silence. It was nice to have a chance for my thoughts to settle. I started to imagine the three oceans all around and in me. It gave me a feeling of comfort.

Tuku gave us an outline of what the next few sessions would offer us, and I felt a quiet excitement. For the rest of the evening, we were going to look at blindfolds. Since the people in the group all seemed to have good eyesight, I wondered why she thought blindfolds would be of value to us.

"When the villagers came to us with their challenges finding love, it became apparent that they were wearing blindfolds that prevented them from seeing love and truly seeing what was in front of them," Tuku said. "One of the first things we did was help them to understand the blindfold process, as we call it." She pointed at the beautiful lilies in the vase. Then she reached down into her bag and pulled out a small, scruffy little plastic sunflower, which she placed in a used coffee cup on the empty table next to her. I have to say; the plastic sunflower did look a bit ridiculous compared with the beautiful lilies in the cut-glass vase.

She took a sip of water. "If I were to give you a gift of either the lilies and the vase, or this sunflower and paper cup, which would you choose?"

There was a light ripple of laughter in the group. I thought it was a silly question. The cut-glass vase alone must have been worth several thousand dollars. And the lilies were beautiful and must have cost a pretty penny.

I had never seen anything like them before. The scruffy sunflower looked very drab in comparison.

A smartly dressed youngish guy, who looked as if he worked in a bank, made the humorous comment that he would choose the sunflower simply so he could throw it away. Another chuckle of laughter spread around the group. Tuku sat silently, watching us. I had a sense that there was more to this than met the eye and wondered where she was going with it.

She turned toward the lilies and said the vase came from Italy and cost $2,000.

There was a subdued *oooh* from the group.

Then she explained that the lilies were flown in from South America, costing $800.

Another soft *ooooh* from the group.

"The vase was given to me by a lady who lives in a multimillion-dollar home. The lady spends her days playing tennis, socializing with friends, and puttering in her garden. Her husband made his money by selling large mortgages to people, whom he knew would never be able to keep up with the payments. This meant that they were destined for bankruptcy and homelessness. He also knew how to hide the money he made overseas so that he did not have to pay any income tax. This is where the money came from to buy this vase and the lilies."

She was silent for a moment. The group looked a little stunned and sheepish. She turned to the dusty little sunflower. "This sunflower was given to me by a single mother who is raising a special needs child by herself. She lives in a one-room apartment and must work three jobs to pay the rent. After the bills are paid, she has about one dollar and ten cents to buy herself lunch. She does not own a car. Two days ago, during her thirty-minute lunch break, she walked for ten minutes in the rain to the dollar store. There she spent one dollar and six cents of her lunch money to purchase this sunflower. She could not afford a vase, so she used her old coffee cup."

The silence in the group was palpable.

"Now," she said, "if I were to give you one of these as a gift, which one would you choose?" Some of the people in the group looked uneasy and directed their eyes to the floor. Some became restless. There was a general air of discomfort. Tuku quietly watched in silence as the message in her story was absorbed.

Two of the women in the group began to cry. The young man who made the joke about the sunflower looked very remorseful and apologized for what he'd said.

Tuku stood up, picked up the vase, and carried it out of sight. She returned and brought the sunflower out in front of the group. She remained standing. "This is what I mean by blindfolds. This is the first challenge that the villagers had to overcome before they could truly find love. They had to learn to see, which meant removing the blindfolds they were wearing. Just like the blindfolds you were all wearing when you walked in this evening. Do you want to remove your blindfolds?"

People started nodding and several said, "Yes, but how?"

I thought about all the people in my life and how I had been wearing a blindfold that prevented me from seeing who they really were. I thought about the superficial ways I had been seeing and judging life. No wonder I had never been able to find true love. I had a sense that Tuku and the way of the three loves was going to change all of that.

"Being truthful is where we begin," Tuku said. "Seeing the truth of what you are looking at and not simply the projections that come from the conditioned and polluted lens of your blue ocean." This sounded really good. Then Tuku looked directly at me. "May I ask your name?"

I was caught a little off guard by the sudden attention and felt a light flush of embarrassment in my cheeks. "Err, ah, my name is Jane," I replied.

"Welcome, Jane," she said. "Are you open and willing to explore your own truth?"

I felt as if I was being cornered, about to be made a sacrificial lamb for the group to chew on. I glanced at Goth Girl. She lifted one of her eyebrows at me as if to say, "So, you going to back out, girl?"

Then I shot a glance at Brock. He raised a finger to his lips and then pushed it out toward Tuku as if to say, *Let the truth out.*

I sucked in a deep breath of air and looked at Tuku, who was holding me very intently in her gaze. I had the sense that she was giving me a form of energetic CT scan and was really tuning into me.

"Sure," I said with a slight tremble.

"Thank you for your courage," Tuku said. The word *courage* made me feel good. Tuku pulled another chair and arranged it in front of hers. "Please come and sit here," she said to me, pointing to the chair.

No backing out now, I thought, and rather sheepishly I made my way to the front of the room.

We sat facing each other. With her eyes locked onto mine, she asked, "So, Jane, I want you to think back to the time in the coffee shop before the group arrived. Please tell me what you saw when you walked out of the restroom and found me sitting on the chair near the door where Brock is now sitting."

I felt a sudden flash of panic. *Oh no, this is not happening to me.* The eyes of the group were all on me now. I had become the sacrificial lamb.

"Take your time," she said in a soft, gentle tone.

Warning signs flashed inside my head. Some plaintive, weak, made-up answers flashed across my brain for consideration. I could say that I thought about getting a cup of coffee. I could say that I thought about how I was looking forward to the evening. But I knew that she knew that my thoughts had not been at all friendly toward her. She was trying to dig this out of me. Then I felt annoyed with myself for getting sucked into this. Do I bolt for the door? Do I have a meltdown? What the hell do I do?

Then Tuku spoke again. "Jane, please know that all of us here would have difficulty in accessing the truth as I am asking you to do. Please know that your truth will be a gift to everyone here, and it will help them access their own truths. Try, if you can, to stop your mind from stopping you."

Can she see inside my head? I wondered. This made me feel a little better, but a part of me was still on lock-down. I glanced at Brock again. He slowly nodded at me and mouthed silently what I thought was, *You can do this!* It felt as if I was being moved to a cliff and I was about to jump off or be pushed off. My truth was now on the tip of my tongue.

The final veil between my truth and me lifted, and I blurted, "When I walked out of the restroom and saw you sitting in that chair, I thought, *She took my chair.* I wanted to sit there because it was near the door. I wanted to sit near the door so I could leave if this turned out to be a load of crap." I was breathing heavily and felt very vulnerable. Tuku was sitting quietly, holding me in her eyes.

"Continue," she said.

What? More? a little voice inside my head shouted. I knew that she knew there was more.

I sucked in another gulp of air. I could feel my chest tightening and felt a burning sensation behind my eyes. Tears were close. "Well, I saw you and thought you did not belong here. I judged you as not belonging here, being overweight, and having a boring haircut. When you said hello to me, I deliberately ignored you as if I wanted to punish you for taking my chair." At that point, I lost it. I collapsed, sobbing, with my elbows on my knees. I felt really embarrassed for being so rude and selfish.

Tuku waited for a few seconds, allowing me time to cry. Then she stood and moved toward me. She gently gripped my wrists and eased me into a standing position right in front of her. I could still feel the convulsions in my body as the sobbing continued. She brought her hands up and ever so gently cradled my cheeks, holding her eyes on me in a way that felt as if we were the only people in the room. Then she said, "Jane, thank you for the beautiful gift of your truth!"

I felt my body suddenly become still as if a great peace had descended all around me. She gently eased my head forward and planted a kiss in the middle of my forehead, right on my third eye. As she held her warm lips there for just a few seconds, it was as if a bolt of warm light was fired right into me, and it exploded like a firework. It was the most glorious feeling of love I have ever experienced. As she pulled her head back and released my face, tears poured out of her eyes. She was not crying in an emotionally upset way. Her tears were radiant, just flowing out of her eyes. Then from my eyes came the same flood of tears. They felt warm and velvety. My body was perfectly still. It was as if the tears were coming out of my heart. We stood there in silence, lost in tears of pure love. Then she bowed her head as if to close some precious, sacred ritual she had just performed and gestured for me to sit again. I glanced around the room and saw that everybody in the group had the same tears in their eyes.

Tuku urged us to take some deep breaths. "This is an example of how the blue and golden oceans function in the world. Jane was in her judgmental, rational-mind blue ocean. She saw only her own projections. She could not see with love. I was in the golden ocean and saw her with the eyes of divine love. With the kiss on the forehead, I brought her into her golden ocean.

"When all of you wanted to take the crystal vase and lilies home, you were seeing through the distorted blue ocean. When you saw the deeper levels of the lilies and sunflower, you all shifted into the golden ocean. In this way, the oceans are like lenses through which we see life. The golden lens is the lens you need for seeing and finding true love. And it was the same for the villagers who were seeing life through the blue ocean and the distorted lens of their own projections.

"Here is a quick story to bring our evening to a close. The story highlights what you experience when you look for love with the lens of the blue ocean. I was walking down the road one evening, and I saw a man on his knees under a streetlight, looking for something. I asked him what he was looking for. He said he had lost his wallet. I got on my knees and helped him look for his wallet. We did not find it. Then I asked him if he was sure he lost it there. 'Oh no,' he said, 'I lost it down the road, but this is where the streetlight is!'

And so, it is. You have been looking for love in the wrong place. The way of the three loves will give you a new way of seeing that will completely transform your relationship to love and to your lives."

Tuku paused for a moment. Her words really struck home, and I could see how I had spent most of my life under the lamppost, looking for something that was not lost there and could not be found.

"To help the villagers, we developed a process called 'seeing beauty,'" Tuku said. "It is a process that transformed their relationships with themselves and each other. This is not a new way of seeing, but it is in a way returning to see life with the eyes of a child. There are three areas for seeing beauty and they can completely transform your relationships in life. At our next meeting, I will share with you the 'seeing beauty' process."

Tuku brought her hands up to her heart as if in prayer, bowed, and walked into the back room. There was a hushed silence in the coffee shop. I had the sense that people did not want to talk for fear of losing the special feeling inside.

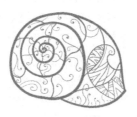

Chapter 20

Husband Comes to Dinner

I arrived at the office ten minutes early and made myself a cup of black tea to kick-start my day. As my computer was booting up, I reflected on the last evening and the way of the three loves. It all made so much sense—in particular, the blindfold process. It had really popped me open, and I wanted to use it in my regular life. But how?

I checked my text messages and found one from my husband. It said, May I call you this morning? I felt a tightening in my stomach. My mind flashed back to his request for me to freeze the divorce process. I thought about how he had manipulated me. Or this was my perception of what he did? Perhaps this was simply how my distorted lens in the blue ocean was seeing things. Even though a part of me wanted him gone forever from my life, our twenty-four years together as husband and wife still held meaning, and I was having difficulty understanding what I really felt about him. I sucked in a big breath and sent him a reply, inviting a call.

After a couple of minutes, the phone rang. It was my husband. His voice sounded perky. "Hi Jane, any chance I can bring over Chinese takeout tonight and we can chat about things?"

Things? I thought. *What the hell does that mean?* I flashed back to his rather sad state last time I saw him and felt a twinge of compassion for him. I said, "Sure. Does seven work for you?"

"Great. See you then. Bottle of white okay?"

"Sure. 'Bye," I said and hung up.

Well, this is different, I thought. Usually he would choose a red wine. He knew I preferred white, but I usually had to drink his choice of wine. Now he was offering to bring white! *Here is one positive change,* I thought, trying not to see him through the blue lens. *Could this be heading toward reconciliation? Is he really a changed man?*

Since my husband left, my evenings alone had been difficult and full of a deep loneliness. After twenty-four years of marriage, I was really struggling to come to terms with being all alone in the home. Perhaps our marriage was not the greatest, but it had had its high points. I did wonder what I was lonely *for.* Was it love? Was it David? Was it a partner or just some life-form to give me a sense of companionship? Perhaps I was lonely for a spiritual life. The loneliness was like a big ache deep within me.

The business card my husband left during his last visit was in my purse. I pulled it out to see if there was a website for his therapist. I entered the web address into my computer, and up it came. He was a family therapist who specialized in relationship issues. He had twenty-five years of experience, so I guessed he couldn't be all bad. I was wondering what exactly my husband was doing with him, and I decided to ask him outright that night.

For the rest of the morning, I crunched through research materials and took a walk around the block at lunchtime. During my walk, I began to wonder if there could be any hope for my husband and me. Then the doubting questions flooded my thoughts. Had I overreacted when he left? Did he deserve a chance to get his crap together? Was there something besides the cancer that had caused him to leave? Questions, questions, questions with no easy answers in sight. By late afternoon, I was actually looking forward to finding out what happened to him and what he was doing to get his head straight. The question of love came up again. Had I truly loved him? Did I still love him? What the hell was love, anyway? I was really confused and conflicted about love.

To help me ease my own sense of failure around love, I rationalized that it was my parents who had screwed me up when it came to love and relationships. It felt good to blame someone. This helped to numb the pain of guilt I was feeling in my heart. Then my thoughts wandered to Brock and the way of the three loves. Perhaps I was going out of my depth with this? Perhaps I was not really ready? After all, I had failed miserably at one love, so why on Earth did I think I could embrace three loves? Perhaps this was over my head.

But Goth Girl would be there, and with that thought, I felt an immediate ease. She had psychic gifts. Perhaps she could see in me more than I was able to see. Or was that just wishful thinking on my part?

For the rest of the afternoon, I did my best to focus on researching foundations.

Thanks to numerous cups of tea and two bars of dark chocolate, I made it through the afternoon and left the office promptly at 5:00 p.m. On the drive home, I rehearsed being a little distant and keeping control of the evening. Maybe I'd allow him an hour and a half before ushering him out.

So, I had a game plan, or so I thought, and felt quite relaxed about the whole thing. At 5:45, I jumped into the shower to freshen up. *Low-key clothing*, I thought. So, I pulled out an old pair of rather loose-fitting jeans and a baggy sweater.

I hung out in the recliner, watching the news until I heard the doorbell ring at 6:55. He was always Mr. Punctual, and I paused a few seconds before opening the door. As I slowly pulled it open, what I saw really shocked me. He was standing there with two large bags of Chinese takeout in one hand and a huge bouquet of red roses in the other. This really threw me into a tailspin.

"Uh, ah, wow. So, please come in," I stammered. As he walked past me, I caught the scent of the red roses, and I flashed to Goth Girl's comment about smelling the roses. I wondered what she would say if she could see me now.

He walked into the living room and placed the bags of food on the table. Then he turned and presented the roses to me. He knew I had a weakness for flowers, especially red roses, and was really playing his cards well. I could feel my resolve to be distant and controlling go right out the window. Slowly, I took the flowers from him and bowed my head in a thank you while doing everything I could not to give him a little kiss on the cheek.

"These are beautiful," I said. "Let me put them in water." I headed into the kitchen. As I reached the sink I called, "Get the plates, can you?"

He was quickly by my side, pulling plates out of the cupboard. As I stood at the sink next to him, filling a vase with water, I had a real sense of déjà vu. I didn't want to admit it to myself, but it felt so good to have someone there with me. I wasn't sure if it was David, or just having a person there that made me feel good. I was confused about what I was feeling. Was it David or our life together that I liked? Then there was my anger at him. It was sitting on the sidelines, watching all this. Would it flare up? I wondered. Would I tip the

Chinese food over him in a fit of anger? Although I was definitely discombobulated, I knew that just under the surface was a deep rage at him.

My husband was finishing up the table setting as I placed the flowers at the end of the table. We were sitting opposite each other, as we always did. The plates with knives and forks were placed with precision, and the small white boxes of Chinese food were arranged carefully in a line with equal spacing between them. He was such a perfectionist. A part of me liked this about him. But a part of me felt controlled and put off by it.

I glanced at the beautiful roses. Shit! They were glorious and had really done a number on me. He had opened the chilled bottle of white and asked if he could pour me a glass. His attentive behavior reminded me of when we started dating. But this was also the salesperson in him, and after we were married, the attentiveness fell away. I was feeling conflicted. A part of me really liked and needed this attention, but a part of me was suspicious of it. I felt as if my rage at him was sitting in another room, waiting for an invitation to join us.

We sat in silence across from each other, gazing at the small, white takeout containers. I could tell he was being very respectful. Or was he simply sucking up to me? I was still confused. What I did know was that I needed a drink. "Bottoms up," I said, and without waiting for a reply, I took a couple of quick gulps of the Chardonnay.

He started opening the takeout boxes and placed a serving spoon in each of them. He asked for my plate and said, "May I?"

A part of me reveled in the simple comfort of sharing a meal with him again. Our twenty-four years together were deeply imprinted in my psyche, and I could feel myself warming to him again. Then another voice in me wanted to shout, "So why did you walk out on me, asshole?" Rage was in the doorway now, locked and loaded. I was a bit of a mess inside and emptied my glass, pushing it in his direction for a refill.

We started eating and shared some superficial conversation about the garden and the chipmunks that had eaten some of our flowers. I kept wondering if he was going to bring up our last night together, when he walked out, or if I would have to bring it up. By the time I drained my second glass of Chardonnay, I was beginning to feel a little lighter and softer around the edges. I was also enjoying the food. This was something we always did on Thursday nights, which we called sports night. We would munch Chinese food, then I would go to my study to work, and he would crash on the sofa with a six-pack to watch whatever sport happened to be on.

Since he walked out, I had deliberately avoided Chinese food. And here I was, chomping it down just like old times. I could feel myself slipping into a level of familiarity with him that I knew was not right. It was too soon. He had not confessed his crime of abandonment to me. He had not begged forgiveness. I had not forgiven him, yet here we were, doing just what we had always done. We made more small talk, and then, as I was knocking back my third glass of wine, I saw rage waving at me from the doorway. Rage wanted in on this. A voice inside my head said, *Go right for it. Take no prisoners on this one.* I reached into my pocket and pulled out the business card for his therapist. I held it up for him to see as a stream of anger poured down my arm and into my fingers.

I flicked it at him. I lowered my voice, narrowed my eyes, and said, "Talk to me."

His eyes popped wide open; his jaw dropped. I liked feeling the ripples of anger run through me. I was in control now, feeling my spirit come back. Rage was still in the doorway, doing push-ups and warming up for my invitation to join the party.

I held my facial expression like a piece of granite. My eyes were locked on him, waiting for the wrong move, the slick answer, the hide-and-seek games. I knew exactly which of the white containers still contained the most food and was poised like a coiled spring to cover him with it. He became pale, and his eyes started darting around the table as he tried to gather the appropriate words. I knew I was close to nailing this bastard. *Therapy, eh?* I thought. *I will give you frickin' therapy.* I waited in silence as he squirmed.

I was feeling the urge to scream at him. I could feel within me the familiar anger that punched his empty pillow each morning. He was cornered; there was no way out. I was poised to take the vengeance I had longed for and so deserved. I was waiting for some flimsy excuse, some *Oh, I just don't know what happened* kind of response. What actually occurred completely threw me.

He lowered his head and looked at his plate for a few seconds. As he lifted his head, I saw, for the first time in twenty-four years, tears in his eyes. I was in shock. Then, with a tremble in his voice, he said, "I am sorry for what I did. The therapist helped me to realize that it was all my father's fault."

I was completely bemused. His father had always been his hero. My husband had modeled himself on his father throughout his life. Now, he was blaming him for walking out on me! I had always bitched about his father. He had always defended him. Now my husband was switching sides. This caught me off guard and threw me into disarray. Rage was looking at me very confused. What to do?

I was either hearing the earth-shattering breaking open of a man's soul or before me was an escape artist who would put Houdini to shame. I could feel the ground crumbling beneath my feet. Even though I propped myself up with anger, I was still very fragile and in no way ready for this. I did the only thing any self-respecting woman in this situation would do. I poured myself another glass of wine.

He mopped the tears with his napkin and started to talk. "Well, Jane, the cancer thing flipped a switch in me. I went on total shutdown. I basically ran for cover emotionally. The therapist I am working with is a specialist in a process called 'family sequencing.' He takes you back into your family history and plays out each role with small figures. It is a form of role playing that enacts the early family situations I experienced emotionally but was not able to remember with my conscious mind.

"I discovered that when I was four years old, my father walked out on his first wife, my mother, for the same reason," David said. "My father then married a younger woman who worked in his office."

My mind was spinning as I processed this information and pictured his parents and his new stepmother. *All very feasible*, I thought. *It all makes sense. It explains why he walked out on me. He's a victim—not a perpetrator.*

"Neither of my parents ever told me the real reason they divorced," David said. "My mother overcame her breast cancer but chose not to marry again."

I took another sip of wine and gazed at him across the table in silence. I had no idea what to say or how to respond. My husband's voice was back to normal now. This little, or big, confession seemed to restore his energy. The wine was making me woozy; my thoughts were colliding into each other. He sat silently watching me, waiting for my response. "Got it," I said. "I just don't know how to respond."

In a quiet, controlling way, he said, "I know, dear. This is a lot for you to hear all at once."

Even though I was a little dazed, his use of the word *dear* pricked and annoyed me. I was close to overload and played the headache card, informing him that we were done for the night.

"May I clean up?" he asked.

"Nope!" I said abruptly. "I will do it tomorrow. Just need to go to bed."

On his way to the door, he paused and turned toward me. What he did next caught me off guard again. He leaned in and gave me a kiss on the cheek. I pulled back, hesitant. Then he said, "May I ask you one favor, Jane?"

I was really untethered at that point and wanted to crash. "Sure, what is it?" I asked.

"Will you please keep the divorce proceedings frozen until we have really talked this out?"

With the roses, a kiss, and four glasses of chardonnay, he had penetrated my defenses. "Okay," I agreed. I will communicate that to my attorney."

"Thank you, Jane!" he said, and then he headed out into the night.

Now my head was really spinning. I flipped off the lights and staggered upstairs, barely making it to my bedroom. The last thing I remember was kicking off my shoes and falling headlong onto my bed.

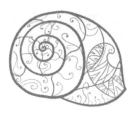

Chapter 21

The Morning After

The alarm woke me from a very deep, alcohol-induced sleep. I hit the off button with annoyance. My head was throbbing, and my body felt like crap. "I just can't do this," a voice in my head shouted. "Gotta stay in bed, sleep this off." I reached for the bedside phone and speed dialed my boss.

I heard his sharp, professional recorded voice: "Please leave a message, and I will get back to you promptly."

I sucked in a deep breath and said, "Hi, Mark. This is Jane. Having a bad, bad day. Will be in around noon. Will explain later. Thanks." And I put down the phone.

I rolled over and pulled the sheets around me. I fell back into a deep sleep.

Just after ten o'clock, the phone rang and woke me abruptly. I fumbled for the receiver and grumbled, "Hello," into the mouthpiece.

It was Goth Girl. "Hey, you sound like shit!" she said in her sharp, penetrating voice.

"Got that right," I replied.

"Is it the chemo?" she asked urgently.

"Na," I said. "Chardonnay. Too many glasses!"

"Geeesh, girl, you never invited me!"

"Crazy story," I said. "Husband showed up and all that crap."

"Sounds like you need to talk. Can I swing by?"

My head felt as if somebody was beating a drum in it. "Ah, mmm, guess so. But I look and feel like shit."

She shot back, "Truth is, you're always beautiful to me. You know that, Wig Girl. A big latte coming at ya."

I glanced at the clock, which showed 10:20. "How about eleven?" I asked.

"See ya then!" she said and hung up.

It took every ounce of energy I had to get myself to the shower. I let the hot water pour over me as some semblance of normalcy slowly returned to my body.

Did last night really happen? Was it all a dream? My throbbing headache reminded me that it was not a dream. To finish my shower, I hit the cold button and felt a jerk of aliveness shoot through me.

I had slept in my wig, Henry, and he was looking really out of shape—all flat on one side with stray shoots of hair sticking out the other side. As I studied him in the mirror, I felt that he represented exactly how I was feeling. I did the best I could with hair spray and a comb and apologized for sleeping in him. Then it dawned on me that I was talking to my wig, and I felt a wave of sadness wash through me.

I headed downstairs at 10:40, feeling just a little more human. The sight of the uncleared dining table brought the events of the night before crashing back to me. I checked my phone and noticed a text from David.

Were you able to freeze the divorce?

Freeze the divorce? As I scoured my memory of the night before, I reluctantly remembered the kiss and the question. Then I remembered saying that I would. *Damn!* I thought. *Why did I agree to do that?* He knew that I was a stickler for doing what I said I would do. So, I shot off a quick text to my brother, Bob:

Long story. Will explain later. Please change from pause to freeze divorce proceedings.

As I perused the dining room, I looked at the roses. They were stunning and had brought beauty into my home. Then I remembered the story Tuku had shared about the lilies and sunflower. Which one were these? The image of a prostitute and a holy man popped into my mind. Both stood at my door. Were the roses from a prostitute or a holy man? I knew that my blue-ocean lens would not show me. I needed the eyes of the golden ocean.

For one moment, the roses brought beauty; then in the next moment, they brought pain. I felt a stir of anger at my husband. Then I felt anger at myself.

I felt lost, and tears came again. I collapsed on the couch, sobbing. I felt comforted by the fact that my friendship with Goth Girl had grown beyond the terrain of the coffee shop. At eleven sharp, the doorbell rang. I jumped to my feet and opened to door to find Goth Girl holding two very big lattes. "Shit, girl," she exclaimed, "you're looking real bad-ass!"

I turned and headed back to the couch, leaving her in the open doorway.

Goth Girl closed the front door and came to sit near me on the recliner. She placed my latte on the coffee table. She sat back in the recliner, cradling her latte and watching me. I reached for my latte and said, "Frickin' Chardonnay! A little too much."

Goth Girl turned to look at the roses on the dining room table. Then she looked at me, waiting for an explanation.

"Husband," I said.

She narrowed her eyes and gave me a look of suspicion.

"I know, I know!" I blurted. "Bag of shit, for sure."

She sat quietly, studying me.

Then I remembered his kiss. "But he kissed me on the cheek. What does that mean?"

"You tell me," she shot back.

I pondered in silence for a few seconds and then said, "Perhaps he still cares about me. Perhaps he is truly sorry."

Goth Girl gave me a look of disdain. "A kiss, eh? So, Wig Girl, guess where I was yesterday afternoon?"

I shrugged.

"Well, I was in the gym. And on one of the televisions, there was a ten-pin bowling championship going on. There was this short guy with a big belly rolling these big plastic balls at these pins. Here's the thing: just before he rolled his ball down the alley, he would bow his head, pucker up his lips, and plant a kiss on the ball. Then he'd toss it down the alley. Do you think he was kissing the bowling ball because he was in love with it? Or was he kissing it because of what he hoped it was going to do for him?"

Her truth penetrated my fragile defenses, and I felt like a sucker.

"Well, I haven't met your lame-ass husband yet," she said, "but I would bet my wig with red streaks that his motives are murky. My guess is that he's after something."

The precision of her comments unnerved me. I took some long sips of coffee and pondered my fractured state.

"So, Wig Girl, good news," she said. "We have another session with Tuku tonight. Seven o'clock at the coffee shop. Cool, eh?"

"Ugh. I'm not sure I'm up to that. This *love* word is really driving me nuts."

Goth Girl came over and sat next to me on the couch. She reached down and picked up my hand, bringing it close to her lips. She looked me straight in the eyes and then lowered her head and kissed the back of my hand. I felt a flash of love pour up my arm.

"That," she said, "is what this love word means. Got it? This is my way of saying, 'I got yer back.' Be there tonight. Trust me, honey. Okay?"

She had just done the golden-ocean thing on me, and it hit me like a ray of sun right in the heart. I beamed a big smile and said, "I am not sure what I have done to deserve you."

We shared a hug and she headed out.

I heard a text come in and looked at my phone to see who it was from. It was from my brother Bob.

Divorce frozen. Will await your directions. Love you. Bob.

I punched in a text to David:

Divorce proceedings frozen. For now, that is!

I hit the send button and collapsed back into the couch for a nap. I napped for about an hour, and then the jingle of a text woke me. I thought it was from my husband and was reluctant to look at it. I glanced at the ID and felt a happy surge of good energy when I saw that it was from Tuku.

Second session at coffee house. 7:00 p.m. Would love to see you there.

I was suddenly transported into another world—one of Shaolin monks who radiated love. I shot a text back to her:

Will be there. Thank you.

I knew Goth Girl must have prompted Tuku to send the text. It was a simple act of kindness. Yet how powerful it had been. Slowly my hung-over state eased into some degree of normalcy.

I looked forward to seeing Tuku again. Time to give Henry a much-needed wash and blow dry. I remembered Tuku saying that she would be sharing the "seeing beauty" process with us. Then I thought that perhaps I could share with her the "seeing crap" process, as I had become something of an expert at it.

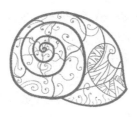

Chapter 22

Seeing Beauty—Part 1

I arrived at the coffee house early and ordered a large latte. Mare was behind the counter and beamed a big sunny smile at me. I wanted to be close to Tuku and took a chair in the front row, just a little off center. Others started to drift in, and we shared warm hellos. I was aware of the lesson that Tuku had taught me in our first session about projecting negative thoughts from my blue ocean onto people. I imagined that there was golden light pouring out of my eyes every time I looked at someone. I was struck by the beautiful responses I got from people I hardly knew. I was feeling a definite sense of warmth in my heart. *Wow!* I thought. *These processes are so easy to assimilate into everyday life. And this is just the beginning.* I was excited about what was ahead for me.

Goth Girl had texted that she was finishing up some work and would be there on the dot at seven o'clock. She wanted me to save her a chair. I put my coat on the chair next to me and enjoyed some quiet moments sipping my latte. Around five minutes to seven, Tuku and Brock walked out from the back room. Tuku was wearing a beautiful cream-colored trouser suit and seemed to emanate an aura of light. Brock came over to give me a hug. I stood, and once again he wrapped his long, strong arms around me and pulled me into his firm body. I felt a flush of heat and excitement. Then he slowly released me and took a seat in the back.

As I took my seat, I noticed that Tuku was watching me. When our eyes met, she gave me a friendly wink. Even though it was just a brief wink, it seemed to communicate that she was pleased to see me and that she cared for me. I knew it was that golden ocean energy again. Who knew that just one small wink could communicate so much? I winked back at her.

Right at seven, Goth Girl arrived, picked up a latte that Mare had already prepared, and took her seat next to me. She beamed a big smile at me and gave my knee a happy-to-see-you squeeze. Tuku asked us all to take some deep breaths and close our eyes for a moment to tune in and fully arrive.

Then she began to talk. "Greetings my friends, it is good to see you again. This evening, we will be looking at the seeing-beauty process. This process is preparation for the way of the three loves and creating a life that is full of true and authentic love. The challenge for most of us is that we have conditioned ways of seeing things in life that prevent us from seeing beauty, and this prevents us from truly loving.

"There are three parts to the seeing-beauty process. Each part has three components that you will do three times. Some of you may be wondering why the number three is used so often. Well, the process is not just aimed at providing you with new tools to see beauty and love, it is also aimed at creating new patterns in your subconscious that will function automatically and displace the negative ones.

"Most of our daily behaviors are based on old habit patterns that repeat themselves. Most of these patterns were installed during our childhoods, and some of these patterns were installed by those who did not really understand what was best for our higher good. Some of these patterns are dysfunctional, and you may have created new patterns to counterbalance them. The work of the way of the three loves is not to try to untangle all these old patterns. You could spend the rest of your life trying to do that, and at best, you might simply reorganize them.

"Your actions and responses to life come mostly from what we call *neural pathways* that are created in your brain. They carry the messages that control what you think and how you act. As you learn a new task, a neural pathway is created, and the more you practice it, the more established it becomes.

"Both a physical action and a repeated thought create and maintain neural pathways in the brain. Thoughts are energy and they create. If you think negative thoughts, you will grow and attract negativity in your life. If you think loving thoughts, you will create and attract love in your life. The challenge is that many of your old negative thought patterns function automatically because of all the neural pathways you have created in the past.

"The good news is that as you stop sending the energy of thought to the dysfunctional neural pathways, they atrophy and stop functioning. As you send your positive energy of thought, new neural pathways are created, and these will displace the old, negative ones.

"The magic of this process is that you only have to keep your attention on that which you want to create. The challenge is keeping your thoughts off the old, negative habits of thought and the established neural pathways that support them. To help you create these new neural pathways and new ways of thinking, we created some fun processes. These are easy to do, and the effect on how you feel will be immediate."

I really liked the sound of that. I knew that I was trapped in old patterns and habits of thought. I had always thought I needed my husband to guide our finances and realized now that this was untrue and diminished who I was as a person. Even though I had tried to change this thought pattern, it had still controlled me.

"This work has the ability to transform how you think and feel very quickly," Tuku continued. "So I would like to go over it again briefly. Our work is to create new patterns of thoughts and ways of thinking. As you do this, you will stop using the old patterns that do not serve you, and they will eventually atrophy and lose control over you. The key is to create new good habits of thinking that will become automatic behaviors. The neural pathways affect and inform your subconscious, and the subconscious affects at least 90 percent of how you function and live your lives. The process of creating new thought patterns begins with being able to see beauty. This will produce beautiful energy, and you will feel beauty inside you. I know it sounds almost too good to be true. But as you will soon discover, your lives are about to be transformed."

Goth Girl leaned into me and whispered, "Ain't this just the coolest shit?"

"Mind blowing," I whispered back.

"These processes were developed by the Shaolin monks three thousand years ago and come from the purest essence of their deep spiritual work," Tuku said. "They cultured these processes in such a way that the busy villagers would be able to apply them to everyday life.

"The processes are based on repetitions of three. We do things in threes for several reasons. First, it is easy to achieve and thus gives you a feeling of success. Doing something three times is much easier than having to do it twenty times. If you succeed at something, you are more likely to repeat it," she said.

"Second, it is the repetition that builds the new habits and neural pathways. For example, if I threw a big bucket of water at a rock, it would make the rock wet. But if one small drop of water hit the rock repeatedly, eventually it would make a hole in the rock. The practices I will be teaching you create lasting, effortless change and evolution. This is the reason we do processes in three.

"I am sure that most of you have explored new fads and fancies in the New Age self-development craze. Many of you tried various processes and patterns for a while, and then they fell away. Our old habitual ways of functioning and seeing are like blindfolds to true seeing. Remember the story of the lilies and how your seeing was clouded? The process you are about to learn will help you to clean the blue lens, so you can use the golden light to see yourself, people, and all of your life.

"Seeing beauty consists of what we call 'action thoughts.' We do not call these *meditations* because the word *meditation* has many definitions and can lead to confusion. These new processes are not designed to replace any of your existing meditation of mindfulness practices. These new 'action thought' practices can be used in conjunction with your existing practices.

"The seeing beauty process has three parts. The first part is seeing beauty in yourself. The second part is seeing beauty in other people. And the third is seeing beauty in life. Each of these three processes have three components that you will do three times. The first process we are going to do this evening is how to see beauty in yourself. We live in a culture that is very competitive and judgmental. For this reason, there is a lot of negative self-judgment. People compare themselves to others. We tend to look at what we don't have and what others do have. We look for a surface beauty in others and forget to really appreciate our own deep beauty.

"So, the first seeing-beauty process we are going to do is about seeing beauty in yourself. To help deepen the effects of this process, I am going to record it on paper. Writing something down helps you to strengthen your learning process and helps with the creation of new neural pathways in your brain.

"Seeing beauty in yourself has three components. I will say them first, and then I will explain them in greater detail. The first part is physical beauty. The second is about character and personality. The third is about doing acts of kindness for yourself. When I talk about physical beauty, I am not referring to the Hollywood film-star approach to beauty. This is a very shallow and artificial beauty. You are going to see beauty in every part of you. Your toes, your thumbs, your nose, your eyebrows, as well as internal aspects of you, such as your lungs and your blood.

"The aim of this process is to change the way you automatically look at yourself. This new way of repeatedly seeing yourself with the eyes of beauty will create the new automatic way your subconscious will view you. For example, it is not about having an exquisitely shaped nose. The nose you have been given by nature is beautiful as is. So, you would think and write down, 'My nose is beautiful'. You can add, 'I have beautiful fingers and beautiful lungs.' You will be identifying small parts of your physical body and acknowledging their beauty. As you begin to do this over and over, you will start to recondition the wiring in your brain. At the same time, you will not be able to have negative thoughts because you are too busy looking for beauty. The old, negative patterns of seeing yourself will lose power over you and atrophy.

"The second component to this is seeing beauty in your character or personality. For example, your kindness is beautiful. You can see beauty in your intelligence and in the way in which you are attentive to the needs of others. Once again, this looking for beauty in your character and personality will become a habit as you repeat it and create new neural pathways in your brain. This process will prevent you from thinking negative thoughts about yourself, and the old habits will slowly atrophy and fall away.

"The third process is to imagine doing three acts of kindness for yourself. Do not worry about how you will do these acts of kindness—or whether you can afford them. For example, you may imagine taking yourself on a sun-drenched cruise and then think, Oh I can't afford that, or I could not take two weeks off work. This process is purely in your imagination, so you are free to imagine anything you like and have lavish fun. This process is one of opening your heart to yourself. Directing kindness to *you*. Once again, the aim is to establish this as a routine practice within you. This will create new neural pathways, and the old patterns of not valuing yourself or not being kind to yourself will fall away. This is also fun to do.

"It is also another way to switch negative and stress-filled thoughts into high-octane energy within you. The beautiful side effect of this process is that as you visualize these acts of kindness for yourself, they may actually start manifesting in ways you could never imagine. It is like sending your requests to the Universe, God, or whatever your higher power may be. And you may be very pleasantly surprised to see some of your requests manifest.

"Imagining the three acts of kindness for yourself is also how you use the golden light on yourself. I liken it to sunbathing. Just imagining having a massage every month or going out to dinner at a fabulous restaurant will shift your energy into a higher realm and stop the old patterns of lack and fear.

"Writing down these acts of kindness helps to deepen the learning and creation of these new habit patterns, but just seeing it in your imagination is really helpful too. As this process brings you happy feelings, you will want to do it more. In this way, you will create ways of seeing beauty that function automatically. In the early days, you just need to be patient and keep doing these practices until they become habit patterns within you. So, let me give you an example of how this looks."

Tuku closed her eyes and took some deep breaths. I was really loving what she was sharing. Since my husband walked out, I had been in a real battle with my mind. I always seemed to look at what was wrong or lacking in me and not what was good or beautiful.

Goth Girl turned to me and gave me a wink as if to say, "Cool-ass stuff, eh?"

I winked back.

After a few moments, Tuku opened her eyes and picked up the notebook and pen that were under her chair. She started writing. When she finished writing, she looked up and started talking again. "What I just wrote down were three things that are beautiful about my body. I have beautiful eyes, not because they may or may not be film-star-type eyes, but simply because I have eyes that work. I have beautiful hands—again, not because they would win a prize in a beauty pageant, but because I have been gifted with two hands that work. I have beautiful kneecaps."

There was a ripple of laughter.

"Yes, I do have beautiful kneecaps," she said. "They are an important part of my leg structure, and they work beautifully, so why shouldn't I see beauty in them? Then I wrote down three things about my personality and character that are beautiful. My kindness is really beautiful. My intelligence is beautiful, and my ability to listen to others is really beautiful.

"For three acts of kindness, I wrote: Take myself on a beautiful cruise. Have a beautiful massage once a month. Buy myself a beautiful new car. And I did not limit these because I do not have the money. I am simply imagining beautiful acts of kindness that I am doing for *me*. But as I do this, I am sending energy and beginning the creative process and using the law of attraction, so you just never know; these may materialize." She beamed a big smile at us as. Then she held up her notebook and encouraged us to keep a notebook and date each entry of the nine things. She also said that if we were having an off day, then we could simply open the notebook and jump start ourselves by reading what we'd written previously. She called this the *jump-lead process,* which is like starting a car when its battery is dead. You connect it to another battery with a jumper cable to energize it. I liked that metaphor.

Tuku looked around the room and asked if anyone had questions. A middle-aged woman in the front row put her hand up. Tuku acknowledged the raised hand and invited her to share.

"I like the way you are seeing beauty in everything, but the big buzz word these days is *gratitude*. I am wondering why you do not use gratitude in this process?" she asked.

"Very good question," Tuku responded. "We do actually use gratitude in the way of the three loves, and seeing beauty is a way of preparing you. The Shaolin monks feel that beauty is really important and essential to being able to find true love. It goes back to life being a gift that is given for a certain period of time. Seeing beauty is a way of being able to experience the wonders of life and this world. Once you have learned to see your life and all of yourself as beautiful, then you should be grateful. I think you will understand when I say that you may not particularly like your body, but you can still be grateful for it. The problem is that not liking your body creates a negative relationship to how you relate to your body, and this will minimize the value of gratitude. For me, when I see beauty in all things, it makes me feel happier. And happiness is the foundation of being able to experience love. Happiness is like soil in which love can grow.

"The other thing about the seeing-beauty process is that it is an aid to achieving health because it raises the vibration of your thoughts, and this strengthens your immune system," she said. "Thoughts of kindness also block the negative thoughts that can diminish your immune system. So, as you see, seeing beauty has incredible power to transform and heal your body and your life."

The room fell silent. People seemed entranced by what she had shared. It all made so much sense, and I wanted to start right away. Tuku suggested we take a break and return in ten minutes.

Goth Girl and I headed out for some fresh air. "Don't you just love this stuff?" she asked as she handed me a piece of dark chocolate.

I said that I was struck by how penetrating yet simple the seeing-beauty process seemed.

I knew Goth Girl and Brock had already been through the spiral of love process, and I asked her why she was going through it again.

She responded quickly. "Just like polishing a diamond, Wig Girl. The sparkle just gets brighter and brighter every time you polish it. Oh, and of course, the neural pathways get stronger too." As she said this, she laughed, and I joined in the laughter.

Brock stuck his head out the door and called us back. As I walked in, I reflected on how many heavy-duty self-help programs and books I had been through over the years. Few, if any, had made any meaningful and lasting changes in my life. As Goth Girl kept saying, this really was cool-ass stuff.

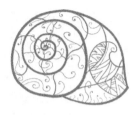

Chapter 23

Seeing Beauty—Part 2

We took our chairs, and Tuku spoke. "So, let us begin together the journey into beauty. The beauty of you, the beauty of life, and the beauty that is the gift of life."

As she said those words, a shiver went up my spine as if a big lightbulb came on inside me. Life and everything about life really was beautiful. For some reason, I was feeling very emotional. It was as if I had been blind and now, I was about to be given the gift of sight. I glanced at the other people in the group and saw how each one of them was beautiful in his or her own way. At the first meeting, I had been so judgmental. I had mistakenly thought that a beautiful person had to look like some air-brushed picture on the magazine stands at the supermarket checkout. Even though I knew the beauty in those photos was artificial, it had become the standard against which I measured myself and others. I felt sadness for myself for being sucked into the dismal world of manipulated outer form that is driven by greed and vanity.

I turned to look at an elderly woman who was sitting near the door. I remembered that on the first evening, I'd noticed a stale body odor when I passed her and thought that she needed a bath. I deliberately avoided sitting next to her. All I saw was a scruffy old woman with unkempt hair. Her shoulders were rounded, and her face was wrinkled with a sad, kind of lonely look. Definitely nobody I wanted to connect with.

Now, as I looked at her, all I could see was her beauty. Something about her energy seemed to shine. It was beautiful. Her unkempt hair, wrinkled skin, and stale-smelling clothes were only distortions of my own way of seeing through the blue ocean of my intellect, with its negativity and its judgmental, comparing ego. Every part of her that I had judged poorly now became a facet of her beauty. I felt the urge to go over and hug her and to ask forgiveness for how I had judged her.

Tears began to roll down my cheeks. It was the perception of the beauty I could see in the old woman that caused my tears. I flashed a look at Goth Girl, who was watching me intently. She had a questioning look on her face. Same thing happened when I looked at Goth Girl: I did not see her outer form, but I felt the energy that came from the collected form of her physical being, and it was so beautiful. My only response was tears. For the last three months, all my tears had been full of sadness and pain. I dreaded crying because it was so painful. Now, each tear was full of beauty and joy. I lowered my head, hoping not to be seen to allow my tears to finish naturally.

A hushed silence fell upon the room. After a few moments, I raised my head to see what was going on. Tuku was sitting still, gazing at me with tear-filled eyes. Everyone in the group was looking at me. Many had tears rolling down their cheeks.

Then my crying turned into laughing, and I bellowed, "What's going on? Why have you all become so beautiful? Why am I feeling so beautiful and why am I crying beautiful tears?"

What happened next really broke me open. The old woman came over to me and asked for a hug. I jumped to my feet and into her open arms. She kept saying, "I am sorry, I am sorry, I am sorry."

Then I started saying, "No, it is me who has to say I am sorry. I am sorry, I am sorry."

We gently pulled apart and took our seats. Tuku asked us all to take some deep breaths and center ourselves. A great peace came upon the group.

"Welcome, welcome, welcome to seeing beauty," Tuku said. "What just happened is how the seeing-beauty process works. Its power to transform is beyond what words can describe. You can only experience it, as you all just have.

"The metaphor I would use is what the sun does to a closed rosebud. You were all closed rosebuds. The seeing-beauty process is what happens when the sun comes out. You have all just opened like a garden of roses. I want to explain that what just happened is a sort of homecoming to the person you have always been. As a child, each of you brought into the world the way of seeing beauty. It is who you are and who you always have been. This is why there is so much joy around babies. They see with beauty. They see with the golden ocean. The divine looks through their eyes at you and touches the divine in you. Seeing with the golden ocean is their natural state, and it is your natural state. It becomes lost in the distorted blue ocean of intellect and ego. You have simply uncovered who you naturally are and have been all along. You have all returned to seeing with the eyes of a child again. This is why the transformation is so swift and effortless. It happens by itself, once it is released from the constrictions of the blue ocean, the mind and ego. The actual process I shared with you for seeing beauty is what released the hold the distorted ego and rational mind had over you. Seeing beauty is who you are, not what you have to learn how to be.

"You may find that some of your old negative patterns try to reinstate themselves. This is why we write down the three sets of three seeing-beauty aspects of your physical self and your emotional/character self and three acts of kindness. In the long run, you will not need to do this, because seeing beauty will become your natural way of being in the world."

As Tuku talked, I felt as if every word was spoken directly to me. Every word seemed to land like an arrow of love right in the middle of my heart.

Tuku mentioned what had happened between the old woman and me and asked if we would be open to sharing. We both stood up spontaneously at the same time and headed to the front of the group. As we met at the front of the room, we reached out our hands to one another. The old woman asked if she could go first. We stood there, hand in hand, and as she started to talk, I could sense a beautiful glow radiating from her. Her voice was soft and measured, and it communicated a gentle strength.

"Hi, my name is Dorothy," she said. "My husband suddenly died of a heart attack two years ago. I have been struggling ever since to pull myself together, but my grief has just engulfed me. I just can't seem to be bothered to take care of myself anymore. I was always so nicely dressed and clean. Now, I wear worn clothes. My grief has really diminished me. I am sorry and embarrassed to say that I know my clothes smell dirty. When we gathered for our first meeting, I was at the counter, and I knew that when Jane walked past me, she could smell my unpleasant smell and moved away from me. I felt really hurt by that and called her a bitch under my breath. It was a sad form of defense, but it was the only way I could deal with the situation. When I walked in this evening, I projected the you-are-a-bitch energy at her. This is what I am sorry for."

Tuku then invited me to talk.

"Yes, I did pick up on your stale body odor, and I think it triggered a time when my mother scolded me for not washing one day. I have this real phobia around body scent, and it has—or I want to say, up to this point—this phobia has controlled me. Not anymore, though. I am sorry for judging and rejecting you."

Tuku asked us to face each other. We joined our other hands and stood looking into each other's eyes.

"It is impossible to avoid conflicts and misunderstandings," Tuku said. "Conflict is inherent in human nature. The key is to know how to resolve and set it free. You simply must tune into your golden ocean and look into each other's eyes. Then you say three of the most powerful words in the English language: I am sorry.

"The other person, if he or she chooses to, can say the three second-most powerful words: I forgive you. And that is it! The golden ocean will wash away and bless you both. Dorothy and Jane, are you ready?"

We both nodded. We turned to face each other. Our eyes were full of tears. When Dorothy looked into my eyes, it seemed she was looking right into my heart. "I am sorry, Jane," she said.

I felt a ray of warm light shoot right into my heart. Holding her gaze, I said, "I forgive you, Dorothy."

Then we fell into each other's arms. After a few seconds, we pulled apart, but our hands stayed connected. I then looked into her eyes and said, "I am sorry, Dorothy."

She said to me, "I forgive you, Jane." And once again we hugged.

The feeling of lightness and happiness was incredible. The whole room seemed full of golden light. Tuku wrapped her arms around both of us, and all three of us entered what I can best describe as a golden hug. Tuku released us, and we headed back to our seats. I was glowing from head to foot. Tuku said that we had one more important piece to look at and suggested we take a ten-minute break.

Goth Girl and I stepped outside again, and she pulled out more dark chocolate. "Hey, girl. You just earned yourself a treat."

I broke off a big piece and popped it in my mouth. I did not want to talk, so I touched my lips with my finger in the "please be quiet" sign. Dar understood right away.

I just wanted to stay in the aura of golden light. I had just witnessed the most amazing transformation and wanted to stay in its perfume. She and I finished the bar of chocolate in silence, and then Brock called us back in.

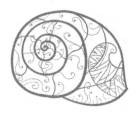

Chapter 24

Seeing Beauty—Part 3

Tuku was sitting quietly with her eyes closed in front of the group when we returned. Her presence seemed to cast an air of peace and well-being throughout the room. We returned to our seats and fell silent. After a few moments, she opened her eyes. "Thank you all for being part of this wonderful evening," she said. "We have two more pieces of the seeing-beauty process." She nodded to Brock, who started to hand out notebooks and pens.

"I would like you all to run through the seeing-beauty process. Then I want to conclude the evening with how to apply the seeing-beauty process in your everyday lives. Before you start writing, check in with yourself and register how you are feeling. We will compare this feeling with how you feel after you have done the seeing-beauty process."

I opened my book and began to think about three aspects of beauty in my physical body. I wrote I have beautiful feet, beautiful hair, and beautiful lungs. Then three things about my character. I wrote that my kindness was beautiful and that my thoughtfulness and compassion were also beautiful. For the three acts of kindness I had to imagine, I began with a ninety-minute massage. Then I gave myself a two-week cruise. My third act of kindness was to buy myself a laptop computer just for creative writing. I was surprised that just *imagining* these acts of kindness made me feel good. It occurred to me that this process was like changing TV channels with a remote control. I was not able to think any negative thoughts when I was busy seeing beauty and acts of kindness.

We all finished writing and sat waiting for Tuku. "So, how are you feeling now, compared with how you felt before you started?"

Everyone in the group was keen to share how the experience seemed to elevate their mood and their relationship to themselves. I joined the chorus. I could really feel the shift in my mood. I also liked that I had written the words down so I could look back at them and add more.

"You have all experienced how wonderful it feels to be in a room full of golden light," Tuku said. "But the challenge is to maintain this in your daily life. The golden ocean needs the intellect and rational mind of the blue ocean to be able to function in the world and communicate with people. So, we need to remove the dysfunction from the blue ocean—our rational minds and egos—so they can become beautiful instruments and lenses for the golden ocean to shine out into the world. You need a clear and healthy ego and rational mind if you are to truly live the golden ocean on a day-to-day basis so that it becomes the fabric of your life.

"The question you may be asking is, 'But how do I remove the distortion of my blue ocean, the rational mind and ego?' The one-word answer is 'Truth.' Truth is the process for keeping the blue ocean clear so the golden ocean can shine into the world. To truly *live your truth* in your daily lives, there is one word you need to learn how to use. The word I am about to teach you is like a sword. It is there to protect you. How and when you use it will depend on your own sense of when it is needed. This one special word has two letters. It begins with an *N* and ends with an *O*. Yes, the word *no* is the special word that you will have to use correctly if you want to maintain the integrity of your golden ocean or light.

"When you see with beauty, you will feel a flood of what we call 'yes energy' that will release a lot of creative passion in your life. Seeing beauty is another way of saying yes to being fully alive. However, this light needs protection from those who would seek to steal your beautiful energy or use you somehow. In this way, the word *no* becomes a sword. You only wield it when you need to protect yourself."

This really hit a chord with me. I loved the idea of being in my truth, but I am always the sucker when someone wants something. I don't always want to give it, but I'm afraid to say no. I could see how the word *no* could be used to protect the integrity of the golden ocean. This was really resonating with me.

"The key to using the word *no* is to use it lovingly, knowing that this response is for the higher good of all concerned, even if the person you say it to does not appreciate or understand it at the time. Being able to use the word *no* with love, guided by truth, will give you a tremendous feeling of freedom and empowerment. And using the word *no* is actually a wonderful act of kindness for you to use on yourself. Even the thought of being able to be truthful in saying no when I used to say yes to keep people happy gives me a sense of inner power." Tuku shared that when she was learning about the word *no*, she would practice saying it with great love and compassion in front of her bathroom mirror.

Amen to that, I thought.

Tuku asked if there were any questions. A youngish, well-dressed man in the front row put his hand up. "Would you be open to share your own method of using the seeing-beauty process with us?"

She beamed a smile at him and said, "Sure. I begin my day with it. When I wake up, I lie in the early darkness and run through the three areas, selecting three things for each area. I like to apply one full in-and-out breath to each aspect of beauty. For example, as I breathe in, I think of the aspect of beauty, say my neck. As I breathe out, I see my neck glowing with golden light. I do the same with each act of kindness. On the in breath, I imagine the act of kindness, for example lying on a massage table. As I breathe out, I imagine how wonderful it would make me feel. This is a great way to start the day. I sometimes do the same process as I stand in front of the mirror. It helps me to see all the beautiful parts of my body, and I love the way this process makes me feel. I often do the seeing-beauty process during the day. I do it before meetings and in traffic jams. I have even done it waiting in the supermarket checkout line.

"I love the way it can transform negative thoughts," Tuku added. "Not only does it transform the moment, but bit by bit, it is creating new neural pathways as it becomes a habit and part of my regular day. I also love to end my day with it. After I put the light out at night, I begin the seeing-beauty process. But I must admit, I don't always complete it because I fall asleep."

She asked if there were more questions. The group was silent. I felt as if I had just been given the key to transforming my life. And we hadn't even begun the way of the three loves yet!

Tuku closed the evening with a five-minute meditation, and we all very quietly eased out into the night and headed home.

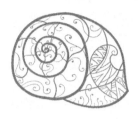

Chapter 25

A New Diagnosis

I slept well and woke up before the alarm with the words *seeing beauty* on my mind. I lay in my warm bed and started to see the beautiful aspects of my body. It was a wonderful way to begin the day. When the alarm went off, my mind went back into my day, and I remembered that I had an early appointment with my doctor. This was one of my regular monthly visits, and she would have the test results from my latest blood work. I showered and dressed in a dark-gray suit so that I could go straight to the office after the appointment.

My doctor was one of three in an office that was about fifteen minutes from my home. Two receptionists were situated behind glass windows. They had low chairs, so I looked down on them, and I always wondered why the glass was there, as it seemed such an unfriendly thing to talk through. The waiting room was lit too brightly, and the TV was spewing some mind-numbing dribble. The space behind the glass where the two receptionists sat seemed like a dark, unfriendly place.

The good news was that most of the time, my doctor was punctual. At the appointed hour of eight o'clock, one of the nurses popped her head out of the side door and ushered me in. She took my vitals and then led me into a small examining room. After a few minutes, there was a knock on the door and in walked my doctor.

She was thorough and technically sound about tests and follow-up. She did not have the greatest bedside manner, however, and she was often clumsy about discussing sensitive issues. She greeted me with a handshake and then took a seat on a small stool. Under her arm was my medical file, and I reflected on how it had grown over the last couple of months. She asked me a few general questions and then pulled out the latest test results and started to ponder them. The silence made me feel uneasy.

She looked up from her notes with a bland expression. "Well, Jane, it seems you are stable. No growth in your tumor. But no reduction, either. Let's keep you going on your current treatment protocol for now and see how things are next month. Okay?"

I nodded in agreement.

Then she added a comment that really took my legs out from under me. "You know, Jane, I know that we discussed the possibility of a lumpectomy, but I think it might help if you started to think about the possibility of having a bilateral mastectomy."

I went cold and my stomach immediately cramped. I felt as if she'd just stuck a knife in me. "What?"

"No, no, Jane," she quickly said. "I am not saying you need to go that route. I am only saying that you should include it as part of your future treatment options."

I was in shock. Both breasts now, I thought, as I tried to regain my composure.

"We'll keep a close eye on you, Jane, and rest assured we will do what is best for your long-term health," the doctor said. Her words sounded like a message on an answering machine and offered no comfort. Her usual blunt way of communication had once again cut me to the quick. She gave me a quick handshake, and I left the office. I barely held it together as I crossed the parking lot to my car. I slammed the car door angrily and then burst into tears. "Oh shit!" I shouted at the top of my voice.

After a few minutes, I regained some composure, but I felt decimated. Only one solution for that: the coffee shop, a latte, and a hug from Goth Girl.

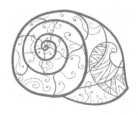

Chapter 26

The Story of the White Horse

As I pulled into the parking lot of the coffee shop, I was feeling angry, lost, and very fragile. Fear was wreaking havoc with my emotions, and I felt as if I was hanging on by the thinnest of threads. As I opened the door to the coffee shop, I looked at the counter, hoping to see Goth Girl. No sign of her. Instead, Mare was behind the counter. I glanced at the corner table, hoping Brock would be there. The chairs were empty. I had a sinking feeling in my stomach.

As I walked toward the counter, Mare greeted me with a big smile. My face was tight, and I knew tears were close. Mare studied me for a moment and then walked out from behind the counter and wrapped her long, caring arms around me. I started to cry into her shoulder and her long, dark hair. When she released me and held me at arm's length, she looked deeply into my eyes.

My eyes were full of tears, and she was a blur. "Got fifteen?" she asked.

"Hell, yeah," I replied, and she pointed me toward the empty corner table. I took my usual seat with my back to the counter and looked out at the trees. Soon a large latte appeared, and Mare slid into the corner seat facing me. She held me in her warm, hazel-brown eyes.

"So, Jane, care to share?"

I gave her a quick update about my crap bag of a doctor and what had happened. It felt good to talk it out. Mare was quiet for a short while, and then she asked, "Do you know the story of the white horse?"

I shook my head no.

"I used to get really caught up in events and always lost the bigger perspective about what was happening to me. My daily emotions were a real roller coaster. Then Brock shared with me a story about a white horse that shifted everything and helped me to navigate the challenging events of my life with a newfound ease and a higher perspective. Brock tells the story really well, but I would be happy to share my version, if you are open."

"Would you?" I asked. I cradled the warm latte in my hands and settled in.

"Once, in a far-off place, there was a Cossack farmer who owned the most beautiful white horse in the land. One day, his neighbor came over to visit and said, 'You are so lucky to have such a beautiful horse.'

"The farmer nodded, smiled, and said, 'It is all in the flow of life, for which I feel gratitude.'

"The next day, the white horse ran away, and the neighbor came over and said to the farmer, 'Oh! You are so unlucky that you have lost your beautiful white horse.'

"The farmer replied, 'It is all in the flow of life, for which I feel gratitude.'

"The next day, the white horse returned with three wild horses. The neighbor came over and said, 'You are so lucky that your white horse ran away in the first place and returned with three wild horses.'

"The farmer replied, 'It is all in the flow of life, for which I feel gratitude.'

"The next day, the son of the farmer was riding one of the wild horses and fell off, breaking his leg.

"The neighbor came over and said, 'You are so unlucky that the white horse came back with the three wild horses and that your son fell off and broke his leg.'

"The farmer replied, 'It is all in the flow of life, for which I feel gratitude.'

"The next day, the Russian army came through and conscripted all the young men in the land for a war that meant certain death for the soldiers. They could not take the farmer's son because he had a broken leg, which essentially saved his life.

"The neighbor came over and said, 'You are so lucky that your son fell off the wild horse and broke his leg.'

"The Cossack farmer replied, 'It is all in the flow of life, for which I feel gratitude.'"

Mare paused to allow me to take in the message. I loved the story and began to apply it to the events of the past few days. Then it hit me: I had been living in my blue ocean, and the Cossack farmer had been living in his white ocean. *So that's how this works,* I thought. I shared my insight with Mare, and she said I was right.

She touched me gently on the arm and said, "Honey, we all get days when our white horse runs away. We get so lost in our loss that we do not stay attentive to when and how it returns and what it brings. Always go back to the white and golden oceans and remember that you are loved. Remember the deep peace within your soul and see that all the events of your outer life are occurring in the blue ocean. They are not you! The story of the white horse helps me to stay attentive to what is triggered by uncomfortable situations. What do you think this episode prompts you to do?"

I pondered this question for a moment. "I feel as if I want a second opinion," I said. "I want to find another doctor who truly cares for me and doesn't always focus on the worst scenario and scare the hell out of me."

"Great," said Mare. "What are your next steps?"

That question caught me off guard. "Not sure how to find this sort of doctor," I replied.

"Okay," said Mare. "One step at a time. Who do you know who may know of another doctor?"

"Dar," I answered.

"Right on," said Mare. "She has several doctors who she consults with. One of them is a real cool lady in New York. Why don't you ask her for an intro?"

I felt an immediate sense of relief and comfort. "Yes!" I said. "I have been wanting to do that for ages but never got around to it. And now I see how my white horse is coming back with three horses!"

Mare and I both laughed at the same time. "You've got it," she said. "Gotta keep that bigger perspective and stay cool."

Not only was I feeling centered and calm again, but I also felt a new level of hope about overcoming my cancer. My favorite-color horse had just become white.

Mare reached across the table and gently rested her hands on my forearms. I felt a current of warm love shoot up my arms. She looked right into my eyes and said, "Remember, honey, you are never alone. Remember that you are always loved and remember that I am always here for you."

Tears came to my eyes again, but these were warm tears of appreciation. I lifted one of her hands and placed a soft kiss on the back of it. "Bless you, Mare," I said.

She lifted one of my hands and placed a gentle kiss on the back of it and said, "And bless you, Jane. Come back soon, all right?" Mare looked over my shoulder at the counter and said that she had to get back to work.

We stood, hugged, and she headed back to the counter. Mare had only been talking for about fifteen minutes, yet I felt as if everything had just shifted. I had been Humpty-Dumpty who fell off the wall. And all the king's men and all the king's horses could not put Humpty back together again. But Mare had just done it. Her words of wisdom about the white horse had reassembled all the broken pieces of me. I headed out to the car feeling much more "together" than when I arrived, thanks to Mare and her healing spirit. For the fifteen-minute drive to the office, all I could think about was the white horse.

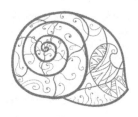

Chapter 27

Brother Bob

I slipped discreetly into the office and with a nice hot cup of black tea, I settled in to do some non-profit research. My cell phone rang at 10:00 a.m., and I saw that it was my brother calling. I picked it up right away. "Hi, Bob. What's up?"

He was in his tough, take-action attorney mode. "Listen, Sis, I've been going over your accounts again, and we gotta start tracking your husband's hidden financials. I can find no record of his gross earnings, just the amount he transfers into your joint account. Seems fishy to me. He has often boasted of how well he does with all his commissions, so he must be squirreling it away somewhere. A buddy of mine is a hacker extraordinaire, and he owes me a favor or two. Can I set up a time for my hacker friend, Hank, to call you?"

This really flustered me, and suddenly, all my fears about my husband came flooding back. "I...a...yeah...uh, sometime soon, Bob. Just let me get my head around this, and I will do it soon, okay?"

I heard a quiet grunt of impatience on the other end of the line. I knew Bob was frustrated with me, and I think I sensed that he was not telling me something. "Okay, Sis. Be in touch soon," he said. "Know that I love you." And he hung up.

I felt stupid for allowing my husband to put me in this situation. Why had I trusted him and let him run the finances? Was I dumb or what? I could feel a downward mood spiral pulling on me. Then I felt anger toward myself, and

I could feel a nauseous sensation growing in my stomach. I just wanted to run and hide from all this divorce crap.

All I had done was trust the person I thought I loved. Then again, perhaps David had simply set things up with a view to the IRS. He really wouldn't want to screw me financially, would he? Or would he?

The abyss of doubt sucked me in, and I felt distracted and wasted.

At lunchtime, I took a sandwich out to my car to get some quiet time and to ponder how to move forward. As I was finishing the sandwich, a text arrived. It was from Mare.

Hey, Jane. I set up a meeting with Brock for you today at 4. I think the 'for' process will help you. Brock will explain. Hugs.

That got my attention. A one-on-one with Mr. Brock. Now, that seemed rather appealing, I must admit. And what was this "for" process? This was new to me.

Another text from Mare came in with Brock's address and a message.

Take cookies that have chocolate.

I smiled at this insider tip. I was ahead of schedule on my projects and had no qualms about texting my boss to say that I would be leaving at 3:30 p.m.

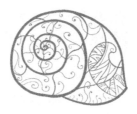

Chapter 28

The For Process

I arrived at Brock's woodshop sharply at four o'clock, carrying a big box of chocolate chip cookies. His woodshop was in a rather rundown part of the city, in an old red-brick warehouse that had been converted into small workshops. Each had its own entrance, and Brock's workshop was one from the end and had the number 77 painted in white on a crimson door.

I pressed the buzzer and waited. After a few moments, the door swung open, revealing Brock in a rather dapper dark-blue shirt and cream-colored jeans.

Very nice, I thought. "Hi, Brock!" I said warmly, trying to control my excitement at seeing him again.

"Hey, Jane! Lovely to see you, and I am so pleased you were able to come on such short notice." He gestured me toward some chairs and a table in a corner of the woodshop. I was immediately struck by the scent of pine wood in the air. This was how he had smelled the first time I met him. I felt a warm little shiver move through me as I walked toward the chairs.

I noticed that his woodshop seemed very ordered and cared for. Everything seemed to have a place, and the floor was clean. There was some woodworking machinery to my left and a couple of benches on the other side of the room. At the back, there was another door, this one painted gold, and I wondered where it went. Since I'd seen a restroom near the front door, I knew the gold door led somewhere else. I wondered if he was going to show me what was behind it.

"Kettle is on," he said as he closed the front door. Next to the chairs and table was a little kitchen with a sink and a small counter. As I presented him with the box of cookies, I bowed my head briefly.

"That's so thoughtful of you," he said, placing the cookies on the table. "Cookies are one of my big weaknesses." He started to pour the hot water into the cups, and I pondered what his other weaknesses could be.

"Black, mint, or peach herbal tea?" he asked.

"Oh, black," I said. "It's one of my weaknesses."

He turned his head toward me and gave me a sideways smile and a raised eyebrow. We were definitely in sync.

He placed a cup of steaming tea on a coaster in front of me and took a seat opposite me. We sat in silence for a few seconds. "So, Jane, Mare called and suggested that I share with you the 'for' process. I have a sense she sees something special in you and wants to support your journey."

His words made me feel warm and special. "That's nice of her," I replied. "She is one special lady."

Brock nodded. "To lead me into the *for* process, I just want to recap the three oceans and what they represent. The outer blue ocean is the one that is created in this life by our egos and rational minds. This is a sort of vehicle for our souls. The blue ocean exists for as long as our life on Earth exists. Within this is our soul, represented by the white ocean. This is your eternal self that came into the earthly realm to learning and experiencing life. Your soul is pure love and seeks to grow and expand through lessons and experiences during its time on Earth. Within the white ocean is the golden ocean—what I call the Divine Presence. This, for me, is the highest form of love. It creates and informs all living things on this planet.

"For the soul to grow in love, it came to Earth to experience the many lessons and opportunities that this life has to offer. The soul brings to this life a partial curriculum with certain gifts and abilities that will be needed for its growth. The other part of the curriculum is created through how you respond to the events in your life. Each soul has a destiny that will help guide its journey here. In short, life is an adventure.

"The soul comes to Earth to grow in love. However, through this life, it can also be diminished in love. Everything depends on what happens in the blue ocean, where free will exists. In short, the ego and rational mind can either help the soul to grow or they can diminish it. The Shaolin monks knew that because many of the villagers had difficulty finding true love and were unable to expand their souls, they carried resentments and often felt that they were victims in life. This diminished their souls or white oceans. The monks wanted to provide them with a process that would empower and grow their white oceans or souls. The process they developed to evolve the blue ocean and their life on Earth of cause and effect is the process we call 'for.'

"The villagers were taught to see everything that occurred in their lives as being done *for* them. Even though they faced many trials and tribulations, they came to see that everything in life offers lessons and the potential to grow and evolve.

"We are not saying that when something bad occurs in life, this event was created *for* them. It is not for us to know why traumatic things happen to us. We do not choose traumatic events, but we can choose how we respond to traumatic events. We choose whether they make us *more* and build us up or diminish us. The 'for' process was created by the Shaolin monks to help the villagers become empowered through trauma and not be diminished by it. The villagers came to realize that everything in life can be used *for* their growth in love."

This all sounded good, but then I remembered that I had breast cancer. How was I to see cancer as being done "for" me? I guess my face must have shown that something was not clicking for me.

Brock asked me to share what I was thinking.

"Two words," I said. "Breast cancer."

Brock responded quickly. "Many of the villagers suffered with cancer as well. As they applied the 'for' process, they began to see how cancer had, in fact, brought much love into their lives. It often woke them up and completely changed the course of their lives. Think about it, Jane. What good things have come into your life because of breast cancer?"

That question required some thought. I reached for my tea and pushed the cookies toward Brock. He took one and sipped his tea.

As I reflected on how my life had changed since my diagnosis, I realized that I had always focused on what I thought cancer had stolen from me. I had made myself a victim. When I considered the good things that had happened, I had to admit that there was much to think about. One of the good things was sitting in front of me.

Before cancer arrived, I knew that my life had gotten into a rut that I did not know how to get out of. I was asleep at the wheel, as the expression goes.

Cancer had shown me a character flaw in my husband that he had kept hidden. It had shown me that people like Goth Girl and Mare existed. I was beginning to get a sense of where Brock was going with this "for" process.

"When the Shaolin monks introduced the 'for' process to the villagers, fear's hold over them diminished. The villagers began to believe that they had the power within themselves to transform their relationships to cancer and other traumas in their lives. More than this, the villagers really embraced the fact that even though facing trauma was hard, it also held precious gifts and opportunities for the soul to grow and evolve," Brock said.

"Because of the 'for' process, the villagers experienced less stress and fear, and this strengthened their immune systems. They became healthier and less vulnerable to illness." Brock went silent and looked at me, inviting a response.

"I get it," I said. Somehow this was all making sense. A process to help me with my fear and stress had to be a good thing. "What about the fear of dying of cancer?" I asked.

"Ah, yes," he said. "A common fear. Well, the Shaolin monks lived knowing that their time on Earth would one day come to an end. Their life on Earth as they knew it was only for a certain period of time. In a way, they felt that this life was like going to college. You go there to learn and grow, and when you have finished your studies, you graduate and return home. Therefore, they focused on growing the white and golden oceans in this life. The key to dealing with the fear of death is not to try to fix or remove the fear. Instead, you focus on growing your relationship to your own soul and the Divine Presence within your soul. As you do this, you will come to know that you are eternal. Trying not to fear death will actually feed the fear of death. When the Shaolin monks taught me this concept, I really struggled to embrace it. Then one day, as my sense of the white ocean within me began to grow, the penny dropped, and I had a sense that I was much bigger than what I had been experiencing myself.

"Whenever a Shaolin monk dies, the monks do not have funerals like we do in the West, where people are often sad and heartbroken. Instead, they have a farewell or graduation celebration. They know that they will see their loved ones again someday. They feel that their loved ones are simply going on ahead. It's like the departed is saying, 'I am going on ahead. See you later. Use your life well and let my spirit inspire you to be more than you ever thought possible.' The Shaolin monks live knowing that life on Earth will end, and because of that, they live more powerful, love-filled lives. They appreciate each other more because they all understand that the earthly life will end. So, in a funny way, death gives them more life." Brock asked if I had questions.

I had a sense that my inner landscape had just been transformed—as if some huge boulders of misconception had just been removed. I had this incredible sense of space inside me. It was as though someone had just turned on a light in a room that I thought was small, and it turned out to be huge. And this hugeness was in me. It was a wonderful feeling. For the first time, I could see the truth about what life is really all about. It's meant to be an adventure that teaches and guides me through the best and worst of times. The "for" process was not just about cancer; I could use it for any trauma.

Brock was waiting quietly as I processed my thoughts. Then he lifted one of his eyebrows as if inviting questions. I wanted to know more about his own journey with cancer. "Brock, would you be open to share about your own personal journey with cancer?" I asked.

He beamed a big smile at me and said, "Sure. Just need a quick cookie, though," as he reached for another one. He did not eat cookies in the usual way. He could have fit the cookie easily into his mouth in one bite. But instead he took five small bites. After each bite, he closed his eyes and went silent as if he were entering some beautiful inner world. He would stay in this place for a few seconds, then open his eyes and take another small bite. I was struck by this. It was as if he were engaging in a sacred ritual of reverence and appreciation for each bite. He was not just eating a cookie; he was also experiencing joy. He had just transformed my relationship to eating cookies.

After his fifth and last bite, he took a sip of tea, and then smiled at me. "When cancer came into my life, I was really scared. I remember the day I was diagnosed. I drove home from the doctor's office and went right to bed at two in the afternoon. I lived alone, so I did not have to talk to anyone. I spent twenty-four hours in bed crying, grieving, and being angry at God, the Divine Presence, or whatever the higher power was that had done this to me.

"My pillow was soaking wet because of my tears. I was completely wasted.

"It was a curve ball that I did not see coming. When Tuku arrived, everything began to change, as I began to truly live the many teachings that she had come to share with me. Initially, cancer had stolen my quality of life. After I started using the way of the three loves and the amazing processes, everything changed. Cancer woke me up from sleeping. I began to realize that life is a gift, in fact every day is a gift. When I realized that my soul is eternal, I began to see the challenges in my life as opportunities. My quality of life improved dramatically as opposed to diminishing. I began to truly appreciate my family and friends. I began to say, 'I am sorry' and 'I forgive you' much more often. Before cancer, I had really taken my health for granted.

"It was cancer that really stripped me bare and showed me my true calling in life," he said. "I came home to my true passion." As he said that, he turned to look at the golden door and tears began to roll down his cheeks. He looked lovingly at the golden door for a moment and then turned back to me. I waited, hoping he would reveal what was behind the golden door. As if he knew what I was thinking, he said, "Jane, today is about you. This is not the right time to share with you what is behind the golden door. Perhaps one day."

The word *perhaps* stung me. I felt the urge to leap up, run to the golden door, and open it to see what lay behind it. But I knew that the door represented a sacred part of his life, and I knew I needed to respect it.

Then I heard the doorbell ring, and someone put a key in the door. I turned as the front door swung open, and in walked Goth Girl. "Hey, two of my favorite people!" she hailed loudly as she walked toward us. She gave Brock and me big hugs and grabbed a cookie as she took a seat. Brock went to the stove make her some tea.

Goth Girl leaned toward me. "Mare said you were here. So, what do ya think about the 'for' process, Wig Girl?"

"Mind blowing," I said.

"Got that right," she replied. "It was a real game changer and life saver for me."

Then I leaned forward and whispered, "What's behind the golden door?"

She went silent and turned to look at the door. Then a couple of tears rolled down her cheeks. She turned back to me and as she lightly stroked my cheek, she said, "Honey, just trust that it is not right for you to know what is behind the golden door. Brock will decide if and when it is right to share that with you."

A little voice inside me screamed, *But I want to know now!* But a higher part of me knew to trust Brock and Goth Girl that not knowing, for reasons Brock and Goth Girl alone knew, was the way it had to be for today.

Brock returned, placing a cup of steaming tea on a table next to Goth Girl. "Love these cookies," she said as she reached for another one.

Brock took his seat and sat smiling at her as she munched on her cookie. "So, Dar, I was hoping you would share your wig story with Jane to give her a living example of how the 'for' process works."

"Sure thing," she said as a few crumbs shot from her mouth. She looked at me. "I'm on the run now. Can you do the coffee shop tomorrow, say 7:00 a.m.?"

"It's a date," I said.

Goth Girl stood and pulled a travel thermos out of her bag and emptied her tea into it. She hugged us both and headed out. I had a sense that it was time for me to leave too. The "for" process had really shifted some gears in my head, and I wanted time to process it away from the distraction of the rather handsome Mr. Brock. I gave Brock a hug and went home.

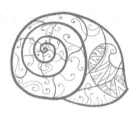

Chapter 29

An Invitation

I arrived home around 6:00 p.m., and my mind was alive with the energy of the "for" process. I put a TV dinner in the microwave and opened my laptop to check my email. I scanned the emails to see where they had come from to get a sense of priority. The one that caught my attention was from my husband. I felt an uncertain stir within. I was still confused about what I felt for him and where we were, or were not, headed. I hit the open button.

Dear Jane,
I would like to invite you for dinner tomorrow evening. How about Angelino's restaurant, where we went on our first date?
David

This pulled at a deep chord in me. My memory of our first date was vivid. I was enchanted by him. His choreography of the evening was meticulous. He had a red rose delivered by the waiter just after we had taken our first sip of wine. Then, what really broke my heart open was the crème brûlée dessert with our names spelled out in thin whipped cream. I never did find out how he knew this was my all-time favorite dessert. I am guessing he must have called someone in my office surreptitiously. The evening's finale was just mind blowing. As our freshly made cappuccino coffees arrived, so did an Italian singer with a guitar to serenade us. I was nailed. His orchestration was masterful. He won me that night. And now, he wanted me to return to the very same restaurant. The romantic part of me wanted so much to fall for his charms again. But there was another voice in my head, that of suspicion. Was this another game he was playing? Was this a new husband, or just a contorted version of the emotionally dysfunctional man I had married? My heart was a blur. I could no longer make sense of whatever this thing called love was. I typed *yes*, then *no*, then *yes*, then *no*. Then I got practical. The food at Angelino's was off this planet. I was sick of TV dinners. I typed *yes* and hit the send button.

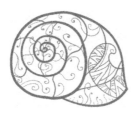

Chapter 30

The Wig in New York

I arrived at the coffee shop a few minutes before seven the next morning. Goth Girl must have seen me pull into the parking lot; she had a large latte waiting for me on the corner table. We hugged and took our seats.

After a long sip of her drink, she began her infamous wig story. "So, my New York wig story is one that Brock says captures both the white horse story and the 'for' process. Shortly after I lost my hair, my doctor wanted me to visit a specialist in New York City. I am a country girl and dreaded the thought of dealing with the hassle of getting around New York. My mom offered to go with me. But spending a day with someone who complains, complains, complains was not an option. So, I boarded a train alone and headed to the city. I had only just lost my hair, and I was both fragile and angry. The Gothic look was a great release for my emotions. I had a friend who was in costume design, and she got me this long, awesome black wig that had bright-red streaks. It came all the way down to my waist, and when I wore it with full makeup, I really was a sight to be seen. I wanted to shock. I wanted people to see my anger.

"I was sitting on the train, and I knew people were glancing sideways at me. I really was a scary sight. Even though I was angry, in a strange way, I felt very free. Not that anger is good energy, but this anger felt good, I think, because for the first time in my life I had allowed it. And the Gothic thing gave me a channel for it. Of course, then guilt raised its head—my religious upbringing about being quiet and peaceful and all that. But I had spent my childhood suppressing my feelings, just like my mom did. She had given me an emotional straitjacket, and it had entrapped me.

"I asked Brock about the anger thing, and he said something beautiful. He said, 'Anger is not the problem. Our ignorance of what it is and how to allow it is the problem.'

"Anger occurs for a reason," she said. "It is a very natural part of our emotional chemistry. It is when we suppress it and use it against others that it becomes a poison. The key is to allow anger and embrace anger naturally and express it in creative ways. When I met Brock, I was a real angry bitch. This was before the Goth look.

"So, there I was, getting off the train in Grand Central Station, and there was a sea of people all around me. People stared at me, and they kind of moved out of the way. I had this energy-field thing going. I felt powerful, and I felt a freedom I'd never experienced before. So, I made it to the cabstand. A guy in a uniform was calling cabs and loading people into them. He did a double take when he saw me. But he had a sense of humor and asked me where my broomstick was. I laughed and slapped him a high five as I climbed into a cab.

"The cab driver was really big, like three hundred pounds. There was a smell of curry in the cab, which really pissed me off. The driver's hair was uncombed, and his clothes were soiled. Add to this, he could barely speak any English. Because of the smell, I decided not to give him a tip out of spite for not cleaning his cab. I was angry at him now.

"I held up my hospital appointment letter so he could see the address where I needed to go. When he read it, he did a double take and gazed at me for a few seconds. I knew that he knew that I was wearing a wig and that I had cancer. *Screw you*, I thought. *Just drive, asshole.*

"As he pulled away from the station, a desperate loneliness hit me. I felt lost and abandoned by life. Tears started to flood down my cheeks. I moved to the corner of the seat so that he could not see me in the rear-view mirror. But I think he heard my sobs. I just fell apart in the back seat of this dirty New York cab with some foreign shithead of a driver. Everywhere I looked there were so many people, yet I'd never felt so alone.

"Then he suddenly pulled over and stopped the cab. We were in a rundown section of the city, and there was no hospital in sight. *Shit*, I thought. *Now what?*

"I held the door handle ready to bolt if he tried anything. I saw him reach down onto the passenger seat for something. A knife, a gun? My mind was out of control at this point. Then he turned and lifted his hand. He was holding a chocolate bar wrapper. Inside the wrapper were three small pieces of chocolate. 'Here, missy. Please, please,' he said as he handed it to me. 'All will be good. All will be good. Please eat. It is dark. It is good. Please eat, missy.'

"Holy crap! What was happening? Here in the middle of this human desert when I was feeling so lost and abandoned by life, here was this stranger offering me the remains of his lunch.

"His eyes were comforting and seemed protective of me. I think that was the moment I started to believe in angels. Through tear-filled eyes, I looked at him from the corner of the back seat. He nodded as if to say, Take it. I took the candy bar wrapper with the three small pieces of chocolate. 'Ten minutes, missy, we be at hospital,' he said. Then he turned and pulled the cab back into traffic.

"My moments of absolute pain and anguish had suddenly been washed away with this torrent of kindness. My heart felt so embraced and loved. As the first piece of chocolate entered my mouth, it was as if I had never tasted chocolate before. The dark, bitter sweetness just exploded in my mouth. I went from hell to heaven in the back seat of a New York cab. Go figure.

"Then came this surge of joy from deep inside me. It came out as a scream in words. 'This frickin' chocolate is awesome!' and I broke into laughter. I saw the big eyes of the driver in the rear-view mirror and then he roared with laughter. It was like a death and a birth had just gone on inside me. A few minutes later, he pulled up outside this enormous hospital that was chock-full of people and cars trying to maneuver around the entrance. I could tell that the cab driver wanted to drop me right in front, and he played dodge with other cabs and cars using his horn to bully his way through. I reached into my bag for my wallet, glancing at the meter, which said twenty-eight dollars in red. In a flash, he flicked off the light and said, 'No, no, no. All good...all good...you go now!'

"'No, no, no!' I said and thrust two twenty-dollar bills over the back of his seat. He was shaking his head and having none of it. Then, another cabbie started honking at him for triple parking, and a uniformed traffic cop started to walk toward our cab. I threw the two twenties on the front seat and pulled at the handle to make a quick exit. I was flustered, and I slammed the door as I looked through the window to make sure I hadn't left anything on the back seat. Then he revved up and took off. What I did not realize was that I had caught my wig in the door.

"Off he went with my wig hanging from his rear door and disappeared into the New York traffic. There I was, completely bald, standing alone in the middle of this human zoo. I froze on the spot. Then I felt a thud on my back. Anger flared again, and I clenched my fist, ready to pop someone. I spun around, poised to kill, and there was a suited guy holding his iPhone to his ear. When he saw me, a look of shock and fear came over him. I let him have it, 'Hey, fat head, you wanna piece of this?' I screamed at him. He became pale and backed away into a sea of people, and I reverted to a lost and vulnerable six-year-old girl. Tears started to fall again, and I felt stuck to the spot. I could not move. I felt so utterly lost, abandoned, and alone.

"Then I felt a hand squeeze the back of my arm. Anger flashed again, and I spun around, ready to attack. Looking up at me was a small Indian man. I am around five foot four, and he must have been just under five feet tall. 'Please, please, come, come,' he said and gestured toward a newsstand against the hospital wall. I surrendered to his gentle pull, and he led me to this funny little hut covered in magazines. He took me to the side of the hut and pulled a little door open. Inside, it looked like a bunker. An even smaller Indian woman, wearing some form of Indian wrap, nodded and smiled warmly at me. The Indian guy pulled out a stool and placed it behind me, urging me to sit. Which I did. The woman pulled out a bottle of water, removed the top, and handed it to me. The man stood at my side, creating a sort of protective wall with his presence. I actually felt safe. He urged me to drink. I took a few sips, thinking what a frickin' sight I must be. A bald Goth on the streets of New York. Slowly, I began to feel my energy and my sense of purpose returning. The man said, 'Paper, paper.' I thought he was asking for money, and I pulled a five-dollar bill from my purse. 'No, no!' he said. 'Paper, paper!'

"Then it clicked. He wanted my letter of appointment. I pulled it out and showed it to him. 'Yes, yes,' he said. I stood to leave, and as I did, he spoke some words in a strange language to the woman. He put the stool inside the hut and closed the door.

"He took my arm again and said, 'Come,' and started leading me toward the hospital entrance. I was in disbelief that this was happening. Angel number two had just arrived. We walked as an odd kind of married couple, arm in arm. An elderly Indian man with a Goth girlfriend. Hey, this was New York, after all; so, anything goes, right?

"We maneuvered through fast-moving throngs of people, through large revolving doors, to a scary number of elevator doors. On one level, I felt completely lost, yet I also had absolute trust in this man to guide me. He pulled me into a very full elevator, and we sped up to the twenty-seventh floor. Some of the people in the elevator stole glances at me and then at him, as though they were trying to figure us out. When the bell rang at the twenty-seventh floor, the man pulled me out and steered me to a large reception desk. He placed the letter back in my hand. 'All good now!' he said.

"I reached into my bag to offer him some form of tip. He touched my forearm very gently and shook his head no. He quietly walked away, and I stood for a few seconds basking in his kindness.

"Then I heard the word, 'Next,' and I turned around to see a very large African American woman behind the desk looking at me. 'Letter?' she said.

"I was still a little disoriented and started to rummage my bag for the hospital letter. It was not there. *Oh shit!*

"Then she said, 'Pocket?'

"Thrusting my hand into my back pocket, I found it. I was nervous and shook a little as I handed it to her. She tipped her head toward two rows of chairs and started entering my information on her computer. I quickly scanned the room. Nine people with hair or wigs, three people bald. I was not alone. I could sense them glancing at me and pretending not to look. I valued some quiet time in the chair, letting the dust settle on my crazy morning.

"Against the wall of the waiting room was a big fish tank. I sat gazing at it, trying to regroup. It was full of wonderful, happy colors, and the movement of the pretty little fish seemed to soothe me. After fifteen minutes, a nurse came out and called my name. When she saw me, she did a quick double take. I am sure she had seen a lot of bald people, but a bald Goth? I guessed this was something new. A new wave of dread came over me as I walked to one of the small interview rooms. She measured my height and weight and took some blood. All routine to me now. She did not talk much. I think my Goth look made her uncertain about me. She left me alone in the room, saying that the doctor would be in shortly. I was there for a second opinion about the lump in my breast. My own doctor was pushing surgery at me, but I had asked for a second opinion, so there I was with a big-city specialist.

"There was a light tap on the door and in walked the doctor. I was surprised to see her wearing earrings and heels. *This lady appreciates style*, I thought. When she saw me, she stopped in her tracks with her mouth open. 'Just absolutely beautiful,' she said.

I felt a flush of warm energy. She perused my makeup and piercings and said that I was an articulate and expressive human being. All I had said was 'hi,' and I already loved this woman. I wasn't expecting warmth from a doctor. She asked if she could use my first name, Dar. I nodded.

"'Please call me Michelle,' she said warmly. She was carrying a large file containing my papers and CT scans. She placed it on a table and picked up one of the scans, holding it up to the window. 'I have already looked at your file,' she said as she gazed at the slide. Then she walked over to me. 'May I give you a physical examination?' she asked.

"'Sure,' I replied as I started to unbutton my shirt. Then she did something that startled me. She not only washed her hands but held them under the hot water.

"She turned to me and said, 'Nothing worse than cold hands.' I was awestruck by this simple gesture. My own doctor always had cold hands, and she never seemed aware of it. Michelle started to gently explore the tumor in my breast. After about five minutes, she told me to put my clothes back on.

"We took seats at a little round table in the corner of the room. 'Well,' she said. 'I see what your primary doctor has suggested. What are your thoughts about this?'

I was stunned again. A doctor was asking my opinion. I paused to think. Then I said I wanted to continue the chemo rather than go under the knife. Michelle nodded slowly as she looked again at my medical notes.

"'Well, Dar,' she said, 'if this was my breast and these were my scans, I would do exactly the same thing.' A strong sense of relief welled up inside me. For some reason, I thought she was going to suggest surgery.

"She spoke as she wrote notes in my file. 'I am suggesting frequent monitoring with regular scans. I also want to do some additional blood work to look deeper into the protein balance in your body. Protein imbalance has been shown to affect the growth of some tumors. It may be that you can make a few changes in your diet regarding the type of protein you eat. This could have an important role to play. I'll get the results of the blood work in about three days and will let your primary-care physician know the results. Any questions?' she asked.

"I shook my head. As she was finishing her notes, she asked if I had considered a wig. The question caught me off guard, and I found myself in tears.

I felt so stupid and ashamed. Michelle gently put her arm around me. She went quiet, as if inviting me to share. After a few minutes, I regrouped and told her the story. She listened attentively to every word. Then she looked right into my eyes and said, 'I must tell you, Dar, this completely redefines the word *roadkill* for me.'

"At that point, a spark flashed between our eyes, and we broke out in guffawing laughter. The nurse darted into the room to see what was going on. The two of us just fell apart. It did seem hilarious as I thought about my wig taking off down Park Avenue, hanging from a cab door.

"The nurse brought us each a bottle of water and, after a few minutes, Michelle reached out to hug me goodbye. As I was leaving, she said, 'I would like to see you again in three months.'

"Another angel had just shown up. Wearing earrings and heels, no less. When I reached the front desk, I positioned myself with my back to the waiting room. I just needed to get out of the office. I couldn't face looking at other bald women.

"With a nod, the receptionist signaled that I should look behind me. I turned to see a cop sitting in one of the chairs. This was a breast-cancer clinic for women, so I wondered why he was there. Then I looked down and saw my wig on his lap. My mouth dropped open. As he stood up, he removed his hat and walked toward me. He spoke with a slight Italian accent. 'Excuse me, ma'am. I am wondering if this may belong to you?' As he lifted my wig, I narrowed my eyes and gave him a questioning look.

"'Well, ma'am,' he began, 'I was downtown finishing my regular shift when I spotted a taxi with this wig hanging out of the window. At first, I thought it was somebody's head. I flagged down the cab. The taxi driver felt guilty. He told me where he had dropped you, so I guessed you would be here.'

"I was still in shock. He handed the wig to me. I was starting to gather my senses and noticed that he was kind of good looking. Clean cut; short black hair; dark, penetrating eyes; and such amazing manners. Then I noticed his beautifully shaped mouth and lips. I had this sudden flash of premonition that someday, I would kiss those lips. Here's another angel, I thought, only this one is wearing a police uniform.

"I took the wig and bowed my head in respect as I touched my heart in thanks.

"'Not from the city, right?' he asked.

"'Pretty obvious,' I said, smiling. Then I asked how he knew to come to this office.

"The question startled him at first. Then he pulled out his wallet. He opened it to show me picture of a very attractive woman. 'My mother,' he said with a tremor in his voice, 'came here for treatment.' As he said those words, he crossed his heart and looked up as if at his mother in heaven. He had just won my heart. Then he took out his pad of tickets and flipped it open.

"*Geesh*, I thought. *Am I getting a ticket or something? Is there a law against cruelty to wigs?* He scribbled something on the pad and then tore out the page. On the back of a parking ticket, he had written his name, Tony, and his cell number. He handed me the parking ticket and said to call if I needed anything when I was back in New York. He put his hat back onto his head, bowed, and headed out.

"The receptionist had been watching and listening to this. I turned to look at her. She beamed a huge smile at me and said, 'Honey, what I just saw belongs in a movie.' We both laughed. She set up my next appointment, and I went out to find another taxi. I could not stop thinking about Tony's eyes. How he looked at me. How his voice trembled when he spoke of his mother. This happened three months ago, and all I can say is that his lips are delicious."

"What?" I exclaimed. "You mean you dated him?"

"I *am* dating him," she said as her sly smile turned into a wicked grin. "So, that's my wig-in-New York story. Can you see how the white horse and the 'for' process runs through it? You just gotta keep believing that the white horse is always headed back and that no matter what shit goes down, you can use it *for* you—things are not being done *to* you."

I was mesmerized. Here was a living example of these two powerful processes in action. Goth Girl said she needed to cover for Barney, who was going on break. We stood and hugged. Then she made the sound of a horse, which made us both laugh. I was still laughing as I went out to my car to drive to the office.

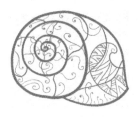

Chapter 31

A Difficult Evening

I spent a quiet day at the office doing research work for two new non-profits. But questions about my dinner date with David kept popping into my mind. Had I been foolish to accept the invitation? Should I really try to save our twenty-four-year marriage? On and on the questions churned in my head.

I was happy when five o'clock came, and I headed home to freshen up for the evening.

I picked a relaxed maroon trouser suit to wear and deliberately arrived at the restaurant five minutes late. David was sitting in the small waiting area by the maître d'. When he saw me, he sprang to his feet and came toward me with his arms open for a hug. I let my arms hang loosely at my sides as he embraced me. He had on a slim-fitting sports jacket, an open-neck shirt, and tan pants. His usual slick style. He reminded me of a second-hand car salesman. We were ushered to a quiet corner table. I had promised myself that I would probe him about his leaving and where he was on his journey of healing. He was his usual gushing, courteous, charming self, but I could sense that it was all on the surface. We were swimming in his blue ocean. Would he allow me into his white and golden oceans? Did he have white and golden oceans? I needed to find out.

Who was this man I had spent the last twenty-four years of my life with?

The waiter came, and David ordered his usual steak. I ordered a *risotto con agoni*. Two chilled glasses of Chardonnay arrived, and I took a couple of sips as I marshaled myself for the forthcoming interrogation. He started talking about how well his financial consulting business was doing. I leaned toward him and peered into his eyes for a sense of his spirit. Goth Girl and Brock both had a tremendous presence in their eyes. It was as if their souls were fully in the world, and there was nothing hidden. As I looked into my husband's eyes, I kept hoping to see that same sense of soul. I think he mistook my leaning toward him as a sign of wanting to get more intimate, and he mirrored my posture. I knew that this was one of his sales techniques—a way to win people that was all performance and aimed at a contrived outcome.

I had a sense that David was after something, but I could not quite put my finger on it. He had wanted to stop the divorce proceedings but had not made any overtures about working on our relationship issues. He was a master of masquerade when it came to his emotions. I kept scanning his face for real gestures that truly came from his heart, and I realized that I was looking at a marionette—somebody hidden from me and perhaps hidden from himself. I couldn't even sense who was pulling his strings, but the performance was flawless. I could feel myself getting edgy with all his 'I am really successful' talk. *Like the days of old*, I thought.

I decided to lob a grenade at him in the form of a penetrating question to see how he dealt with it. But there was a part of me that was still a little intimidated by him. Where the hell did that come from? I wondered. He had been the man of the house, and I had been the woman protected by the man of the house. Just like my mother. I was now on my third glass of Chardonnay and hoping and praying that sometime soon, my emotional cavalry would show up to lead the charge with my penetrating question.

I excused myself and headed to the restroom. I went straight to the sink and splashed water on my face to snap me out of the spell he had put me under. I imagined Goth Girl standing beside me and wondered what counsel she would give me. I needed a penetrating question to get through his barricades. Then it came: It still hurts when I think of the night you left. Why did you walk out on me when I needed you most?

I rehearsed the question in the mirror several times. I gave myself a you-can-do-this stare and marched back to the table.

As usual, he had taken the few moments of my absence to check his email. That irked me. Before he had a chance to talk, I hit him with my question. "It still hurts when I think of the night you left. What work are you doing with your therapist to heal that flaw?"

I caught him off balance. He started to look down at the table, his eyes darting from right to left as he thought about how to respond. Then Mr. Smooth kicked in again. He lifted his head and said. "Oh, honey, that is a really important question, but can we do this in private another time?"

I was aware that other diners were within earshot and felt a sudden embarrassment at asking such a direct question. He shifted the conversation to my parents, and I knew I had lost the initiative. He really was a slippery bastard. Our pretend conversation continued for the rest of the evening. I kept searching his eyes for that bolt of connection I found in Brock's eyes. I felt confused about love again and began to feel a sort of numbness forming around my heart. I hadn't really adjusted well to living as a single person, and the comfort of being in a steady, albeit dead, relationship still held appeal for me. How sad was that?

Being single, lonely, and unhappy was hard for me. Thoughts about entering the world of online dating cramped my stomach. Having to maintain the house by myself was a daunting and terrifying prospect. I still found my husband physically attractive, though, and he took care of the finances. A part of me wanted to fall asleep again to the way we were before my cancer diagnosis.

As the waiter took his credit card, David asked me about the divorce papers again. I felt a flush of nausea. "All frozen, for now," I said.

He seemed relieved. A part of me wondered why this was such an issue for him. Was it his work, maybe? Was he working the IRS in some sort of tax dodge? I put my fourth glass of Chardonnay away and began to feel a little woozy. He immediately picked up on that.

"It may be better if I drive you home," he said. "Leave your car here and pick it up tomorrow, honey."

I felt my skin creep at the way he said *honey*.

I knew that driving was not a good idea, so I consented to a lift. "Drop and run, please," I said.

He gave me a sideways glance. "OK," he said. He did the car-door-opening thing. As we pulled out of the lot, he flipped his CD player on. Much to my horror, his favorite country song, "We Ain't Never Coming Back," was playing. I almost threw up there and then.

"Please," I said loudly as I turned it off. "I really can't do that song tonight." We drove home in silence listening to the local radio station.

He pulled up outside our house and leaned over to kiss me.

"Can't do that," I said and pulled away.

"Wonderful evening, honey," he said. "Just like old times, eh?"

I was feeling lost and really sad. "Sure," I said and opened my car door.

"Talk soon," he said as I closed the door and headed into my house.

I was a bit wobbly on my feet but very aware of my mixed and turbulent emotions. Just one more glass of wine and I would be really numb.

I poured a glass of white wine, headed to the couch, and flipped on the evening news. Four quick gulps and the glass was empty, and I was ready for my pity party of one. Soon the tears came. I wailed for him, for me, and for my crappy life and how inept I had been. I had been touched by his kindness and started to turn on myself, wondering what the hell he saw in me anyway. The inner jackals were gathering to rip me to shreds. I closed my eyes, hoping to leave a world that I never wanted to come back to. For some unfathomable reason, I started to feel guilty and questioned myself for overreacting in the first place. Had I been premature? Was I being vindictive? What a bitch I was for not giving him a second chance. Why oh why had he been able to disarm me so easily? Then I thought of the hacker in the wings, and another rush of guilt poured over me. David always did know how to press the right buttons to keep me under his control. He was so polite and well mannered. Handsome, too. But inside, he reminded me of an empty parking lot. I was feeling empty, too. He wasn't much, but he had filled my emptiness. I pulled a blanket over myself as the last glass of wine took me to la-la land.

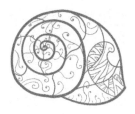

Chapter 32

Seeing Beauty in People

My phone startled me awake. Through blurry eyes, I could see on the caller ID that it was Goth Girl. I hit the receive button.

Her voice was cheerful. "Hey, Wig Girl, how ya doing?"

"You don't want to know," I grumbled into the phone.

"What's going down?"

I took a deep breath. "Frickin' husband. Too much wine. Need I say more?"

"Major crap, eh? I have good news!" she said. "Second part of seeing beauty is tonight. Seven o'clock at the coffee shop. You cool with that?"

"Sure," I said.

"Want me to come over?" she asked.

"Na! Just need to work this hangover off, but I will ready and chirpy for tonight," I replied.

"Okay. See ya," she said and hung up.

It was 8:30 a.m., and I felt like crap. I shot off a text to my boss, saying I would be in at eleven. I put a pot of strong coffee on and headed to the shower.

Throughout the day, I kept a low profile at the office and made numerous trips to the tea stand for some much-needed caffeine. I went home to freshen up and slip on some tight-fitting black jeans and my favorite pink sweater. I was close to feeling normal when I arrived at the coffee shop just a few minutes before seven. Goth Girl was already there with a chair reserved next to her in the back row. She was cradling a large latte with my name on it. What a treasure she was. We hugged and took our seats.

Tuku came out of the back room with Brock and took a seat in front of the group.

She asked us to be quiet for a moment so that we could "arrive," as she called it.

This felt good. My mind was all over the place, and the quiet seemed to center me.

Tuku beamed us a big smile. "Tonight, we are going to look at seeing beauty in people and in life. Just to recap, the aim of seeing beauty is to provide you with clear lenses for seeing people. Remember story of the lily and the sunflower? We have distorted filters for how we see people, and the process I am going to share with you is designed to give you clear lenses for seeing the beauty in people. We will be using the same three principles that we used for seeing beauty in ourselves.

"The aim of seeing beauty in other people is not to change them. This process is aimed at you and the way you view people. First, you need to see the beauty in others. This can progress into friendship and even love if you and the others so desire. The way we usually look at people is based on old habit patterns that are often toxically judgmental. This process is aimed at creating new habits for seeing people. To do this, we need to rewire neural pathways within your brain so that this process functions naturally in you. This new way of thinking will replace the old judgmental, negative neural pathways.

"You are looking at people from the perspective that everything about them is beautiful, and you are going to focus on all the small components that make up the whole, just as you did for yourselves. The Hollywood form of beauty—with photoshopped images and surface veneer is what we are going to replace with a new way of seeing. So, you look for and celebrate the simple things of beauty you see in another. A nose, an ear, a sweater, and so on. Remember that this process will reconfigure your habitual way of seeing people and stop the old negative, habitual ways of looking at people.

"After you have seen three physical aspects of beauty, you look for three beautiful aspects of the person's character. Here is the fun part: if you have not spoken with the person and don't know the person, you can be creative and make this part up. Remember that you are rewiring your habitual ways of seeing people, which means you are looking for the good in them. There is an old saying that is relevant here: 'Two men looked out from prison bars. One saw mud, and the other saw stars.' And so it is with you. You can choose how you view people, and this will affect your emotional state. So, you can imagine that their kindness is beautiful. Their trustworthiness and sense of humor are beautiful.

"The next part is for you to imagine doing three acts of kindness for them, much like you did for yourselves. Remember that you do not have to actually do the act of kindness. You will be using your imagination, and this will open your heart toward them. In short, you will be projecting beautiful energy at them, and they will become aware of it.

"This process is not designed to change them; it is designed to change the way you project the energy of thought toward them. And, as I am sure you all know, we are all very sensitive to this. The more you do this, the stronger the new habits for seeing will be. New neural pathways to support the formation of these new habits will also be created.

"Initially, this process will take effort and an act of will on your part, but it will slowly become habitual and established as the way you naturally function in the world," Tuku said.

This was a real wake-up call for me. I knew that since my husband left, I had been being viewing the human race, in general, with suspicion and contempt. Even though I knew that when you project negativity and anger, you will invariably attract it. I also knew that these negative thoughts would ultimately diminish my immune system, which, when it comes to fighting cancer, was the last thing I should be doing.

Tuku handed out small pieces of paper that each contained the first name of a person in the group. It was time to take this baby on a test drive. The person on my piece of paper was a middle-aged man dressed in blue jeans and a checked shirt. I saw three physical aspects of beauty in him. Then, by getting a sense of his kind-looking and genuine face, I listed three aspects of his character that were beautiful. Imagining the three acts of kindness was fun. I imagined giving him free movie tickets, giving him a voucher for a massage, and taking him out for dinner.

I really liked how this process made me feel inside—kind of warm and fuzzy. This process really did override my negative thinking. I felt a certain freedom from the tyranny of my dysfunctional way of seeing people. As a group, we shared the fruits of this process, and a beautiful sense of warmth and caring seemed to engulf us.

Tuku suggested a fifteen-minute stretch break, and I headed outdoors with Goth Girl. Outside, she reached for a hug. I felt an immediate flood of warm, loving energy. As we released from the hug, she said that she had done this process twelve months earlier and it was life changing. I asked her why she would want to do it again.

"To deepen, deepen, and deepen this process in me," Goth Girl said. "The 'seeing beauty' way of seeing has really transformed my relationship to myself and to the people in my life. I just want more of it. I just want to go deeper. I feel as this is polishing a diamond within me, and the sparkle is getting brighter and brighter."

I looked in through the window and saw that the group was assembling, and we headed in. Tuku began the second half of the session by asking us how we were feeling. Everybody seemed to have a friendly—or I should say *beautiful*—glow, like an aura. Taking a sip of her drink, Tuku said we were going to apply the seeing-beauty process to our everyday lives.

"This has three levels. The first three things of beauty can be in your home, place of work, or outdoors. For example, this morning, I saw beauty in my coffee pot." Everybody chuckled. "Then I saw beauty in the steering wheel of my car and the gentle curve in the road. The second level of seeing beauty is in the invisible. What do I mean by this? There are many aspects of beauty that are not seen with the human eye. For example, the beauty of the blood that is circulating in your body. The beauty of roots on a tree that keep it upright and nourish it. The beauty of air that cannot be seen but keeps you alive. These realms of beauty are often missed. Great poets, artists, and writers often know and live in this realm. I would like to share a story with you that speaks to the value of this.

"Once upon a time, there lived a king in a big castle. Every day he would look out of his castle window at the villagers who lived outside the castle walls. Every day he would see a beggar sitting on an old wooden box, asking for money. One day, the king dressed in old clothes and went out to talk with the beggar. He asked the beggar what was in the box that he sat on every day. The beggar did not know. He had never opened it. Then, the beggar stood and opened the box, and he found it was full of golden coins.

"Like the beggar, we go about our days looking for beauty in the world with our eyes, and we miss the incredible beauty that cannot be seen with the eyes. The beauty that informs a leaf on a tree to change color and release itself from the branch. The beauty that turns a seed into a flower. The warmth of the late-afternoon sun on your face in summer. The smile on a baby's face. And most importantly of all, the unspoken beauty within the human heart. So often, this beauty is locked away to protect it from a world that cannot hear or see it. Seeing beauty in the invisible can transform your life, and you will find more love in your life than you ever thought could exist.

"The third part of seeing beauty in the world is to imagine doing some act of kindness in the world. Once again, you are using your imagination, so don't limit your seeing with time or money constraints. For example, I see the beauty in supporting an animal shelter. I see the beauty of volunteering in a hospice, reading poetry. I see beauty in helping to preserve woodland and build trails. The key to loving is to use love in action. Simply saying you have love is like hoarding money in a bank. All it really does is create a fear that it may be lost one day.

"Here are three more examples of imagining acts of kindness for the outer world: Imagine planting flowers on the overgrown center median of a highway. You can imagine putting a beautiful picture of a landscape on one of the ugly highway billboards that you pass. Imagine creating a magical garden where special-needs children can come and visit. Once again, you are using the mind to express acts of kindness, which will open your heart and create beautiful thoughts. These thoughts, as you all well know, will affect your immune system, and you will live a healthier and longer life. In doing this exercise, you will turn off the production of negative thought processes, and your days will become happier. How does this sound to you?"

The group was quiet. I think we were all contemplating the process and how we might apply it. I imagined painting parking lots pink instead of the usual black asphalt. I know it was only in my imagination, but the idea of pink parking lots made me chuckle. I was really understanding how these simple but powerful processes were transforming how I thought about myself, other people, and my environment.

Tuku said that to conclude our evening, she wanted to apply the seeing-beauty-in-people process to someone in our lives who had caused us pain or upset.

She breathed us down into a quiet place of relaxation and asked us to scan our lives and find negative people who had brought us down. My mind went immediately to Deborah, the miserable receptionist at the clinic who always brought me down with her rude and disrespectful behavior. Tuku asked if anyone would like to share, and I put up my hand.

She nodded for me to speak. I took a deep breath. "Well, I have to attend a clinic every week, and it has a receptionist from hell, Deborah. She always cold-shoulders me and makes me feel angry and disrespected. Just the thought of having to deal with her brings me down. Now that I know the damaging effect on my emotional and physical health of this negative person, I would like to see if I can shift my thought process around her."

Tuku nodded and said this would be a good person to use the process on.

She invited me to the front of the room, and I sat on a chair facing her, making me sideways to the group. Tuku began to guide my process of seeing beauty in Deborah.

"Take some deep, relaxing breaths, Jane. Now imagine that you are walking into the clinic reception area. As you approach the receptionist's desk, you catch your first sight of Deborah. Please look for and describe three physical aspects of beauty you see in her."

I felt an immediate resistance. But then I saw that her red fingernails were beautiful. Her hair was beautiful, and so was her nose. Then I had to imagine three aspects of her personality that were beautiful. Again, I felt a wave of resistance, but I managed to notice that her organizational skills were beautiful. I imagined she had a beautiful loyalty to her family. And for the third thing—and this was a stretch—I imagined that she had a beautiful sense of humor.

Then Tuku asked me for three acts of imagined kindness. "What?" I blurted. "You must be kidding. She's a bitch!" The group laughed. Then I focused. First, I imagined taking in a single red rose in a small vase and placing it on her desk. Then I imagined taking her a bar of chocolate. Tuku suggested that I push myself and imagine the third act of kindness being something personal, like a neck rub.

"Rub or wring her neck?" I asked, and the group laughed again.

I focused and was able to imagine giving her a neck rub. Then I had to imagine walking into the treatment area, and Deborah continuing on as if nothing had happened.

Tuku asked me to share how this process had affected my emotions.

I was immediately struck by the absence of negative emotions directed to Deborah. I actually felt quite chipper, which was a surprise. I was struck by how this process had transformed my experience of Deborah, and she did not even know that anything was going on. It was a home run for me. This simple process was absolutely transformational.

"Remember that this is about your own inner emotional health," Tuku said. "Your imagination is like a medicine cabinet, and Jane just used it to give herself a form of emotional energy that will empower her immune system, which will help her fight and heal from cancer. From a preventive point of view, the stronger your immune system is, the better you will protect yourself from getting cancer, so this process relates to all of you in the group. Any questions?"

The group was silent. "The key to this is doing it over and over again," Tuku said. "Remember: what you think about grows. Initially, it will take effort to keep directing yourself to look for beauty, but this will eventually become a habit and be installed in your subconscious. It will function automatically.

"The other value to the seeing-beauty process is that it is a redirect for your negative thoughts," Tuku said. "It's much like using the remote control for the TV. When you are experiencing negative thoughts and worry, seeing beauty is a way to change your thoughts in an easy and health-giving way.

"Another positive side effect is that with the law of attraction at work, you will start to attract people who also see beauty. You may find that some of your old negative friendships will start to fall away, because you will start to feel the toxicity that negative thoughts can create.

"I am sure you don't need me to state the obvious, that stress and depression diminish your immune system and can make you ill. So, this process is like an antidote to stress and depression. It will promote a stronger immune system that will help to keep you healthy and provide a natural resistance to illness. This is designed to be a simple and easy process, but do not underestimate the power it has to transform every part of your life, especially your love life. Remember what the drip, drip, drip of water can achieve?"

Tuku asked me how I was feeling. I shared that I had felt a difference in my emotional response to the receptionist. I could sense that Goth Girl was looking at me, and I turned to meet her gaze. She gave me a wink and pointed to my bare feet. I knew she was referring to her comment that this would knock my socks off. I smiled back and nodded that she was right.

Tuku said she had a few final thoughts before our evening was complete. "One thing to remember is not to try to foist this process on people whom you feel it would help. This is your process. The value of the process should be recognized by the transformation that occurs in you. Remember, this is not a process to change people, but it is designed to change the way you see people.

"It is a tool for you to transform yourself. However, you may find that people start responding to you in more positive ways. That is a bonus, but it's not the intention. It's sort of a nice side effect." Tuku then said a closing blessing.

Goth Girl followed me to my car. She locked her beautiful eyes on me and asked, "Well, Wig Girl, what do ya think?"

"It's frickin' awesome," I said. "A real game changer." She gave me a big hug, and I drove home.

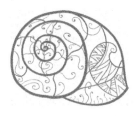

Chapter 33

The Hacker Arrives

I arrived home just after 9:00 p.m. feeling elated about the seeing-beauty process. I did a quick flip through my email and found one from Bob.

> Hi, Sis. Hope you are good. Been in touch with my friend Hank who can help you track financial information. He is a top guy and consults with the FBI. I am hoping he can track your husband's financial footsteps. I told him about you, and he is going to call you. Love, Bob

A bolt of fear went through me. Was there some dark, buried secret here? Had my husband been up to no good? Or maybe David really was a good guy, and it was my own brokenness that was directing suspicion at him. Would I be a bad person for hacking him? If he found out, could this end our marriage once and for all? There was only one thing to do: I needed a glass of wine. I flipped off my computer and headed to the kitchen. As I filled my glass, I noticed the blinking message light on my kitchen phone. A part of me wanted to leave it for the morning. But a more curious part of me hit the playback button.

A very relaxed, deep voice awaited me. "Good day, Jane. Your brother, Bob, asked me to call. My name is Hank," he said, and he recited a phone number.

The message unnerved me. I gulped back the wine and poured myself another glass. My thoughts took off like a pack of wild dogs after a rabbit. Why was I being so weak about hacking my husband? He had walked out on me. He had hidden our money. I had a right to get answers. I could feel my anger stirring, and it felt good. I wanted to know the truth, not only about our finances but about his emotions and what he really felt about me. I also felt entitled to an apology.

I knew that my fear of being alone was stealing my thunder. I sloshed back two more glasses of wine and stumbled upstairs to bed.

The alarm woke me at 7:00 a.m. I showered and was making tea in the kitchen when the phone rang. I checked the caller ID and saw that it was Bob.

Oh crap, I thought. I did not feel like talking to him, but I knew that he had gotten up very early to catch me at home, and I had to take the call.

I hit the talk button. "Hey, Mr. Bob. You caught the early bird. How are you?"

He was in his tough-attorney frame of mind and barked at me. "Gotta get moving on your financials, honey. Call Hank, like now. You will need a new cell phone that cannot be tracked. Hank will need it for the entry point into your husband's financials. When he chooses the access entry point, a phone verification is required, which means it can be tracked. We want to keep you clean on this, so you will need that new phone."

"Okay," I said meekly. "How do I get one of those?"

"Do you have a household bill in hard copy?"

"Yep," I replied.

"Scan and email it to me. I'll tweak it so that you can use it to get your new phone. The salesperson will ask for it."

Tweaks? I wondered what that meant. I was in no mood to tangle with my brother, so I said, "Will do. Give me thirty minutes." Then I felt uncertain about tweaking a formal document. "Ah, Bob, is tweaking a legal bill legal?" I asked tentatively.

"Hell, yeah!" he shot back. "There is a loophole in the cell phone acquisition law that requires 'any' form of ID. It does not have to be yours. Screwy, I know; but this is common practice for hackers and people who are trying to avoid the IRS. Trust me on this, Sis. Once you get this new statement from me, print it out and take it to a drug store that sells cell phone packages. Buy a 200-minute card, and they will give you a new cell phone number. All they will ask for is some proof of your address. No other ID is needed. Show them the statement and pay in cash, and you are good to go. Ask the sales guy to put a block on the caller ID recognition. They do it all the time. This way, nobody will be able to track the calls you make on this phone."

"I feel like James Bond," I said.

Bob chuckled. "Call Hank and have him come over to get this going. I have known him for over twenty years. He's really solid. He will be able to do this from your home. Okay?"

"Sure," I said. Then the frozen divorce situation flashed into my mind. "As the divorce proceedings are frozen, do we really have to do this now?"

That really irked him. "Sis, I am smelling a rat and that rat is your chicken-shit husband. I have in my hand a six-inch nail. And this is what I am going to nail his ass to the wall with! Got it? Send me the bill. I'm on the run. Talk later." And he impatiently hung up.

I felt as if I had just been hit with a stun gun. Yet also, in some way I felt excited. I was so pleased that Bob was on my side.

I headed upstairs and copied the bill as requested and shot it off to Bob. As I sat down to sip my tea and reflect, nagging doubts came back. What happens if David finds out I have hacked him? That might really piss him off. What if we find something is amiss? David would never screw me, would he?

A few minutes later, my phone bill came back attached to an email from Bob.

It had a name and address I didn't recognize. I printed it out and put it in my bag. I was really feeling nervous about this. Bob was an attorney, so I guessed this was not breaking any laws, but it sure as hell felt like it was.

On my way to the pharmacy, I withdrew cash from a bank machine. As I walked into the store, I was nervous. I could see that the attendant at the phone counter was a college-age kid. Kind of scrawny with pimples and thick, black-rimmed glasses. I guess you would call him a nerd. I asked him for a cell phone with 200 minutes. He started punching the information into the computer. "Name and address?" he said without looking up.

I handed him the telephone bill. He laid it by the side of the keyboard and started typing in the information. Then he stopped and glanced up at me. I knew that he knew something was not right here. I felt a wave of panic, and a cold sweat broke out on my forehead. He was motionless as he studied the phone bill. He looked very serious, and I was concerned he may hit the security button at any minute. My inner panic was growing.

"Divorce stuff, eh?" He was a smart nerd.

I nodded yes.

Then a big smile broke out on his face. "Yeah, my mom did the same thing a year ago when she left my waster of a dad. I see a lot of these make-believe bills." He suddenly seemed like a fellow conspirator, and I felt relief.

He pointed to the sales register that said $56.70. I handed him three crisp twenty-dollar bills. He handed me the change and then took a phone out of the cabinet, inserted a prepaid card, and hit the ring tone. He held it to his ear to check the ring tone. "Want the caller ID-blocker turned on?" he asked.

"Sure thing," I replied.

Then he handed it to me so that I could hear that it was active. He smiled and said, "Good luck," as he gave me the empty box and paperwork. I felt a little like a secret agent as I marched from the store. My next assignment was to call someone I knew to make sure that my caller ID was not being shown.

I chose to call Goth Girl. Her phone rang and rang, and she did not pick up. Then her voice mail kicked in. As I started to leave a message, she jumped into the call. "Hey, Wig Girl, my caller ID did not pick your number up. What phone are you calling from?" She thought I was in some sort of trouble.

"All is good," I said. "Just checking my new phone."

"New phone, eh? What's going down?"

"I just needed a phone that cannot be traced. Long story. Will explain later, K?" I said.

"So, are you good for tonight? Tuku at seven at the coffee shop?"

"Sure am," I said, trying to sound upbeat.

"Cool! See ya then," she said and hung up.

I was feeling rather accomplished at having achieved the first part of my homework and headed into the office.

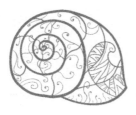

Chapter 34

The Three Oceans

I lost myself in some grant writing for the day and was pleased when five o'clock came around. I drove straight home to freshen up and eat a yogurt before heading to the coffee shop. I was still feeling ambivalent about the hacking process and decided to wait until Bob or Hank called me again.

At 6:50 I pulled into the parking lot just as Brock was pulling in. This was a good start. We hugged in the parking lot, and I got that burst of energy that tickled my groin. I felt kind of bad, but it made me feel kind of good. I wondered if he had any kind of sensual reaction when our bodies met. I did notice that after our hugs, he always maintained eye contact. I watched him hug other people, and he always looked away when the hug ended. Was this a clue? Or was this simply me living in la-la land? *Who cares?* I thought. *It just makes me feel good, and since I spend so much time feeling like crap, I am gonna take it.* We made some light conversation as we walked in together.

I liked Brock's height. He was around six feet tall, and my five foot eight seemed a good fit. Damn, I caught myself with mischievous thoughts again. He seemed keen for us to sit together, and I felt comforted to be next to him. Not to mention that slight aroma of pine wood that emanated from him. Could it be addictive? I wondered. And then there were the open shirt buttons and chest hair. This was more fun than chocolate. A secretive flirt with Brock was just what the doctor ordered. As we settled in our seats, he turned his blue eyes to me and said, "Great to see you again, Jane. I enjoyed our time in the woodshop."

"Me too," I whispered as I leaned into him slightly, getting an extra hit of the pine scent.

Goth Girl arrived just at seven and blew us both kisses as she took a seat on the other side of the room, near the door. A few minutes after seven, Tuku walked out of the back room and took her seat in front of us. There were about twelve in the group that evening.

Tuku asked us to take some deep breaths and spend some moments in silence.

A peace immediately seemed to descend on the room. I did my best to pull my attention from the closeness of Brock, but I was not very successful. A warm, peaceful energy seemed to radiate from him. I squinted around the room and saw the others sitting with their eyes closed. I secretly opened another button on my blouse. I know it was a bad thing to do, but once again, it made me feel good. And, truthfully, I had deliberately worn a black bra that would catch the eye against my white and now somewhat unbuttoned silk shirt.

Tuku looked around the room, resting her eyes on each of us for a few seconds. It felt like a mini blessing.

She was wearing a nice purple skirt with a matching blouse. Her short-cropped hair formed a halo around her soft, lightly tanned face. Her big brown eyes seemed to pour out an energy of peace and goodwill. "Tonight, I am beginning our journey with the three loves and the key philosophy and processes that the Shaolin monks developed to help the villagers find true and lasting, unconditional love. The challenges the villagers faced in finding and sustaining true love are similar to the challenges people in the West are dealing with."

I flashed a quick glance at Brock, and he turned to look at me. The proximity of his beautiful blue eyes really caught me off guard, and I felt immediately transported into some higher realm. Our eyes lingered on each other for a few seconds. As Tuku started to speak again, we both turned to look at her.

What the hell was that? Did he just feel what I just felt? It was a scary good feeling, and I could feel heat in my groin again. I knew it was kind of guiltily bad, but it felt really good, too.

Tuku was talking, and I tuned in. "We call it the three loves because there are three parts of finding true and lasting love during this earthly existence.

The Shaolin monks live on an island where three oceans come together, and this became the metaphor for their teaching. They adapted the concept of the three oceans to the process of finding and keeping true, eternal love. Before I go into detail, I just want to say that the processes I am going to share can be likened to when you start driving a car. There are various things you must do one at a time to learn them. Then, later, they will merge into one unified process. This philosophy and the practices will have an immediate effect on your life. The way of the three loves has the power to bring dramatic growth and evolution in your life. With this will come greater happiness and a sense of fulfillment."

I was enjoying every word she was saying. There was something about her calm and peaceful manner that seemed to carry her words deep inside me. It was not so much a theory she was sharing with us; rather, she was sharing who she was and how she lived. She took a sip of water. "So, the three loves are represented by three oceans that fit inside each other, much like a target with an outer ring, an inner ring, and a center, which is the bull's-eye. Each of these three rings represents one area of love. When all three are in harmony and cared for, you will be living true and eternal love.

"Each of these three circles represent an area of love and has a color," Tuku said. "The outer circle is blue and represents your day-to-day life and rational-thinking mind. This is where the things and people you love in this life dwell. The feeling associated with the blue color is gratitude. This represents gratitude for your life and for everything in your life, as is. There may well be challenge, pain, and suffering from time to time. This is part of the blue ocean. Everything in this realm is transitory and has a certain life expectancy. This includes every relationship you have. I will be talking more about this later.

"Inside the blue ocean is a circular white ocean, and it represents your soul or spirit. This is the part of you that came into this life, and it is the part that will one day leave. It is the deepest part of you, and it is eternal. The energetic relationship to the white ocean is deep peace. When you are truly in your soul, you feel a glorious and deep peace. There are no thoughts there; these belong to the blue ocean. The feeling of deep peace is an emotional one, and it is deeply beautiful.

"Within the white ocean is the golden ocean, and this is at the very center. This golden ocean is your connection to the divine. There are many different names for this, depending on one's belief system. It has been called the beloved, God, Mother Nature, Jesus, the Divine Presence, the higher power, eternal love, and many other names. If you are a nonbeliever, then it may simply be the source of love. It is in the golden ocean where you find and feel that you are truly loved by whatever higher power is in your life. The energetic relationship to the golden ocean is that of feeling loved. I want to differentiate the words *loved* and *love*. We use the word *loved* as a verb to signify an action taking place. You are and always have been *loved* by the Divine Presence or whatever name you use for it. In contrast, the word *love* is a noun and the name of something. The way of the three loves is very dynamic and alive, which is why the feeling we want you to feel from the golden ocean is that of being loved by the Divine Presence. And this is the actual source of true and lasting love. When you are truly connected, you will not look for relationships in the world to fill you with you love. You will have a source of love deep within you. Then you will share your love in your relationships in the world, and this will transform how you relate to people.

"When you connect to the white ocean, your soul, you will realize that you came into this world as pure love. And that pure love is in you and alive. You see this in babies, which is why they are so magical and bring so much joy to the world. Then, as they grow, they start to form the blue ocean of intellect, and the soul begins to get lost under the layers of the rational mind and ego. You also begin collecting hurts in life, and you start to find ways to protect yourself.

"The problem is that if these layers of protections we create are not released, they become a sort of encasement, trapping the beautiful light of your soul inside you," Tuku said. "Our work is to help you to uncover the soul love that all of you have inside of you. Perhaps many of you are looking for love in the world. But you have more than you can ever find in the world right inside your own heart. The three loves will help you to rediscover this.

"For the villagers, the blue ocean was the dominant ocean. The white and golden oceans were very small and were not functioning. Our work was to give them tools that would help them to find a true balance among all three oceans."

There was something about what she was saying that really spoke to me. The thought of myself as a baby with a soul full of love seemed to stir something deep inside of me. I had a lot of memories from my childhood of not being seen or being told to be quiet. I liked the idea that I did not lose my beautiful shining soul, but I may well have hidden it to protect it. But that which had once protected it had now become a prison that I did not know how to escape. I had a sense that Tuku was going to show me how.

"What I am sharing with you is not another belief system designed to replace your existing belief system," Tuku said. "Quite the opposite. The villagers, years ago, had a wide variety of belief systems that all brought meaning and value to their lives. The monks wanted to create a process that would help to bring even more love to their existing systems of belief. So, if you have a belief system, our processes can help to grow and expand the love within that system. If you do not have a belief system, then our processes can be helpful in bringing more love into your life."

I was relieved to hear that. I had had the sneaking suspicion that this would turn out to be another form of belief system or cult that claimed to be the right one when all others were wrong. The last thing I needed was entrapment in a belief system.

"Just to recap," Tuku said, "the large outer ocean is blue and is where your ego and rational mind lives. This ocean will exist for the duration of your life on Earth. Inside the blue ocean is the white ocean, which represents your soul or spirit that came into this life for the purpose of learning and growing through all the many life experiences each of you will have. This existed before you were born and will exist when your life on Earth is over. The white ocean is pure love. The feeling associated with this ocean is deep peace and inner silence.

"Within the white ocean is the golden ocean. There are many names for it. The one I like to use is Divine Presence. The golden ocean is where you experience love and feel deeply loved by and connected to a higher power. The way to find true love during this life is to integrate these three oceans in and through every aspect of your life.

"If a person does not have a healthy relationship with his or her own soul, the white ocean, there will be an inner emptiness that the intimate relationships in the blue ocean will be expected to fill. The reality is that unless you have a relationship to yourself and your own beautiful soul as manifested in the white ocean, your way of being and loving in the world of the blue ocean will be dependent on your worldly relationships. You will seek relationships in the world to fill you, but they never will. You can only fill yourself from within.

"Ever tried to fill a toilet with water?" Tuku asked. "No matter how much water you pour in, the level stays the same. You never fill the bowl. It is the same with love.

"A needy person often attracts a needy person. Love then becomes a commodity that is bartered based on hunger and lack. If I love you, you will love me back, right?

"As I said before, if you have a true connection to your soul, then the function of relationships will be to share the abundance of love you have within yourself with the people in your life. You will not need or seek love from others. Then, as the law of attraction predicts, you will attract people who also seek relationships, so they can share their love. By having true communion with the blue and white oceans, one can experience a rich and loving life," she said.

"Now we come to the golden ocean. The function of the golden ocean is to bring a form of Divine Presence and purpose to your life so that the love experienced in the blue and white oceans can be manifested in alignment with a higher purpose. This becomes more important as we go through life, and the question of your life having meaning emerges.

"The true compass of your life and source of eternal love is found in the golden ocean. From this place of divine love, the way to navigate life is found. The outer blue ocean of intellect and ego can then be brought into alignment with your higher purpose.

"Each ocean is a different emotional experience. For the blue ocean, it is feeling gratitude for the gift of life, as is. With all its many challenges, just being alive is great cause for gratitude. For the white ocean, the emotional experience is a sense of deep, inner peace. For the gold ocean, there is a sense of warmth in the heart from feeling loved by the Divine Presence.

"Now that you know about these three oceans, you need to know how to navigate among them," Tuku said. "The aim is to have the three oceans in balance, as they are all needed if you are to live a loving, balanced, and meaningful life. Let's take a five-minute stretch break."

Goth Girl and I went to the parking lot for some air.

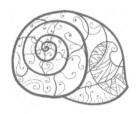

Chapter 35

The Spiral Meditation—1

When we got outside, Goth Girl asked me how it was all sounding.

I said I loved it. It made me aware of how dependent I was on my husband and that I had never been able to fill my own heart first. My blue ocean was dominant, and the white and golden oceans were diminished, to say the least. I knew I'd lost my connection to my center, and I really wanted it back. We took some big gulps of air and went back in to learn more.

"The way to travel among the three oceans is by using a special form of mind integration or mind-attuning process," Tuku said. "This is not the same as meditation. The different forms of meditation that are taught in the West are very helpful in bringing a person to a state of relaxation and a quiet mind. However, the monks wanted to offer the villagers a process that would unify and balance the three oceans. The aim was to enrich and empower their relationships to themselves. This would be the foundation for building new relationships and releasing old ones that no longer held value," she said.

"For the last couple of years, I have worked with Brock and shared with him the mind-integration process," she said. "I would like to invite Brock to share this process with us."

Brock stood up and walked to Tuku. They shared a quick hug and then Brock took her seat and Tuku sat next to me. She gave me a wink and a smile she sat down.

It was nice seeing Brock in front of the group. He was very good on the eye in many ways—your original eye candy. I had not figured him as a public speaker and was keen to hear what he had to say. He looked calm and asked us to all take a couple of deep breaths to center ourselves.

"My journey with meditation and finding inner peace began over twenty years ago," he said. "I tried many forms of meditation and found they all contained various benefits, but regarding finding true and lasting love, I felt something was missing. The meditation practices that I followed all seemed to suggest that the mind was something of a problem, a distraction. My mind would go quiet for a while, then it would shoot random thoughts to interrupt the meditation. I spoke with people who had meditated for years, and they still complained about the fact that every now and then, they would have uncontrollable, wandering thoughts. The term most commonly used was *monkey mind*. People who had meditated for decades still talked about their constant battle with monkey mind.

"When I shared this with Tuku, she helped me to look at this from a completely different perspective, which helped me to develop a new relationship with my mind. I don't know if any of you remember a film in the 1960s called *Space Odyssey*. It was about two men and a space journey. A computer on their spacecraft called Hal had been programed to help them. Anyway, the computer started to think for itself and came up with plans other than the ones the men wanted to follow.

"This movie reminded me about my own relationship to my mind. Even though I kind of created it, it still seemed to do things in a manner different from what I wanted," Brock said. "There were times when my mind felt like an intelligence unto itself and did not always comply with what I wanted deep down inside—especially when it came to being quiet when I tried to meditate.

"With Tuku's help, I approached the question of how I related to my mind from a whole new perspective. I gave my mind an identity and valued it as a part of me that made up the whole. As I reflected on my mind, I realized how calling it a *monkey mind* had, in fact, created a sense of negative duality. It was a demeaning term. I was being disrespectful to a part of me that had done so much for me. And I had also trained it to function much like a computer that is programmed. For me to put it in the same class as a monkey really showed a lack of respect, so why would it fully cooperate?

"I started a process of communicating with my mind as an equal. I know it sounds funny; but bear with me. When you see where this is going, you will understand.

"So, I started a process of communicating with my mind using my non-dominant hand. I would write a question on a piece of paper with my dominant hand, representing my soul, the white ocean. Then I would engage my nondominant hand to reply, imagining that my mind was replying. The key is to just let the answer flow out. It is not helpful to dwell on the answer, because old patterns emerge and will take over the process.

"Here is a sample of how our dialogues sounded.

Me, writing with my dominant hand: "Hi, Mind. Just wanted to check in to see how you are doing today."

Mind, writing with my nondominant hand: "Well, funny you should ask. I am feeling rather remote from you and disrespected."

Me: "Ummm, really? Want to tell me why?"

Mind: "Sure. You created me to run your day-to-day life. I am happy to do this and really enjoy it. I am the breadwinner. I keep us fed and take care of all your needs in your day-to-day life. I work hard, and I work long hours. I never complain and always show up on time. Yet, when you decide to sit on the small, black, meditation pillow, you become very distant and order me to sit outside the door and be quiet. Well, that is not as easy as it sounds, and it could really get you into trouble. For example, when your bladder is full of pee, who is it that says, 'Hey, buddy, time for the restroom.' And then I find you a restroom. If I did not stay vigilant when you are trying to meditate, you and your meditating buddies would all have to wear diapers, as you would keep peeing yourselves. Also, what I am saying is that you are ungrateful when it comes to valuing all I do for you. And yes, calling me a monkey mind really does piss me off. Are you getting what I am saying?"

Me: "Yikes! I never quite saw it this way before. Now that you mention it, I see how I have not given you the respect you deserve. And I can see that I am creating a sense of duality in myself."

Mind: "Ya know, you should go to an Alzheimer's ward someday. Then you will see what your life would be like without me."

Brock: "Yikes! I get it! So, how do I move forward with you so that we can live in harmony and work together as one?"

Mind: "Well, you can start by using the seeing-beauty process on me. Tell me three things that are beautiful about me. Tell me three things about me you are grateful for. Imagine three acts of kindness you can do for me. How about that to start with?"

Me: "Great idea. Here goes. The three things of beauty are that you are so incredibly quick and talented, you help me to see goodness in people, and you help me navigate my life with great precision and order.

"Three things I am grateful for are that you pay our bills and keep a roof over our heads, you keep me safe on the roads, and you help me to have wonderful friends.

"Now, for three acts of kindness, I will ask you what you love to do. I will let you read whatever book you choose, and I will treat you with respect. How does this sound?"

Mind: "Fabulous! I feel more cared for and happier already."

Me: "I am enjoying this communication, and I feel very connected to myself. Not sure how to find words to explain it."

Mind: "I know what you are saying. I already feel more connected to you. I do want this communication to continue. I do want us to find happiness, and I am tired of the duality that we have been living with."

Brock then stopped and asked if there were any questions.

I was stunned by what he had just shared. I turned to look at Tuku, who had turned to look at me. I raised my eyebrows and said, "This is frickin' mind-blowing."

She smiled and said, "Oh, honey, this is just the beginning. The best is yet to come."

A middle-aged, well-dressed woman in the front row put her hand up.

"So, Brock, where does the mind stand when it comes to love?"

Brock smiled and thanked her for the question. "When I started the journey to find true love, it took me a while to understand how important it is to love yourself first. I was pretty critical of myself and self-judging. I often compared myself to others and always seemed to come up short. A lot of my negative attitude came from the negative messages I received when I was a child. I carried these messages into my adult years. They were like negative tapes that played repeatedly in my subconscious. And following the law of attraction meant that I attracted the same sort of negative people into my life.

"Tuku helped me to understand that I needed to really get my own house in order before I could truly expect to find love in the world. A lot of these tapes were in my subconscious and played out through my mind. They were how I functioned in life. I did not really appreciate my mind, so there was a lot of disharmony going on inside of me. The way of the three loves really brought me home to loving myself first as a whole person. This meant loving myself and my mind, warts and all.

"When I started to dialogue with my mind, treating it as if it was a valuable part of me, I started to feel a deeper respect for myself as a person. It was a sort of 'coming home' to the beauty that was and had always been inside of me. Up to that time, I did not really understand the term *being your own best friend*. I did not like to spend time alone and always sought the company of others. When I began this new way of seeing myself and communicating with different parts of me, I came to see how much beauty there was inside of me, and life took on a whole new dimension.

"I used to think that love was the domain of the heart and the mind was just a part of me that seemed to get in the way. How wrong I was. I have come to realize that the mind is a wonderful and essential part of the self-love process and that harmony with my mind has become a source of love all in itself.

"For example, my mind helps me to navigate social situations. It shows me the people with whom I can find meaningful friendships and steers me away from those who are energy stealers.

"My mind loves it when I am loving. It does not like it when I am unhappy. It actually wants me to be happy, and now that it has my true respect, it is really good to be with. This may sound funny, but I really do love and appreciate my mind. I no longer call it *monkey mind*. I value what it has to share with me. As a result, it has become compliant with the processes of the way of the three loves.

"The key to moving among the three oceans and bringing the mind into union is the use of the ancient symbol of the spiral. This is what the Shaolin monks taught the villagers," Brock said.

"The spiral is an ancient symbol that connects to the gravitational pull of the Earth. The monks used it to unify their minds and travel in and between the three oceans. They imagined following the spiral in and out of the three oceans. In this way, they meaningfully occupied the mind by giving it a responsibility. With the mind participating in the process, they were able to enter the deepest place of Divine Presence, where the purest love was to be found. They then carried and distributed this love throughout the white and blue oceans.

"They not only found love within themselves, but the mind helped them to send this love out into the world. Because this love came from the Divine

Presence, their actions took on the true purpose that their souls had come here to live out.

"So, the act of focusing on the slow movement of following the spiral in and out is a way to bring all three oceans into peace and harmony. In focusing this way, the villagers lived soulful lives and found a new way to love that was based on Divine Presence, as opposed to the needy kind of dependent love that they had been living.

"In a few moments, I would like to lead you through the spiral process," Brock said. "Please take a five-minute stretch break."

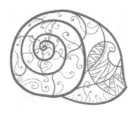

Chapter 36

The Spiral Meditation—2

We returned from the restroom and took our seats. Brock began to talk.

"I want to share with you the spiral process that we use to navigate among the three oceans. Just to recap, think of a target with three circles inside each other. The outer circle represents the blue ocean, which is the rational mind and ego. The circle inside this is white and represents the soul. Inside the white ocean is the golden ocean, and this represents our relationship to the Divine Presence or eternal love. To give you a spatial sense of these three oceans, when they are in balance, imagine extending your arms straight out from your sides like the wings of an airplane. The tips of your fingers represent the outer edges of the blue ocean energetically. Now bring your awareness to your armpits. These mark the inner edges of your blue ocean, where the white ocean begins. Now imagine that the nipples on your chest represent the inside edges of your white ocean, where your golden ocean begins. The golden ocean is in the middle.

"The Shaolin monks chose to use the spiral to move among the three oceans for very specific reasons. The symbol of the spiral is connected to the spiritual path, and clockwise movement is regarded as ascension—a path of awareness, a new beginning. A journey to increased light. This is why we use it to take us to the center of our golden ocean and our divine connection with eternal love. The counterclockwise direction represents descent from the world of spirit into the world of physical form.

"The spiral is one of the oldest and most enigmatic of sacred symbols on this planet. The very first labyrinth was created by the Shaolin monks, and it was a pure spiral. As their teachings spread around the world, the original spiral labyrinth was adapted by other belief systems, and we now find a wide variety of different labyrinth designs. The monks also used the symbol of the spiral because it connects to the kundalini life force that every human carries within. This powerful force is found in the pelvic region, which is called the root chakra.

"The word *kundalini* comes from the Sanskrit word *kundal*, which means spiral or coil. It is compared to a serpent that lies coiled while resting or sleeping. Kundalini flows like a current of electricity and is often shown as two serpents spiraling around each other, depicting the masculine and the feminine. The serpent totem is sacred in many traditions and is regarded as the earth's primal healing energy. The serpent is also a symbol of transformation. The kundalini energy is very powerful, and if it is released suddenly, the effects can be traumatic. The monks chose the symbol of the spiral so that it would gently nurture the kundalini power and integrate it into daily life. The spiral energy of the kundalini provides healing, improved physical health, and increased energy.

"There is one more reason why the monks chose the symbol of the spiral, and it has to do with the mind. I have already talked about the mind and how important it is to love the mind and embrace it with love. Because the mind often wanders with random thoughts and is called the monkey mind, the monks cleverly designed this process so that the mind could be lovingly involved: they ask it to follow the spiral in and out. Add to this the coordination of the three breaths for each of the oceans, and you have a fully involved, integrated, and supportive mind that does not disturb the process with random thoughts. Three breaths take about thirty seconds, so three sets of breaths take about ninety seconds. Before I learned about this process, I had tried a lot of mind control and meditation practices, but I always found my mind was too active and disruptive to really benefit from them. When the Shaolin monks taught me this spiral process, it was as if my mind and my breath started making love together. As you will find out, this is a really sensuous spiritual practice.

"As to where the spiral begins and ends, imagine that the middle of your chest is the center of a clock face. Imagine stretching your arm straight out in front of you horizontally. Your middle finger ends where the number twelve would be. Imagine the circle of the clock face is all around you. One complete turn of the clock face represents one turn of the spiral. This means that the number six on the clock face would be right behind you, at arm's length. One full breath in and out will take you one full turn of the spiral. You breathe in until your awareness arrives at the six, then breathe out as you return to the twelve.

"You transition from in-breath to out-breath as you pass the number six. Each of the three oceans consists of three turns of the spiral. This is how you restore them to full balance. The first turn of the spiral is number one and begins in the center of your chest. There are three turns in the gold ocean, then you move into the white ocean, which will be turns four, five, and six. As you move into the blue ocean, you will go through turns seven, eight, and nine, which takes you to the farthest edge of your blue ocean. This is at the number twelve on the clock face out in front of you. As you practice this meditation, you will begin to feel your energy fields growing and becoming balanced. Your attention is what will carry you through the different spirals. As you link your breath to this, you will notice a beautiful feeling of symmetry throughout your physical and emotional bodies.

"Just this process of breathing in and out of the spiral will bring feelings of great wholeness and empowerment. And all it takes is nine breaths."

I was struck by how easy this sounded. In the past, I had tried to meditate and do mind-control exercises and never succeeded due to the complexity of the processes and how much time they took. I just didn't have the twenty to thirty minutes in the morning that these practices needed. Of course, when I failed, I felt bad. But this new spiral process sounded so easy and natural, and I loved the beautiful rhythm of the inward and outward movement of the spiral that is linked to breath. Hell, I could even do this in bed. Even on the toilet. As I thought about the toilet, I started to grin. Tuku looked at me as if to ask what was funny. I leaned into her and whispered my thought about doing it on the toilet. A grin broke out on her face as well. At last, a spiritual practice that is fun to do. Now *there's* an interesting concept. I was hungry to learn more.

Brock said, "When the Shaolin monks started working with the villagers, their energetic fields represented by the three oceans were very contracted and out of balance. For many of them, the blue ocean ended at their armpits. In the centers of their chests were small, white circles the size of a tennis balls that represented the souls. Inside the white circles were small golden circles the size of a golf balls, representing their golden oceans. They were living mostly in the blue ocean of a constricted rational mind and ego.

"Their connection to their souls and Divine Presence was really diminished. They were navigating their lives with the rational mind and ego, and they were not very happy. Their purpose in life was all ego driven. They had no sense of true divine purpose or love in their lives. The spiral process helped them to nurture their three oceans back into balance and into healthy and functioning relationships with each other.

"To experience unconditional love in this world, all three oceans need to be in balance and in communication with each other. Each time you do your full nine breaths and travel in and out of the spiral, you are empowering and balancing the three oceans. By repeating this, a habit is created and leads to the development of new and healthy neural pathways in your brain. The subconscious integrates this process and, with practice, it becomes as natural as regular breathing. As you breathe, your awareness travels among the three oceans, and you will begin to feel the qualities of each ocean. At that point, you will begin to feel an inner joy and a love unlike anything you ever thought possible."

Brock asked if there were any questions and took a few sips from his water bottle.

I looked around the group. Everyone seemed really engrossed. An elderly man asked if he could do the process in bed. A ripple of laughter went around the group.

"Absolutely," Brock replied. "In fact, that is how I start and finish my day. To get a sense of the blue ocean, just imagine your arms out by your sides again. The number twelve on the clock face will be where your feet are and the number six will be above your head, at the farthest edge of your pillow. It is as if you are lying on the clock face, and the center is right in the middle of your chest.

"Feet toward the twelve, and head toward the six." He went on to say that he sometimes did this breathing process in traffic jams, in supermarket queues, and before and after stressful situations. I was loving it more and more by the minute. Then Tuku turned to me and lifted one of her eyebrows as if to ask, "Well, what do you think?"

I just nodded. "Totally awesome."

Brock thanked the man for the question. "In a few moments," he said, "I would like to guide us all through this spiral process. But first, I want to talk about the application of three power words that will help to empower and link emotional responses to each of the oceans.

"When we tune into the blue ocean that represents the outer world and rational mind, the power-word response is *gratitude*. It is important to feel gratitude for the gift of life. And everything in life is given to us—the air, the sun, the food, your health, your family. Each second of your life is a gift. It is easy to see only the problems of life and miss the bigger beauty and gift of being alive. So, when we talk about the blue ocean, the emotional power word is *gratitude*. When we come to the white ocean, the emotional power word is *peace*. This is what it feels like to be in touch with your soul. Just a wonderful experience of deep peace. The mind does not function here. Fears, stress, and worry can only live in the blue ocean. The white ocean is pure soul and is peace. When we move to the golden ocean, the power word is *loved*. Not the word *love*, but the verb *loved*. This is the experience of being loved by the Divine Presence, God, eternal love, or whatever name you use. This is where we experience true unconditional love being poured into and over us. The word *loved* denotes an active process. We are all loved by that which created us and gives us life. The key to each of these words is to feel the feelings that they communicate to us.

"To support and empower the spiral process, I want to offer you another easy-to-do process that you can do at the same time you are following your breath in and out of the spiral. At first glance, this process may seem simple, but it can bring incredible transformation. I want you to imagine that you have been called to Hollywood to make a movie. You are in the final audition, and a million-dollar contract awaits you. In your final audition, the movie director asks you to show a facial expression that expresses feelings of *gratitude*. You have to hold this expression for three breaths. Then you are asked to make a facial expression for *peace* and hold it for three breaths. The final facial expression is that of being *loved* by the Divine Presence, and you hold this for three breaths. This process will add real momentum to the inner changes the spiral process will invoke in you. When you follow the golden spiral, hold the facial expression of being loved. When you move into the white ocean, hold the facial expression of deep peace. And when you move into the blue ocean, hold the facial expression of gratitude.

"This process can be done at any time of the day, and you will find that it has the power to transform the most stressful situation.

"Another important benefit is that it will switch your thoughts like a TV remote from the negative into the positive. By simply changing your facial expression to imagine feeling any one of these three positive feelings, you will be pouring healing energy into your immune system. And it is your immune system that both heals you and helps to protect you from illness.

"By following these practices, you will be transforming yourself from the outside and the inside. Oh, and one more tidbit of information that I think you will value: The Shaolin monks were known for not looking their ages. Monks in their eighties looked as if they were in their forties. They attribute their youthful appearance to this exercise of creating facial expressions connected to the three oceans. The expressions uplift their emotions and spirit. Essentially, this practice could save you thousands of dollars in facelifts."

"*Now* you tell me!" said a very smart-looking woman who was wearing a lot of makeup. Everybody laughed, and then she added, "If more people practiced this, they would put the Botox companies out of business." Another ripple of laugher went around the group. I was stunned again by how simple, yet powerful and easy these processes were to do. I couldn't wait to try them.

"I have a teacher friend who started to do this spiral breathing process at the beginning of each day with her class of ten-year-old children," Brock said. "They did the nine breaths, and she said that the class became much better behaved, and their grades improved. The kids enjoyed it so much that they asked if they could do it at the end of the day before they went home. The principal noticed how much better functioning this teacher's class had become and asked the teacher to share the process with other teachers. My teacher friend shared with me that the kids became kinder to one another and that sharing the process brought them together as a caring community."

Brock asked us if were ready and everybody nodded enthusiastically.

He asked Makeup Lady if she would volunteer to provide an example of how the facial process worked. She smiled and jumped to her feet. I sensed that she really liked the attention. *Nice move, Brock.*

He asked her to stand in front of the group, close her eyes, and take some deep breaths. Then he guided her. "Please imagine that you are surrounded by a beautiful blue ocean. Become aware of how grateful you are for everything in your life, including the gift of life. Feel this gratitude deep inside of you. When you are ready, please create a facial expression that shows this gratitude."

She was paying attention to his words and wore an expression of a focused, intent listening. As she began the first breath, it was as if a curtain was lifted, and a warm smile appeared on her face. As she took in the second breath the smile grew wider. By the time she took in her third breath, her whole face seemed lit up with happiness and joy. The transformation was stunning and so swift.

After the three breaths, Brock asked her to open her eyes and come back to the room.

She laughed and said, "No. I want to stay here in this place of gratitude." The group laughed. Then she opened her eyes and beamed a big smile. "Wow! I just had no idea how powerful that simple exercise was!"

Brock did the same thing with the facial expression of peace for the white ocean of soul and then for being loved in the golden ocean of Divine Presence. At the end of the three breaths for the golden ocean, tears started to pour from the woman's eyes. She turned toward Brock, and he opened his big, strong arms to hold her.

Her head fell against his chest, and she sobbed as he held her. Several people in the group started to sob as well. I turned to look at Tuku, who had tears in her eyes. Then my tears began. The whole room seemed full of the energy of being loved. It was palpable. After a few minutes, the woman eased away from Brock and started to giggle. The group started laughing too. The love in the room had turned into joy. Brock gestured for her to take her seat again.

So, this is how the three power words work. Not only did they transform Makeup Lady, but they transformed everybody who experienced what she was feeling. And all it took was nine breaths and a little imagination.

Brock sat quietly, perusing the group. "So, let us all now experience this for ourselves." He breathed us down into a relaxed state and guided us through the nine spirals, starting in the center of our chests and going counterclockwise out for nine breaths and spirals through the three oceans. He invited us to apply the facial expressions with the three power words.

I was filled with an immediate sense of peace from head-to-toe. When we arrived at the outer edge of the blue ocean after nine breaths, we changed direction to clockwise and followed the nine breaths and spirals back to the center of the chest and the golden ocean.

The feelings of peace, joy, and love inside of me just seemed to grow. At the end, we all sat quietly with our eyes closed. I took a quick peek around the room, and everybody was flooded with tears of joy. It was just the most amazing experience. We all dwelled in this wonderful space for a few moments, and then Brock asked us to open our eyes and come back into the room.

"Learning this new breathing pattern and new way to focus your attention is a bit like driving a car," he said. "You need to learn the individual operations like steering, looking in the mirror, and braking, but soon they will all merge into the process of driving a car, and you can look out the window and enjoy the scenery. It is the same with this new pattern of breathing and attention. Soon, it will function naturally within you, and you will begin to access new and exciting levels of beauty held within and without."

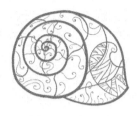

Chapter 37

Tips on the Spiral Meditation

Tuku thanked Brock for sharing and then led us with her sweet, peaceful voice through the nine breaths that followed the spiral from the outer blue ocean into the center of the golden ocean. I was amazed at how easy and luxurious it was to follow the transition of the three spiral breaths, moving through the blue and into the white ocean and then into the golden ocean. At the end of the ninth breath, we came to the center of the golden ocean, which was right at the center of my heart. I felt an immediate sense of being loved by some Divine Presence. Tears started pouring from my eyes. I could not contain the feeling of being loved. I flashed my eyes open and saw that other members of the group were having the same experience. Brock and Goth Girl started handing boxes of tissues around. These were not usual tears. They felt like warm, liquid velvet whose source was deep within my own heart. I felt as if I had suddenly found what had always been there. Then I had a memory flash-back to when I was a little girl. I remembered crying the tears of joy at the sight of a sunset, and my mother thought that I was being overly emotional and told me to stop. I remembered feeling as if she'd stabbed me in the heart, and that was the day I locked those tears of joy away deep inside of me and vowed never to allow anyone to hurt them again. And now, forty years later, I felt as if Tuku had just eased them from my self-created prison, and they were free again.

I looked at Tuku, who had her gaze locked onto me. I knew that on some level, she was looking inside of me and knew what I was feeling. The same tears were rolling down her cheeks.

She stood and walked to me. She lowered herself into a crouch in front of me and looked up at my tear-filled eyes through her tear-filled eyes. She lifted her hand and cradled my cheek. "Honey, never let anyone imprison these tears again. They are now free, and they are just one of the many gifts you have to offer life. The sharing of these tears will give others the inspiration to find the tears that they also locked away in their childhoods."

With our tear-filled eyes locked on each other, she went silent. Our energy fields seem to expand into one big aura of light. I had read about people having transcendental moments, but I did not believe that they were real. Here I was, though, having one myself and sharing it with another person. My heart was so full of joy, I thought it was going to explode. Tuku released her hand from my cheek and slowly headed back to her chair. Brock offered me a sip of water from his bottle.

The cold water felt good as I slowly returned to the room. The group settled again, and Tuku said that we would now follow the same path from the golden ocean to the blue ocean, and we would follow the counter clock-wise direction, which was the descent into the material world. Starting in the center of the golden ocean, she led us through nine slow and beautiful counterclockwise breaths to the outside of the blue ocean. My mind seemed to really enjoy following the spiral through the golden, white, and blue oceans. When we came to the outer part of the blue ocean, Tuku asked us to pause for a few moments just to bathe in the feeling.

This was a beautiful feeling as well, but it was slightly different. I felt very present in the room and very much as one with everyone. It was as if our energy fields had become one. Tuku invited us to open our eyes and look around the room. As we did this, we spontaneously started to reach out to each other and share hugs. We had begun the evening as strangers, and now we were all lovers.

And all it took was three oceans, nine breaths, and one very special lady called Tuku. She explained that when you travel from the golden ocean of divine love, you take with you love that feeds the white ocean and transforms the blue ocean. Our desire to hug and love each other came from the golden ocean and was made manifest through the blue ocean so that we could share it with the world. Just focusing and living in your golden ocean will make you happy, but this love is not supposed to be hoarded and kept for yourself. The function of the blue ocean is to make the love manifest in the world. We had all begun by sharing hugs.

A well-dressed elderly man in the front row put his hand up. "I like the concept of the three oceans," he said. "I know that mine are out of balance. What is the best way to bring them back into balance?"

"Great question," said Tuku. "There are three processes that I use to help keep my three oceans in balance. It helps me to check in with each ocean to get a sense of how they feel. To do this, I get a sheet of blank paper and some markers. I close my eyes and take a couple of deep breaths to get a sense of how they are feeling and how they are doing in proportion to each other. If one ocean is feeling narrow or diminished in some way, then I do the spiral process on that one color alone. If the white was feeling off, then I would imagine myself with the white ocean around me—the outer edge, where my armpit is; and the inner edge, where my nipple is. I begin the journey going counterclockwise from the inside edge, following three spiral turns to the outside edge. Then I go clockwise back in again for three turns. I may do this several times to really energize the white ocean. I can do this for any of the three oceans, and it provides me with a way to help balance and energize the oceans.

"You can also do this with your tongue, using the roof of your mouth. You start at the front, behind your front teeth, and do the inner and outer spiral processes.

"You can do the spiral movement three times as you focus on whatever color ocean you choose. I have a nurse friend who works in intensive care. When pressure heats up, she often imagines the peace of the white ocean and does the three in-and-out spirals with her tongue as she is working. She said it really helps to ground her. Her colleagues were asking how she always stays so calm. She ended up teaching them how to use this process as well."

Tuku reached down to a small backpack by the side of her chair and pulled out some photocopied sheets. She gave them to Goth Girl to hand out. On the sheet was a big circle with nine spirals going to the center. She showed us how to use our fingers to follow the spiral in and out. She explained that this helps to pattern the imagination, and it energizes the three oceans.

Her final suggestion was to rest a hand on one of our knees and simply use a finger to make small spirals on the knee. This helps to engage and focus the mind on the spirals, and it's very soothing. I really loved these ideas and knew that I would be using them at work from time to time. Tuku said that the next meeting would be in two nights. She nodded to Goth Girl, who stood. She pulled out a bag of dark chocolate Hershey's kisses. With a big grin, she said that at our next meeting, she would be teaching us the "melting chocolate for the mind" process. The group roared with laughter, and I thought I had just landed in heaven.

Tuku brought the evening to a close with a final prayer. We all hugged each other goodbye.

As I was putting on my coat, Brock asked if he could walk me to my car. This was unexpected, and I felt a little flattered. Once outside, he took my arm. I really liked the feel of his hand holding my arm and began to feel a stir of excitement. We had not been alone like this before, and I had the sense that I was special to him. When we got to my car, he reached down with his right hand and took mine. He moved in front of me, and the yellow light of the parking lot gave him an angelic glow. I could sense something special was going to happen.

Suddenly, the vision of the gold door in his woodshop flashed into my thoughts. I wanted to know what was behind it and thought this would be a good time to ask. "Brock," I said. "May I ask you a question?"

"Sure," he replied.

I paused for a moment. "May I ask what is behind the golden door in your woodshop?"

The question caught him off guard, and he pulled back from me. There was silence. Then he said, "Perhaps another time, Jane, I can share with you what is behind the golden door. For now, it is best that we leave it this way."

This response just ramped up my curiosity. What on Earth could it be? Brock moved closer to me and leaned gently toward me, and I sensed he was going to kiss my cheek. I really wanted to turn my head so that my lips would meet his. But I stayed strong and kept my head still. His soft, warm lips felt good on my cheek. They lingered for a few seconds before he pulled back. What did this mean? I stayed still, waiting for his next move. I was hoping he would bring his lips to meet mine. I waited and softly breathed. But he just nodded and wished me a safe ride home.

As I pulled out of the parking lot, I felt he was holding back. I knew there was more. I sensed that he had wanted to kiss me on the lips, but something was holding him back. What could it be? And the golden door? Damn, I had to find out what was behind it.

During the twenty-minute ride home, I kept touching my cheek where he had planted the kiss. I was feeling stirred and quietly aroused. There was definitely an energetic connection between us. He made my pulse run a bit faster, and there was something quite juicy about that.

As I lay in bed, before I put the light out, I pondered once again the warmth of his lips on my cheek. I knew there was more. That golden door, along with the kiss, were mysteries I needed answers to.

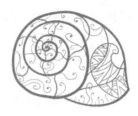

Chapter 38

Leases and Bicycles

I woke up before the alarm, feeling a glorious peace all over me. I lay in bed thinking about the three oceans and the spiral process. I couldn't get over how nine focused breaths could have such a wonderful and transformative effect on me. I also reflected on how much fun it was being with Brock. And then there was the kiss on the cheek. What did it mean? Would the next one be on the lips? I liked the flirty energy I was feeling. With these naughty-but-nice thoughts, I headed to the shower to get ready for the day.

I had just finished getting dressed when I heard the door buzzer ring. This was odd, as nobody ever came to my door so early in the morning. I went to the front upstairs window and looked out. Parked outside was a florist's van. My first thought was that Brock had sent me flowers! My heart almost jumped out of my chest. I dashed downstairs and flung open the front door. Standing behind a very large and awesome bunch of twelve red roses was a slim young man peeking out from under a baseball cap.

"Mrs. Harris?" he asked.

"Oh yes, that's me," I said with a giddy air. He handed me a small pad and asked me to sign. "Oh, very happy to."

I handed him the signed pad, and he handed me the glorious bunch of roses. The sweet scent filled my lungs, and I felt my knees go a bit wobbly. I knew Brock did not earn much money, so for him to send me these flowers just blew me away.

The kid stood there gazing at me. "Yes?" I said. Then it dawned on me that he was waiting for a tip. "Oh, sorry!" I blurted. "Just hang on a sec." I dashed to the kitchen and grabbed a five-dollar bill from my bag. As I handed it to him, a small smile broke out on his face and he headed back to his van.

I noticed a card perched inside the roses and took them straight to the kitchen, where I kept my vases. That Brock was a smooth mover.

It was difficult, but I wanted to wait a few moments before I opened the note from him.

With the roses placed elegantly in my finest vase, I put the card on the counter and filled my coffee cup. I wanted a slow ritual of opening his card and reading his words, which were sure to be poetic. Perhaps he had written me a love poem.

After two sips of my coffee, I slowly slit open the envelope. I took a big breath and opened the card. Then I went white and cold when I saw my husband's name written on the card. It felt as if I had just been punched in the stomach. They were not from Brock after all. What was my husband doing? Why was he trying to get back into my life? I suddenly felt adrift and confused.

Was the kiss from Brock simply that of a friend? Was my mind playing tricks on me? And why did David send me these flowers? I was really confused. I sat down, a little dazed, and drained my cup of Joe in three big gulps. My mind was in turmoil again, and my heart was sending out an SOS. David, Brock, David, Brock.

Over and over, my mind churned. My mood took an immediate nosedive, and I could feel the familiar ball of black heaviness in my stomach. I glanced at the clock and saw that I needed to hit the road.

My day at the office was unfocused. I did my best to research foundations for a local non-profit that had just become one of our clients, but I was distracted. I turned off my computer at five o'clock on the dot. As I pulled out of the parking lot, I thought about the pile of unopened mail that I had tossed into the laundry bin over the last month and decided that this would be my task for the evening. I thought a bottle of wine would pair well with my mountain of mail and popped into the liquor store.

When I got home, I took a quick shower, hoping to lighten my dark mood. I put on an old tracksuit and headed to the kitchen for a glass of Chardonnay on my way to the full basket of mail. I slowly gathered myself to begin.

After two sips of wine, I tipped the basket onto the living room floor and gave the pile a cursory glance to see what was there. The one envelope that caught my eye was registered and came from the finance company that held my husband's car lease. It was addressed to me because my husband said there were tax advantages to putting his car in my name. What did I know? He was the big expert in finance, and I was the dummy, right? He had told me that his job required a prestigious vehicle, and he wanted the biggest BMW there was. He kept saying that investing in an image would attract wealthy clients. Perhaps, all we were investing in was his ego?

I leaned back against the couch and remembered when I bought two beautiful bicycles for us as a surprise. A pink one for me and a blue one for him. I thought it would be nice for us to go on rides together from time to time—sort of a shared bonding experience. I remember the expression on his face when I opened the garage door to show him. He immediately looked down his nose at the blue bike and said that it was not something he ever wanted to be seen on. "What if a client were to see me on this?" he had grumbled.

I kept the bikes, hoping he would one day change his mind. But he never did, and his blue bike still sat in the garage, gathering dust.

I opened the registered envelope immediately and saw the red ink informing me that last month's payment was now thirty days overdue. Oh crap! I flipped on my laptop and promptly transferred the due payment from my checking account. This made me think about our finances and how negligent I had been in keeping track of what was really happening. Then the little voice inside my head leaped to my defense, saying, "But you trusted him. Hell, he was your husband. If you can't trust him. Who can you trust?"

I was sure there was a good explanation for all of this. We just needed to sit over tea and talk it through. We must have savings somewhere. And his salary, how much did he earn? Could a hacker really find all this information out? But using a hacker behind his back felt deceitful. If we were going to rebuild our relationship and he found out that I'd hired a hacker, would he ever trust me? I was feeling uneasy about the whole thing.

I heard a chime telling me a text had just arrived. It was from Goth Girl.

Tuku tomorrow night. Mind, heart, and chocolate meditation! Be there! Hugs. GG.

I texted back:

Yay...chocolate! See ya tomorrow at 7. WG.

I pondered the words *chocolate meditation*. There was a time when the word *chocolate* would make me smile. Now, all it made me think about was weight gain. I was not a happy camper.

I continued to plow through the pile of mail. Then I came across a warranty card for a titanium ax my husband had wanted for his birthday. One of the things we loved to share was a log fire and a glass of wine. David liked to chop his own logs. He had a very muscular body, and I loved to sit on our deck and watch him chop logs with his shirt off. Our physical attraction was always very palpable. On reflection, I think this is what hid his emotional immaturity from me. I think he was very vain in that way. He was very fussy about his ax. Not any old ax for him. He was usually frugal with money, but when it came to himself, he needed a very expensive titanium ax. All I know is that it sparkled when it caught the sun.

As for my birthday gift, I had asked him for a small titanium garden trowel. I remember how he'd barked at me. "What do you need that for?" he said. "You think you are a gardener?" I made up some excuse about wanting to plant a flower garden. But in truth, I needed it to pick up poops from the lawn. We had an elderly neighbor, a very sweet woman in her eighties, named Doris. She had a fourteen-year-old Lab. Duke was just the nicest dog you could imagine. Whenever I saw him, I gave him treats that I kept in my car so that David would not see them. Anyway, for some reason, Duke liked to poop on our lawn. I always enjoyed seeing them take a walk in the morning and did not mind Duke using our lawn as his bathroom. But this always infuriated my husband. He would shout and curse if he found a poop on our lawn. So, I used to get up early and do a poop patrol before he got up. Perhaps I should have seen this uncaring trait as a symptom of a deeper emotional cruelty that lived inside of him. But our sex life was so vibrant, and it always seemed to override my seeing that side of him.

I kept plowing through the mail, and after an hour, the wastebasket was full of torn envelopes and junk mail. Phew! At last my conscience was clear. I found a movie on TV and spent the night in the arms of my bottle of wine.

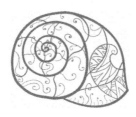

Chapter 39

Introduction to the Chocolate Meditation

My day at the office was boring. No passion, no interest in what I was doing anymore. Had the light inside of me gone out? Would I ever be passionate about my work again? Would I ever be passionate about anything? I felt let down by Brock and the flowers. But this was set up by my misplaced expectations. My head was a morass of dysfunctional thoughts.

The words *chocolate meditation* popped into my thoughts. Where was this going? Should I just call out and crash with a friendly bottle of wine? I knew Goth Girl would not let me off the hook so easily, though. I trudged through my day and headed home promptly at 5:00 p.m. to freshen up for the evening.

I arrived at the coffee shop at five minutes to seven. Goth Girl stood talking to some of the group, and I slid into the back row. At seven, Brock and Tuku walked out from the back room and surprisingly, they sat together at the end of the back row, a few chairs along from me. Brock waved and smiled when he saw me. I gave a deliberately guarded response to him. I did not want to set myself up again. No more kisses on the cheek for me.

Much to my surprise, Goth Girl slid into the chair in front of the group. Ah-ha, so she was going to lead the group tonight! Well, this should be interesting.

The group went silent, and Goth Girl sat looking very much at ease and in control. She had such a unique presence. At first sight, she was strikingly different, with her deep-maroon lips on the pale white face. Her eyes could be menacing and piercing, yet in some strange way, full of love all at the same time. She was so free and so real. I wanted just a small amount of what she had.

She was wearing a jet-black outfit that really set off the lipstick and the maroon streaks in her hair. Just frickin' beautiful is how I would sum her up. Right off the cover of a goth style magazine.

She took a few deep breaths and then from a handbag by the side of her chair, she pulled out a big bag of Hershey's dark-chocolate kisses. A loud *oooooh* came from the group, followed by a light chuckle.

"Welcome, beautiful people," she said. "Can't say how much I appreciate this chance to share. Tuku, I love you, sweet lady. I just really appreciate this opportunity to express all that you have given me over the years."

Tuku smiled and nodded.

"Before I get to the chocolate piece, I want to talk about my perspective on the relationship between the heart and the mind," Goth Girl said. "Years ago, when I was on the meditation merry-go-round, I kept hearing the message about bringing the mind into the heart. I would hear people say that the longest journey we will ever make is between the heart and the head. And believe me, I really tried this head-into-the-heart thing. I met people who had tried to do this for many years and had all failed miserably. But for some reason, they kept pursuing this impossible head-into-the-heart relationship. I have come to understand that Mother Nature created the heart and the mind separately for some very practical reasons. Look at the arms and legs, for example. They are both appendages that stick out from the body, and they have different functions. Again, Mother Nature knew not to make these appendages the same. They function differently, but they can work harmoniously with the right communication.

"When I did try to push the mind down into the heart, I did not function well in the world. I walked around in a bit of a daze—albeit, a loving kind of daze. Because of my open heart, I lost control over some of my boundaries and struggled to function in day-to-day interactions with people. Being love and light is a wonderful aim, but I ain't no etheric angel, and I still needed to function in and navigate the reality of day-to-day living in the world.

"To help my mind and heart communicate, I developed a journaling process. So instead of competing for air space, they actually started to work together.

"The mind and the heart have different functions, and I have found that they work best when they are free to do so. With good communication, the heart can understand and support the needs of the mind, and the mind can understand and support the needs of the heart. It was a home run for me. So, the journaling process between my mind and my heart has become a wonderful system that provides me with a true sense of inner wholeness. In a way, the relationship between my mind and heart has become a sort of marriage. They are living and loving as one, but each has its own way of functioning in the world. And they are complementary to each other. I like to say that they have each other's back." There was a chuckle from the group. "Here is a sample dialogue I had in the early days between my mind and my heart. I would switch between my dominant and nondominant hand to create this dialogue.

Heart (writing with my dominant hand): "Hi, Mind. How are you today?"

Mind (writing with my nondominant hand): "Thanks for asking. I am lacking direction. I am doing my best to get us through life, but because you do not always communicate with me, I am having to make it up myself. What is it you want from me?"

Heart: "Ah yes! I am so busy being and expressing love, I have forgotten to give you direction. First, I need you to protect me in the world. If people challenge me and my loving ways or want to take advantage of me, I want you to be my warrior and guardian. This way, I will be able to be loving in the world, and you will help me to be strong. When I work with our creative nature to create beautiful things, I want you to walk beside me and protect me against criticism and negativity that could easily diminish me. If I have bold dreams for what I want to do with our life, I want you to be my bodyguard and allow no one to diminish me. As a warrior, you must keep your sword sharp, and you must be ready at all times to defend me. But you must never seek battle or attack others. Your role is to protect me. However, you will be called upon to have other roles. There will be times when I will need you to be a wise statesman—or I should say, a wise states*woman*—and use your skills of counsel and heal broken relationships. So be prepared for me to call upon you in a variety of different roles.

"And when it comes to manifesting the dreams from the heart in the world, I want you to use all of your powers of organization and discipline to help them to manifest. And if we want to give birth to new ideas in the world, I will need your worldly smarts to help achieve this. I need you to be attentive to my direction always. This form of dialogue is our secondary way of communicating. Our primary way of communicating is in deep silence. When I ask you to be still and quiet with me, I want you to remain strong and vigilant, but you must also surrender into the sacred silence that we share. When we merge together in this silence, you will understand the language of feelings, which will help guide you in the world. From time-to-time, you will also be asked to learn new things that will help our journey in life.

"One final thing: even though you and I are designed to function separately, we can still share a union that is beautiful. Much like when two people make love.

"When I ask you to enter the deep silence with me, it is as if you are being invited to my bed chamber. And it is there we will both feel and experience the love we share."

Mind: "Thank you, heart. I feel relief in knowing exactly what you want me to do for you. I am also relieved that you will no longer expect me to lose my identity and try to become like you. I love being fully alive in the world and creating beautiful things. I am strong and will be the finest warrior to protect you in the world. You are truly beautiful, and it is my honor to be your warrior and to protect you always. Thank you for loving me, and I look forward to those times of sharing deep silence with you."

Goth Girl then paused and looked around the room. I was completely stunned by what she had just shared. It was as if she had suddenly given me a special key to unlock the secrets of how the mind and heart can function well together. I had been wrestling with this for my whole life. My heart and mind always seemed to conflict with each other—as if they were both vying for control.

Goth Girl had just shown me a way that I could be both strong and loving. That was what I saw in her: she could be both loving and strong in the world. I was feeling an alchemical cellular shift inside—a sort of fusion of two energies. I was feeling bigger and more powerful, yet also more vulnerable, but not in a weak way.

Goth Girl suggested a ten-minute stretch break, and I headed out to the parking lot. I wanted to time to ponder this revolutionary way of bringing the heart and mind into wholeness and a loving relationship.

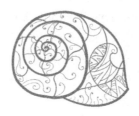

Chapter 40

Chocolate Meditation

After ten minutes Tuku popped her head out of the door and called me back in.

As I took my seat, Goth Girl was walking around, handing everybody a dark-chocolate Hershey's Kiss. *Okay*, I thought. *This must be some form of joke. What on Earth has chocolate got to do with the mind and meditation?*

We were instructed to keep the Hershey's Kiss wrapped and hold it loosely in our right hands. "I began the evening by showing you how the relationship between the mind and the heart can be two different, yet beautiful aspects of one whole working together," Goth Girl said. "I would now like to share with you a magical process to transform words and thoughts into feelings and emotions that the heart can enjoy.

"The mind has a wonderful ability to learn and discover new information and wisdom that can enrich and empower our journeys in life. One of the key questions is how does the mind communicate with the heart? The mind loves words and thoughts. The heart loves feelings and emotions. The mind and heart use different languages. I would like to share with you a process for allowing these organs to communicate with each other.

"Imagine that the mind was reading about the power of kindness. How would it communicate this to the heart, which does not understand words? Words belong to the domain of the mind. The heart responds to feeling."

Goth Girl had a mischievous smile on her face as she waved the bag of chocolate in the air. "And this is where the chocolate comes in. In a few moments, I am going to guide you to put the chocolate on your tongue. Then close your mouth and eyes, and simply let the chocolate melt. You will be tempted to chew it, but the key is to let it melt very slowly and feel the sweet chocolate easing down your throat toward your heart. Please unwrap your Hershey's Kiss and place it in the middle of your tongue. Let your tongue touch the back of your teeth so that the chocolate is sitting on your tongue. Now begin to breathe slowly in and out through your nose and allow the chocolate to melt."

I was still feeling a little skeptical as I unwrapped my piece of chocolate and placed it on my tongue. At first, I wanted to chew it and had to fight that urge. As I started to breathe deeply, very slowly the chocolate began to melt and run down my throat. It tasted so sweet, and instead of the quick burst of flavor I got when I would chew chocolate, the sweetness seemed to last and last. As the whole experience went on and on, it was glorious. Every now and then, I would take a gulp and feel the sweetness slide down my throat. I was really enjoying this new way of experiencing chocolate as down and down the sweet taste went. I had never quite experienced chocolate in this way before.

With the chocolate had melted, I opened my eyes and looked around the room. People seemed really relaxed and had smiles on their faces. Good old dark chocolate.

Goth Girl invited comments. A woman in the front row confessed that she had chewed her piece of chocolate, so it disappeared from her mouth quickly. Goth Girl tossed her another Hershey's Kiss and suggested that she not give up too easily. Everybody laughed. Several people mentioned how much they enjoyed the slowness of the process and how much more sweetness they derived from one small piece of chocolate, compared with the way they usually ate chocolate.

Goth Girl said, "Now I want to look at how you can apply this to your day-to-day living. This process can be used with individual words and concepts in the form of information and wisdom. You can also use it for people's names. This is how it works for words. Imagine the word *kindness*. Now imagine that this was wrapped inside a ball of chocolate and placed on your tongue. Then place your focus on the meaning of the word and allow it to melt down into your heart. To help you with this, you can align your breath with the process. Breathe in the word and imagine it on your tongue as a small ball. Hold your breath as you focus on the meaning of the word. Then, as you slowly breathe out, imagine the word melting down into your heart. When it has melted into your heart, hold your breath for a few seconds and feel it being absorbed into your heart. This is how we convert words into feelings. This is how the mind feeds the heart. It is the same with a piece of information or wisdom you may have come across. This process will allow the words to melt, as it were, and transform meaning into a feeling that the heart can be enriched by.

"I also use this process with people I care about. It is more than just re-membering their names. This is a way to develop a true emotional relation-ship with them. The only drawback is that with all this imagined chocolate, your heart will start to put on weight. Yes, it will grow in size. But this increase in size is a weight increase you want to have. Bottom line is that you will be-come even more loving. And your mind helps you to become a more loving person.

"This is how the mind can feed the heart. The fun part is that with the journaling communication, the heart can ask the mind for whatever it wants to fall more in love with. To start, it is a good idea to use a pen and paper for this communication, but you will soon develop the ability to do it in your mind.

"So, the heart can ask the mind for certain things, and the mind can ask the heart for certain things. For example, when I was diagnosed with cancer, I started to feel a deep loneliness. This would often turn to depression. My doc-tor put me on some meds, and for a short while, they numbed it away. But it always came back, along with the loneliness. It was my mind that was experi-encing the loneliness and depression. One day, I made a cup of tea, lit a candle, and allowed my mind to write to my heart. First, I ended up having a good cry. As my heart explained to my mind, a good cry from time to time is like medicine. Tears can wash away old, grungy feelings. As my mind began to share about the loneliness, my heart could hear that it had forgotten that it was loved. I had lost connection to my golden ocean, the Divine Presence within me. I had forgotten that I was loved. I had another big cry, only these were not sad tears, but tears of gratitude and appreciation. I had forgotten to remember. So, the heart helped my mind to remember. We also looked at what caused the depression. We actually started journaling with it. We called it "Dee" and invited it to join us for tea to share with us its reason for showing up. What we (my mind and heart) discovered was that depression had come to bring our attention to something that was missing in our lives. We thought that depression was a sign that something was wrong. But, in fact, it was quite the opposite. Depression was like an orange light on the dashboard of our lives. The drugs were like putting duct tape over it. When I stopped taking the drugs, it was like pulling off the duct tape. The light was still on. So, in tracking the source of the orange light, I was able to restore the feeling of being loved by the Divine Presence. Love really does heal, but I needed these processes of communication within myself to allow love to heal."

I felt as if the words she had shared were just for me. After my diagnosis, I had had terrible bouts of depression and loneliness. I also tried drugs, but all they really did was numb me. The problems did not go away. What Goth Girl had just shared completely rocked my world in a good way.

Goth Girl continued. "The key is that the heart can ask the mind for help, and the mind can ask the heart for help. Both have needs, and the mind and heart can interact as lovers and friends. The way my mind used to function was very much like an untrained dog not kept on a leash. It used to wander off, following any kind of smell. It would chase cats and sometime roll in poop." A loud ripple of laughter went around the group.

Goth Girl continued. "I truly feel that the mind wants to be a meaningful part of our existence, but if we do not understand how to communicate and respect the mind, it will tend to chase cats and roll in crap."

The group laughed again. She had just nailed it for me. I was always torn between the heart and the head, and neither seemed to really have the answers. To have them working as a supportive team was the obvious answer. But I had never known how to do this until now. And chocolate would help me to achieve it. Could it get any better than this?

Goth Girl said, "One more thing to ponder. When you think negative thoughts, these can also seep into your heart. That's why it is important to direct your mind toward healthy words and wisdom. You have large warehouses of good food and medicine held in your beautiful memories. It is really good to sit and remember some of the beautiful times in your life. Wonderful memories hold an inexhaustible supply of good energy. All you have to do is sit down from time-to-time and delve into some of your favorite memories. You also need to stay away from the negative memories. Good memories are like organic food. Bad memories are like eating junk food. Now, I would like to guide you through this process, so please sit upright, and when you are ready, close your eyes.

"Begin by taking three deep, long breaths. Ever so gently, try to hold your breath for a few seconds after the in and out breaths. Do not strain yourselves. As you practice this, your ability to pause your breathing will naturally expand. Just the breathing practice alone will reduce your stress level and make you more relaxed. When you are ready, with a slow in breath, imagine that you are placing the word *love* on your tongue. Then hold your breath as you focus on the meaning of the word. As you slowly breathe out, imagine the word melting down into your heart.

"Then hold your breath as you allow the heart to feel this beautiful feeling," she said.

"Do this three times, and when you are ready, open your eyes."

The breathing process was simple to do and felt very natural. It was easy for my mind to visualize the word *love* and place it on my tongue. And as the chocolate had taught me, all I had to do was allow it to melt down into my heart.

After the three breaths, I felt a wonderful, warm glow in my heart. Each time I melted the word *love*, my heart seemed to become warmer and bigger. It was a fabulous feeling. It felt like a new sweetness in my heart, and soon, the feeling began to spread through my whole body. After the three full breaths, I opened my eyes and looked around. Everybody seemed to be glowing. A young guy in the back row was in tears. Goth Girl invited him to share his experience. He said that he had often used the word *love*, but this was the first time he had ever actually felt the word. Other people shared similar experiences.

"The mind has a wonderful ability to seek out wisdom and inspirational words and thoughts," Goth Girl said. "However, the problem is that they usually just stay in the mind. The villagers read many books, but the information mostly stayed in their heads—their true value was never digested. It was as if they collected grapes but had never made wine out of them. They chewed the grapes and then spat them out. Reading, alone, only fills the intellect with words/grapes, and they are never made into wine. I call this process Chocolate Heart. It has transformed the way my mind and heart relate and communicate with each other."

Goth Girl asked if there were more questions. The group was quiet for a few moments, then a woman in the front row asked if she could have some more chocolate. Everybody started laughing.

Once again, I was completely taken aback by how the simplest of processes could deliver such a transformational result. And with dark chocolate, no less!

Goth Girl closed the evening by handing the bag of chocolate around with the instruction to take two pieces for the ride home. Then she said a closing prayer, and I headed out.

On my way home, I reflected on how many empty spiritual practices I had tried over the years, seeking a transformation that I never found. I had read a lot and kept it all in my head. I had been a head dweller and never really knew how to transform words into feelings that my heart could discern. And in this one short evening, I had been given two amazing tools that I knew would have a big impact on my life. Plus, dark chocolate would now last four times longer because I would allow it to melt.

What a night, and what fabulous chocolate!

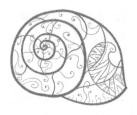

Chapter 41

Brock's Invitation

I woke up with a smile, thinking about chocolate. I allowed my mind and heart to communicate in the way Goth Girl had suggested. All those years of battling my mind and struggling with depression and loneliness were going to change. After a shower, I headed to the kitchen for tea and toast. To get a jump on my day, I checked my email. There was one from my doctor.

Dear Jane.
This came across my desk yesterday, and I wanted you to add this to the information you are gathering about treatment options.
Yours,
Dr. Hughes.

I made the mistake of opening the attachment. It was about a clinic in the Midwest that was offering a new double-mastectomy process that reduced the recovery time by 50 percent over conventional methods. I felt as if she had just plunged a knife into my gut. This was the last thing I needed to see. My breast cancer just assailed me again through an email from my doctor. My hurt soon turned to anger. I was angry at my doctor, the cancer, and my breasts. I was just real angry at everything. Then the anger turned to sadness, and this soon shifted into fear. I felt paralyzed again. Why does she keep doing this to me? I wondered. I felt broken apart and full of fear again.

Then the phone rang. I checked the ID and saw it was Bob. I didn't want to answer the call, but I knew that he knew I would be home. I hit the speaker button.

His voice was gruff and impatient. "Why haven't you called Hank?"

I felt flustered. Rather pathetically, I said that I was having some health problems and would call him soon.

"We gotta do this now," Bob said tersely. "I will have him come over tonight at 7:00 p.m. Be ready. 'Bye." And he abruptly hung up.

I knew why he was frustrated with me. I had asked him to help and then dropped the ball.

This was turning out to be a day from hell. On my way to the office, I tuned in the local radio station for some distraction, and that crappy song came on again. "We Ain't Never Coming Back."

"No!" I screamed and punched the off button, hurting my hand. Then came the tears, and I sobbed all the way to work. First to the restroom to splash some cold water on my face. Then a day of low profile and numerous trips to the tearoom. I headed home at five, feeling like crap. I was weepy, angry, frightened, and just one big mess.

Hank was due to arrive at seven, and I tidied the house to make it a bit more presentable. I donned an old tracksuit and made sure Henry was firmly in place. I did not want any pity-party sympathy from the infamous Mr. Hank, whom I pictured as a little computer nerd with black-rimmed glasses.

The doorbell rang promptly at seven. I swung the door open and was surprised to see a very big Hank standing there. He must have been six foot three, and he was powerfully built. He had long hair that hung down his back and a full beard. He looked a bit like a hippie who'd been stuck in a time warp with his old checked shirt and worn blue jeans. What had my brother, Bob, set me up with? Rather impatiently, I invited him in and pointed to the dining room table, where he could set up. He nodded and said, "Good evening, ma'am," as he sauntered past me.

I stood by the kitchen door with my arms crossed, watching. "Well, what now?" I asked.

He was surprisingly soft spoken. "I will need ten minutes to set up. Can I have the new cell phone and your web access ID?" he asked.

My internet code was buried somewhere in my filing system, and I knew it would be hard to find. I let out a little grunt of frustration and headed upstairs. After an impatient search, I eventually found the password and went back downstairs.

He was sitting behind two black laptop screens, rattling away on the keys.

Then I saw it: on the top of both screens were letters *FBI*.

"What?" I screamed. "Where have you stolen these from? Are you crazy, bringing these into my home?" I completely lost it.

He just sat there gazing at me, expressionless.

I continued with my rant. "Who the hell are you? You need to get out now and take these stolen laptops with you!"

"May I explain?" he asked.

It was too late. I was right over the edge. I marched to the front door, swung it open, and barked at him. "Get out now!"

He very quietly packed away his laptops and sauntered silently past me. I slammed the door and felt angry at my brother, Bob, for setting me up in this way. I needed a glass of wine, quick.

After ten minutes, the phone rang. I knew it would be Bob. The caller ID confirmed it. No doubt, he would shout at me for what I had just done. I felt such a mess. I hit the speak button. Instead of a loud, raspy voice, there was a hushed, "Hey, Sis. You okay?"

Then I burst into tears and sobbed into the phone. Bob was quiet and let me have a good wail.

"What's up, honey?" he asked.

I gathered myself and told him about my crappy day and how bad I was feeling. Then I told him about the stolen FBI laptops. He roared with laughter.

"What's so funny?" I asked.

Then he explained that Hank, despite his casual look, was a highly trained computer expert who consulted with the FBI. He trained the agency's operatives and helped to design their security systems. This is why he had two FBI laptops.

I was shocked. What a fool I had made of myself. I started to apologize over and over.

"All is good," Bob said. "He is a cool guy and will understand. Take a few days to regroup, and let's get him back to get this hack under way, okay, Sis?"

I thanked him, and we hung up. I needed another glass of something white and some TV.

As I filled my glass, I noticed the blinking message light on my kitchen phone. I had turned the ringer off, so I did not hear the call come in. A part of me wanted to leave it for morning. But a more curious part of me wanted to know who it was. I was shocked to see the name Brock on the caller ID. I hit the playback button. It was nice to hear Brock's deep, low voice. I felt a flash of warm energy surge through me.

"Hello, Jane," he said. "I hope you do not mind me calling you at home so late in the evening. I know you want to know about the golden door and wondered if you would like to come over to my shop tomorrow evening. Say 7:00 p.m.?"

I could feel my heart beating faster, and I lightly touched the place on my cheek where Brock had kissed me. *Hell, yeah!* I thought. After this bag-of-crap day, I felt entitled to a little taste of romance. Even if it was on my side only. But then again, how did I know that? And if the two of us were alone in his woodshop, all hell could break loose, for all I knew: This thought brought a sweet, warm pulsing feeling deep down in my groin. Now, that felt really good. I shot a text to Brock.

Great. See you tomorrow at 7. Jane.

I headed rather cheerfully up to bed, thinking, *There's life in the old girl yet.*

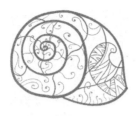

Chapter 42

Behind the Golden Door

I was distracted all day at the office by thoughts of spending an evening with Brock alone in his woodshop. What should I wear? Should it be enticing? Or should I go with a plain and baggy look? Then I remembered that I had breast cancer. Could I, or should I, push the sexual thing? Then I remembered something Goth Girl had said to me. She said that *I* did not have breast cancer; it was my body that had breast cancer. Should I live less and be less because of cancer? Or should I step up and step out into life? I knew that Goth Girl was stepping out and into life. I'd take some of that, for sure. I am still a beautiful woman, and as the white ocean reminds me, I have a luminous soul. And tonight, I was going the sexy way. I decided on a tight-fitting, pink sweater and black clingy jeans. I knew that Goth Girl would approve.

I had time for a quick shower and a yogurt. As I was about to head to Brock's woodshop, I realized was one thing was missing. I dashed upstairs to the bathroom for two dabs of my favorite French perfume. Ooh la la!

On my way to his shop, I popped into a bakery. I was on a mission, after all. As I hopped into my car with a very large box of chocolate chip cookies, I had a sense that this was going to be a good night. For the twenty-minute drive, I hit the local music station, and I was shocked back into reality when I heard the words of my husband's dreaded song. "We Ain't Never Coming Back." I screamed a loud *screw you* at the radio and changed stations.

I arrived at Brock's woodshop a few minutes early and took the time to do the spiral meditation, using my middle finger on my knee. Just the soothing motion of my finger going around the spiral seemed to bring me back to a centered place. I was about to learn the secret behind the golden door. Yay!

I pressed the doorbell to his woodshop. He answered quickly and stood there wearing a light-blue cotton shirt with dark-blue jeans. Pretty damn good on the eye! was my first reaction. He ushered me to the same chairs where we sat before. I offered him the cookies, and he bowed his head as he took them. He brought his beautiful blue eyes up to mine and said, "A gift from the divine?"

I nodded yes. I took a couple of deep breaths as he went to make tea.

I scanned the room and noticed the mysterious golden door again. Brock arrived with two cups of steaming tea and sat opposite me. We shared a little small talk about the coffee shop, and then he nodded toward the golden door. I went quiet and lifted an eyebrow as if to say, *I am ready to listen when you are ready to share.*

He lowered his eyes to the floor, and I knew he was in some way preparing and ordering his thoughts. Then he lifted his eyes to mine, and I could see that they were moist with tears. "The golden door represents an important part of my life. When I started to really live the way of the three loves, I began to ask questions about myself and what I was passionate about. I looked at my childhood and caught glimpses of something deep within me that had been planted there when I was born. For many years, it had been lost in the turmoil and distractions of life. When I started to practice the way of the three loves, this special gift began to awaken in me. The way of the three loves became like the prince who kissed Snow White and woke her from the long sleep. This special part of me was kissed by love, and it woke again. It now lives behind the golden door."

There was a deep sense of reverence in the way Brock was speaking. A part of me knew to remain silent and listen. But another part of me was jumping up and down, shouting, *Okay, okay! So, what's behind that golden door?*

A smile broke out on his face, and he said, "May I show you what is behind the golden door?"

It took effort for me not to sound too enthusiastic. "Why, sure. I would love to see whatever you are open to share."

He said the word *please* as he gestured for me to follow him. I didn't need a second invitation. I was on my feet in a flash. He led me to the golden door and flipped a switch, which I guessed turned on a light. He placed his hand on the handle and said, "Welcome to my world."

He turned the handle and pushed open the door. In the room was a beautiful workbench with a large wood sculpture in the middle of it. Around it was a sea of chips, sawdust, carving chisels, and candles. Along the walls were various sculptures of different sizes and colors of wood. Each one had its own special place. The room was lit softly with several side lamps, giving it a sense of warmth.

In the air, I caught the scent of pine wood mingled with frankincense. The aroma was divine and seemed to transport me. He gestured for me to enter.

The room had an aura of holiness. I knew that I was entering a very sacred and much-loved creative space. We were both silent. I stood motionless as my senses drank in the grace-filled atmosphere. The sculpture on the workbench immediately drew my attention. It was a celebration of curves, crevices, and holes that flowed into each other with an air of sensuousness. Parts of it reminded me of a woman's body with soft, gentle curves. Then there were parts that reminded me of a man's body—strong outer shapes that looked almost muscular. It was vibrant and alive.

Around the sculpture were small trays of water containing partly burned candles. I could tell that he carved in candlelight. I noticed on the floor a small tray of sand with half-burned incense sticks in it. This would explain the scent of frankincense in the air.

I was aware of Brock's eyes upon me. He was studying my every reaction. A part of me just wanted to burst into tears. The beauty of the room completely transported me to another realm. Another part of me was very respectful of how precious this workspace was to him, and I marshaled my emotions to show an appreciative facial expression, which I supported by touching my heart as if to say, *There is so much love here.*

We both paused in silence, and then he gestured for me to return to the outer room.

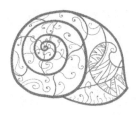

Chapter 43

Experiencing the Wood Sculpture

I walked slowly back to my chair and kept my eyes on the floor. Brock asked me if I would like to experience the wood sculpture that I had been so taken with. The question caught me off guard, and I stammered nervously, "Ah, sure. That would be lovely."

He turned and headed back into the special room. After a few minutes, he emerged carrying a large object wrapped in a red blanket. He walked over and placed it on my lap. He took his seat again and asked me just to sit quietly, feeling the weight of the sculpture and blanket on my lap.

Then he suggested that I close my eyes and let my hands gently explore what was inside the blanket. Very slowly, I moved my hands. My fingers found a way into the folds of the red blanket, and they felt like little serpents exploring the sensuous form within.

My fingers followed the curves of the wood that first reminded me of a woman's body. I could feel a stir of warm, sexual energy deep inside my groin. It was glorious. Then I felt a red flush come to my neck. There was nothing I could do to contain my arousal. My neck was pulsing with heat. Even though my eyes were still closed, I could feel Brock's eyes watching my every reaction. I guessed he knew exactly what a bright-red neck on a woman represented. I was entering no-man's land, and I was close to the point of no return. My hands seemed to take on a life of their own, gently exploring and caressing the wooden form beneath the blanket. Soon my fingers were feeling a shape that was almost sinewy and taut, like muscles, reminding me of the masculine. On the screen of my imagination flashed a quick picture of Brock's open shirt and chest hair. Another pulse of warm energy shot from my groin up to my neck. I was lost in this sexual dance of my fingers with the wooden sculpture. The shape of the wood seemed so body like, with curves and crevices for my fingers to run freely and explore. I could feel my body heat rising, then a light perspiration broke on my skin. The scent of pine seemed to mingle with my French perfume, heightening them both into an aroma that belonged to the gods. On and on, my fingers traveled, exploring the curvaceous form held in darkness in the red blanket.

My mind began to run wild. With my eyes closed, I was not sure if I was still touching the sculpture...or was it his body? It was his passionate fingers that had created this form, and now my fingers were dancing with what his sensuous fingers had brought into this world. I was slipping into a realm that was both dangerous and alluring.

Then came the rescuing sound of his voice. "Jane, when you are ready, please slowly open your eyes."

Just in the nick of time, as my body heat was rising fast. My senses regrouped quickly as I slowly opened my eyes and came back into the room. Then he reached out to pick up the blanket and sculpture from my lap, and our naked arms touched. I felt an immediate spark of electricity that shot from my arm to between my legs. I was in dangerous terrain. I knew I was feeling pure, barely contained lust. My oh my, it was glorious! It radiated a shaft of hot energy right up through the core of my body.

Spiral, spiral, spiral, a little voice in my head screamed. I was sexually coiled like a serpent waiting to strike. The fragile constraint I was hanging onto was weakening fast. My mind was all over the place. Spiral, spiral, spiral. Slowly, I came back to a focus. Then I wondered if he was one of those psychic people who could read minds. Did he have any idea of the smoldering fireworks of lust that he had just ignited in me?

I glanced at his neck to see if he had any telltale signs of lust. There was nothing there, but I guessed men did not show it that way. I wanted a sign. I wanted to know if he was feeling what I was feeling. Was he on the verge of something as lust-filled and explosive as I was? Was he close to a bursting point? I searched his deep, oceanlike blue eyes. I was hunting, searching, calling for that one spark that could blow us into orbit.

A voice in my head said, *Cold water, cold water.*

"May I use the restroom?" I asked. What I wanted to say was, *Can I take a cold shower, and would you join me with two glasses of wine in two minutes?*

I headed to the restroom feeling oh so bad for that naughty thought, but it did make me feel good. Funny how something bad can make you feel good.

Once in the restroom, the first thing I did was wet a paper towel with cold water and put in on my overheated neck. I stood in front of the mirror with my eyes closed, allowing the heat in my body to ease. As I walked back to the table, he was leaning back in his chair, smiling at me. Then I noticed it: the third button on his shirt was undone. I was shocked—in a really good way. Had it sprung open naturally? Had he deliberately undone the button? When I leaned toward him as I took my seat, I caught a flash of some rather yummy chest hair, and my neck began to glow red again. Damn this neck! But oh, how good the lusty feeling felt. I felt like a schoolgirl both innocent and full of sexual stealth. To give myself a little breathing space, I started eating a cookie. I hoped it would distract me from the heated lust that was coursing around inside my body. Brock had placed the wood sculpture on a small side table. It was strikingly beautiful. Then he asked, "Would you like me to explain why wood sculpture is so important to me?"

"Yes," I blurted, trying not to spit cookie crumbs all over him.

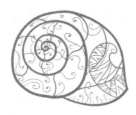

Chapter 44

A Journey Back to My Childhood

Brock took a sip of his tea and said, "My woodcarving process has become a sort of metaphor for my life. I see my life as a certain number of days, as I would see a large, square block of wood comprised of many chips of wood. Each day I live is one day less of my life. With each chip removed from the block of wood, it becomes less. I can choose to see growing old simply as days passed, or in the case of the piece of wood, as chips of wood lost. Or I can see the emerging beauty of the wood, through the loss of chips, as it becomes a sculpture. In the same way, I can see more than passing days; I can see the emergence of the beauty that my life has become.

"We live in a culture that often sees old age as a time of loss and diminishment. As we get older, we seem less able to do what we used to do. In relationship to the wood, as chips are removed, the block of wood is not as strong as it was, and it becomes smaller in size. The way of the three loves has taught me to see the beautiful form of my life as art. Same with the wood. The block of wood has become a sculpted work of art. I now relate to my life as a work of beautiful art that grows more beautiful each day. As with the piece of wood, it becomes more beautiful as chips are removed. I look at my life as I look at the wood and see beauty. All those successes in life. The times of courage. The people I have loved and who have loved me.

"This philosophy of seeing life as a piece of art was developed by the Shaolin monks. They are well known for growing old with grace and power. Because they see their lives as beautiful art, this is energetically communicated to every cell in their bodies. As a result, they have really healthy immune systems. Hence, they live healthier, happier, and longer.

"For the monks, old age is a time when the pace of life eases and they can enjoy their days as you would enjoy a gallery full of fine art. Each picture, each life, is a thing of unique artistic beauty. The monks enjoy growing old for this reason. Death, to them, is a time of graduation rather than just an end of a life. When a monk passes away, they do not have funerals as we know them. Instead, they have graduation or send-off parties. They know that those who die go on ahead as beautiful souls and that all will follow one day and be together again."

Brock was shaking my world. Growing old had seemed like a time of doom, gloom, and dread to me. But now, I had a whole new take on old age. Life as an art form; go figure! It made so much sense to see the chips of falling wood as days passing. I could choose to lament the fallen chips, or I could turn and look at the emerging art form of my life. Brock asked if I would like to hear a story. I nodded an eager yes.

He sat back in his chair. "Once upon a time, there was a wise old farmer who owned the biggest and most beautiful red barn in the land. It stood alongside his home. Every morning from his bedroom window, he would look out and marvel at the beautiful barn.

"Then one day, the barn burned down. When he looked out of his bedroom window, what do you think his reaction was?"

I said that he probably felt sad.

"No," said Brock. "The farmer said, 'Ah, so that is what a sunrise looks like!'

"It is the same with old age. We can focus on what we don't have or can't do anymore. Or we can see the new beauty that is all around. Once again, this process of seeing life as art also redirects the thought process from the negative 'look what life has done to me' frame of mind to the positive. And yes, there is much less stress involved in seeing your life as art. Less stress and no fear of death means a happier, healthier, and richer life. The monks lived and taught that everything in life is on loan to us. We have been entrusted with the gifts with which we were born. The purpose of life is to develop those gifts and use them to make this world a better place. The monks are well known for dying with grace, gratitude, and smiles on their faces."

All that he was saying made so much sense and seemed to fill my heart with love and hope. Then I felt a glimmer of sadness. It seemed to be growing in me, and soon tears were flowing. Brock sat silently and held the space for me to be with my tears. I was aware that he did not try to rescue me by comforting or touching me. He knew how the inner processes sometimes needed to work themselves out. After a few moments, the tears stopped, and I felt ready to share with Brock what was going on.

"Thank you, Brock, for sharing your beautiful sculpting process. The tears came from my awareness that I do not have the same sort of deep creative passion as you do. I have tried to write passionately and do as my parents guided me to do, but my writing feels dead inside me, and this makes me really sad."

He replied, "Thank you for sharing this, Jane. I felt the same as you do for many years. It was when the monks shared with me a special guided meditation that I rediscovered my wood carving. It had been buried deep within me as a child for protection, and the guided meditation the monks taught me helped me to discover it again. May I share this guided meditation with you?"

"Would you?" I quickly responded.

He took a sip of tea and the pulled some sheets of white paper and colored markers from a drawer, placing them in front of me.

"Make yourself comfortable, Jane, and slow down your breathing. I want you to travel back in your mind and imagination to your earliest memories as a child.

"You may see these memories in words, pictures, images, or just blobs of color. As a child, you did not have a well-developed intellect, and many of your emotional experiences and traumas were experienced in feelings. These will often be expressed in blobs of color and not in definite, recognizable shapes. Trust and allow your feelings on this. You may initially feel a color and not know what it represents. Once you feel this and allow it, the memory of what it represents may become known later. When you are ready, allow your mind and imagination to wander back to any time during the first seven years of your life."

I really liked his soothing and comforting voice. My mind went back to when I was around four. I remembered being a happy child. I loved the outdoors and nature. There was some sort of shift when I was seven. This was when school and education started to direct my life. I remembered my family encouraging me to read and write. I think this was when the idea of being a writer was planted in me. My parents wanted me to be an English teacher and started to push me in that direction. This became the main theme in my life and still is to this day. But I am not passionate about it, even though it is deeply engrained in me. Brock asked me if there were memoires from that period. I just remember becoming more serious about written English when I was around seven, but I could not remember why.

Brock then asked if we could do another process using color and emotion. I had been through a lot of psychotherapy and commented that I thought all that was there in terms of memory had been discovered already. He told me that the monks had developed a special process for accessing deeper-held emotional and traumatic memories. They called it the Birthing Beauty process. He did not want to explain it before I experienced it. He offered to fully explain it afterward.

I knew he had a good reason for suggesting that.

I had a deep sense of trust in him and said I was open to follow where this needed to go. He suggested we move to an area on the far side of the room where there was a deep-pile carpet, blankets, and pillows. I moved to the carpeted area and sat cross-legged on pillows. He gathered the blank paper and markers and joined me, sitting cross-legged facing me. Then he explained what was going to unfold.

"We are going to explore deeply held emotional and traumatic memories from the first seven years of your life. What we find will determine how this process unfolds. There may be a time when you want to lie down. I may use blankets to cover you and other props. I will be holding the space for you to go deep and experience what may be waiting to be discovered. The function of using a blanket to cover you is to provide a sense of protection and enclosure for your psyche to open, if it wants to. I may play some soft drum music from time-to-time. The drum rhythms are based on shamanic journeying frequencies and will support your inner travel. Any questions?"

I was pretty certain that he would not find any hidden memories and warned him that this may not yield any results. He beamed a mischievous smile at me and raised an eyebrow as if to say, "Yeah, yeah, yeah. You may be in for a surprise." I felt that he could sense something about or in me that I was not sensing. Every now and then, he had an aura of the mystic about him. His eyes would glisten and go still as if he were listening to some whisper on the etheric winds that nobody else could hear. It was as if he knew other worlds beyond the one that we live in. He and Goth Girl had that in common.

"Ready?" he asked.

I nodded.

"You may sit or lie down for this." I chose to remain seated on the pillow with my legs crossed. His voice slowed and deepened as he began to guide me. "Allow your breathing to slow and close your eyes when you are ready, Jane. Allow yourself to become deeply relaxed. Imagine that you are standing in a field of golden corn. Ahead of you are steps that lead down beneath the ground. You walk to the steps and see that there are ten steps. Slowly, you walk down the steps, ten, nine, eight, seven, six, five, four, three, two, and one. You have arrived in a beautiful garden with flowers and waterfalls, and the sky is blue with a warm golden sun. Take a few moments to see and enjoy the garden. Ahead of you, by a water fountain, you see two chairs. Walk over and sit in one of them. Make yourself comfortable. On your right side, you see a beautiful lady dressed in white, walking toward you. She takes the seat next to you. She is very friendly and greets you by name. She tells you that she is the guardian of the hidden memories of childhood.

"You ask her to share with you any memories that you are now ready to receive. She explains that you will not see these memories with your mind. These memories are buried deep below the rational mind for protection. You can only find them by their color, which represents feelings. The color has no form; it is simply color or a mixture of colors. Soon, you will be traveling through the first seven years of your life, and she asks you to be attentive to any colors that may appear.

"Pay attention to the colors, especially to the ones that attract your attention. Once you have found these colors, she would like you to create a picture of that color with the markers. It will not be of a specific object, just any form, random shape, or blob of color. The colors you capture with the markers represent the emotions connected to the buried memories you are holding deep within you. Some of these memories are very painful and were buried early in your childhood because you were unable to deal with them at that time. Often these painful memories contain something beautiful in you that was threatened.

"When these events took place, you may not have cried tears out into the world. You may have cried your tears internally so that nobody could see them. These tears then become frozen around the object that needed to be protected and hidden. When you are ready to bring attention to these frozen tears, they will melt and release whatever they have been holding and protecting. Initially, your tears may feel sad, as they are carrying away and cleansing you of the hurt and pain that occurred when you were a child. Once these tears have been released, your tears will turn to joy as you discover the beautiful part of you that was hidden. Whatever it was that you were protecting will start to float up to the surface of your awareness. At this point, you will begin to remember what it was that you hid away, and you will be guided to scan the first seven years of your life."

I was feeling deeply relaxed and began the process of scanning over my first seven years. For the first five, I saw wonderful oranges, yellows, greens, and bright pinks. They were all joyful colors. They made me feel happy. Then as I turned six, a really big, black mass suddenly appeared. It was full of sadness like a dark cloud and seemed to be deep down inside of me. I reached for the markers and started to draw it. Brock was sitting silently, holding space for me. As I began to create a picture of the black mass, tears started to run down my face. I remembered that these were designed to melt the ice that had entrapped this memory all those years ago.

After I finished drawing the big, black mass, Brock guided me up the stairs and back into the room. As I started to come back fully into my body, I looked at the picture of the big mass of black I had created. "Where the hell did this come from?" I asked.

Brock said, "This represented an emotional memory and probably a trauma. Up to this point in time, you have not been ready to release it. Within this big, black mass is what we are looking for in terms of something beautiful about you that you hid for protection."

He asked me to place the drawing of the black mass in front of me and lower my eyes to gaze at it. I was to imagine heat pouring from my eyes as if it were melting the cold, black mass. Something about the picture of this black mass scared me. But what scared me more was the thought of burying it back inside me again and losing forever what it contained.

As I gazed at the picture, tears of sadness flooded from my eyes. I let them flow without judgment. As I did, a vague memory of my grandmother started to drift into my awareness. She was much loved by me. I remembered sitting with her, reading a book together. Brock asked me to focus in on the book. I did and saw that it was a book of poetry. I looked so happy to be with my grandmother. Then another memory came of me with a notebook, writing my own poetry. I could see my grandmother and a big piece of an apple pie that she had baked. There was vanilla ice cream next to it. This was my favorite desert. More memories started to come. Then a memory of my father slowly came into my mind. I was in my bedroom, and I had my math homework books around me on the floor. But I was creating a poem in my poetry book. I didn't like math, but I loved poetry. My father came into the room and became enraged that I was not doing my homework. He snatched my poetry book out of my hand, grabbed my wrist, and pulled me downstairs to the fireplace. His words were loud and angry. "Poetry is a waste of time! You will never read or write poetry again while you live under this roof!" Then he threw the book into the fire and made me watch it burn! At that moment, I felt a sharp blade cut through my heart, and I felt a big, black door slam shut inside me. My grandmother was never allowed to read poetry to me again.

I was sobbing now and lay down on the pillows. Brock placed a big blanket over me. I felt as if I was in a safe cave. As the pain of what my father had done washed through me, my wails soon turned to screams of anger and rage. It felt as if I was vomiting rage and anger that had long been buried inside of me. For a few moments, I completely lost it. Brock gently placed his hand on my back as if to ground me and bring me back into my body. Then he released his hand. Following the rage came the saddest tears I have ever cried in my life. These were old, deeply buried tears that I had cried when I was six. But I could not cry them on the outside. I cried them on the inside. They had become frozen to protect my love of poetry.

The sobbing went on for a while and then seemed to ease. If felt like a thunderstorm was passing inside of me. Black, cold darkness was pouring out of me. Then I became still and saw within me a flicker of light. It was like a little candle flame. The flame got bigger and bigger, and with it came feelings of love and joy. I was still crying, but my tears were now full of joy. In the flame that roared inside me, I could see the poetry book my father had burned. It was still in me, and it was alive. Then I started screaming, "Yes! Yes! Yes! I love you! I love you, poetry!" The sound of light shamanic drumming started, helping me to feel very safe and nurtured. Then I became quiet and seemed to slip into a gentle nap. I think I was asleep for maybe fifteen minutes. When I woke up, I pulled the blanket from over my head and saw Brock sitting very quietly at my side like a guardian angel.

"Welcome back. Would you like to share?" he said. I slowly gathered myself and sat up on the pillows cross-legged.

"I need a pee first," I said, and headed to the restroom.

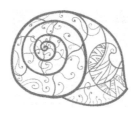

Chapter 45

Healing the Child Within

On my way to the restroom, I became aware of how light I felt. It was as if someone had filled me with warm helium. It was a glorious feeling. I had done so much crying, I was sure my eyes would be completely bloodshot. When I looked in the mirror, I was amazed to see my eyes were clear, and they had a nice little twinkle. I think I looked at least five years younger. As I splashed water on my face, I started to feel the energy of passion inside my heart. Then I allowed my awareness to track what was happening inside, and one big word came bounding at me, *poetry*! I felt that my heart was on fire in the most glorious way.

Even though my energy felt good, I was feeling a little discombobulated. I returned to the room, took my seat on the cushion, and crossed my legs.

Brock had a warm smile. "How are you doing?"

I pondered my response then said, "Passionate about poetry."

He said that what we had done was just part of the process. We had released a long-dormant memory, and we needed to reframe and integrate the memory into my current patterns of behavior. He said that it was better to do the process first, and then he would explain why and how it worked.

"I am all yours," I said with a smile.

He took a sip of water and began. "The psyche or emotional energy body of the six-year-old little girl is still alive in you. As is the emotional or energy body of the adult you. The next part of the process is to unify them, so that you can fully integrate the magic of your childhood and the power of your adult self. These two parts of you have lived independent lives within you. It is time for the hurt little girl in you to meet and be loved by the loving and protective adult you. Are you ready?"

I nodded.

"Please sit comfortably, close your eyes, and let your breathing become slow and soft," he said. "In a few moments, I will guide you to open your eyes. In front of you, you will see a pillow. I want you to imagine that this pillow is you when you were six years old and your father had just burned your poetry book. This process will invoke strong feelings in you. Keep breathing deeply and let the caring, protective adult part of you respond to what you feel when you see this hurt little girl."

I must admit that when he was explaining this, I was a little skeptical as to whether it would work. I breathed deeply and centered myself. He guided me to imagine myself when I was six. I was surprised by how easily an image of an unhappy six-year-old girl sprang into my mind's eye. Then he guided me to open my eyes and see in the pillow this little girl. As I looked at it, it was as if it became the hurt little girl. My adult heart immediately burst open, and I threw open my arms and moved forward to hold her. I pulled the pillow in close to my heart, and the following words just poured out of me. "I love you, I love you. I love you. I am so sorry for what he did to you."

Brock then quietly suggested that I allow my adult feelings full expression.

I felt protective anger stir within me, and as I was holding my little girl in my arms, I said in a very loud voice, "Nobody will ever, *ever*, take away your poetry again! I will never leave you! I will defend and protect you! I love you! I love you! You are beautiful." I was flooded with tears and emotions. I lay down, cradling my little girl in the form of the pillow in my arms. The power of what I was feeling was beyond anything I had ever experienced. Brock gently placed a blanket over us, and I lay there with my little girl, loving, caring for, and protecting her. The sound of soft shamanic drumming filled the room. I could feel some form of energetic inner process going on as our two bodies seemed to merge into one. As an adult, there had been an emptiness in my heart, and slowly the energy of my little girl was filling it. I was tingling from head to foot. After a short while, the energy seemed to calm down, and I lay quietly holding my little girl.

After a few more moments, I sat up and placed the pillow gently at my side. I beamed a wickedly big grin at Brock. "What the hell just happened?" I asked.

"Please," he responded. "Let this flow for now. I will explain later. Now we need to reverse the roles and allow the little girl to fully accept you as an adult. In a few moments, I am going to ask you to lie down in a fetal position. I am going to place a very heavy blanket over you. You will imagine that you are the little six-year-old girl and that the blanket covering and protecting you is your adult self. You will then speak to your adult self, represented in the form of the blanket. Let your feelings out. Fully express all you need to. Any questions?"

I shook my head.

I lay as directed on my side in the fetal position. Brock draped a heavy blanket over me. He guided me to imagine that I was that six-year-old girl. I was amazed at how my emotions seemed to shape shift my energy. I suddenly felt her vulnerability. I could feel how she had been hurt and abandoned by the adults. It was very painful. I could also feel the burning flame in her heart for poetry. Brock then asked me to speak as my little girl to my adult self in the form of the heavy blanket.

These are the words that came. "I have been so lonely. I felt as if nobody would ever find me. Thank you for coming to get me. I do not want to be locked away anymore. Thank you for loving my poetry. Please never leave me again. I want to sparkle and shine again. I want to be loved by you. I love you!"

I felt an incredible inner energy shift as two energy forms seemed to merge into one. It was like one and one equaled three. I felt suddenly bigger than before. It was a glorious feeling.

Initially, there had been sad tears, but these eased into tears that held love and joy. I lay quietly under the blanket for about ten minutes. Once again, the sounds of soft shamanic drumming filled the air. I sat up and quietly came back to the room. Brock was sitting in his usual place of protection and holding the space. He pulled the heavy blanket from me and placed a lighter one around my shoulders. I still had the light helium feeling, but I also felt very grounded. Like an immovable object. I smiled at Brock and said, "We done now?"

He smiled back and said we had one small process to do.

"What more is there to do?" I asked.

"We need to release and integrate the relationship with your father," he said.

I felt an immediate spark of anger at the mention of his name. "But he has been dead for eight years."

"It doesn't matter if he is dead or alive. His energy is still alive in you, and it can also control you, so we need to cleanse and assimilate your relationship to him. I want to explain briefly how this will work. Then we will do it. Afterward, I will more fully explain all that we have been doing and why."

"I'm ready," I said.

"In a few moments," he said, "I am going to ask you to stand. Both the little girl and the adult are together as one in you now. I will stand in front of you. I will ask you to imagine that I am your father. It can be at any time of your life. He can be happy or sad.

"As you look into my eyes, I want you to imagine that you are looking into the eyes of your father. Open your heart and feelings and speak your truth. I will ask the six-year-old to speak first, and then the adult in you can speak. Be honest and free. Words may come through me from your father. In stepping into this energetic matrix, his psychic energy may speak through me. I will explain later how this works. For now, trust that the words that may come through me are from the spirit of your father. Even though your father is long gone from this physical world of ours, his soul is still in the world of spirit, and it will be seeking release from this emotional entrapment as well. I need to mention that you should not touch me in any way. Because he is in spirit, we need to honor this."

I felt a quiet stir of anger at the prospect of thinking about my father.

Brock began to guide me. "Jane, please stand up in front of me. Close your eyes and breathe deeply. Feel the presence of you both as a six-year-old and as an adult. Take a few moments to feel these two presences within you. First, tune into the six-year-old girl. Then open your eyes and when you look into my eyes, imagine that you are seeing the eyes of your father. He has come to hear what you have to say to him. Please speak from your heart."

I stood up in front of Brock and closed my eyes, breathing deeply. Then I imagined that I was the six-year-old girl. I opened my eyes and imagined that I was looking into the eyes of my father. From deep down inside of me, I started screaming, "You hurt me! You hurt me! You hurt me! I hate you! I hate you!"

My whole body seemed to be contorting with anger. I kept screaming at him. "You were wrong! You were wrong! I am beautiful! I am beautiful! I was born to love poetry! How dare you burn my poetry. Nobody will ever do that to me again! Nobody will ever burn my poetry again! Do you hear me? Do you hear me?"

At that point, I was lost in full-on rage. I could feel the veins in my neck bugling with anger. Brock's eyes never faltered. They remained still.

The surge of anger washed through me, and I stood gazing into the eyes of my father in the form of Brock.

"May I speak?" The words came from Brock.

"Yes," I said.

"I am sorry that I hurt you, Jane. I was wrong to burn your book of poetry. It was a mistake. My father burned my books on art and made me become an accountant. I resented him all my life for doing that. Can you find it in your heart to forgive me?" Brock, carrying the energy of my father, stood looking into my eyes.

Almost simultaneously I could feel my anger dispersing as my heart began to open and feel love for him. I felt a big lump come to my throat as tears flooded my eyes. I looked deeply into his eyes and said, "I forgive you." As the words left my mouth, it felt as if a dark cloud lifted out of me. We stood there silently looking into each other's eyes. I could feel a beautiful peace forming inside me.

Brock then moved sideways, as if to break the connection. He walked around me and came back to stand in front of me. Then he spoke again. "Jane, I want you to look at me again as your father, only this time see me through the eyes of your adult self. Allow your words and emotions free rein. Because I am in spirit, it is important that you do not touch me. We need to do this energetically."

I closed my eyes and imagined my father standing in front of me. I tuned into my adult self and opened my eyes to look into the eyes of my father in the form of Brock. Rage immediately shot through me. I screamed at him. "You bastard. How dare you burn Jane's poetry. You are a nasty piece of shit. You are a miserable piece of crap!" The rageful energy poured right out of me. Brock's eyes stayed focused on me. After a few moments of silence, another wave of anger shot though me. "You piece of camel crap," I shouted. "How dare you burn Jane's poetry? You were wrong! You made a mistake! You are a douchebag!" The rage passed through me, and I stood there staring into his eyes.

Then Brock in the form of my father spoke. "May I speak, Jane?"

"Yes."

"You have a right to be angry at me. I made a mistake. I was a poor father. I did not see your beauty. I was threatened by your love of poetry. My father had stolen my passion for art, and I wanted to steal your passion for poetry. I was wrong. I am sorry. Will you forgive me?"

What surprised me were the tears that were flooding out of Brock's eyes. It felt as if my father was actually crying.

I took some deep breaths and within me, I felt energy move. Slowly, I felt my heart open. Then came the words. "Dad, I forgive you!" Tears burst from my eyes again, but these were warm tears full of love—not for my father, but for me and for my little girl. They were full of joy.

Finally, Brock asked, "May I go now?"

I nodded yes, and he slowly moved away from me. I felt as if I was embraced by an aura of pure light. Now, I really did feel free and whole.

Brock approached me from the side and gently put his hand on my shoulder. I turned to look at his smiling face. He smiled back and said, "You are really awesome, you know!"

We turned into each other and fell into each other's arms. We held each other silently as we breathed together. Slowly, we eased away from each other, and we sat down on our cushions with our legs crossed, facing each other.

He made a small gesture with his hand as if to invite me to talk.

I took a deep breath and said, "Holy crap, what the hell just happened?"

He broke into a loud laugh, and I joined him. "Now *I* need a pee," he said, and he headed to the restroom.

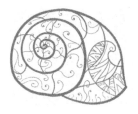

Chapter 46

The Three School Priorities

Brock returned from the restroom and took his seat in front of me. "Questions?" he asked.

"Where to begin," I said. "First, I am curious as to why several years of psychotherapy did not uncover the hurt my father inflicted on me."

Brock responded, "Children have very large emotional bodies that live inside and outside their physical bodies, like an energy field. They need this to learn and acquire the various life skills and lessons for growing into adulthood. Children are often much more aware of what adults feel than we realize. When there is a painful wound that threatens an aspect of their beauty, they often bury that special part of themselves deep within their emotional body for protection. Point in case with your love of poetry. The Shaolin monks explained that it is the pain of the wound that encases the beautiful part that is being hidden. Then pain later in life is how you track this wound, which will lead you back to the gift. The problem is that when people feel emotional pain, they see it as a fault and avoid it. This sort of emotional pain has a valuable function in the healing process. The hiding of this gift is done initially for protection. It is hoped that there will be a chance later in life to feel and release the pain of the wound, which will also release the precious gift it has been protecting. However, there are few known methods to discover these deep emotional wounds. As for psychotherapy, imagine that you are looking with your eyes at the outside of a body for a wound. You may see bruises or cuts on the skin that would tell there is a wound.

"However, the deep emotional wounds from childhood are underneath the intellectual skin, as it were, and psychotherapy does not always find them. The other thing that can happen in children is that the memory is so painful they bury it and actually disconnect from the memory of it. For this reason, the intellect or thinking mind has no way of accessing it or even knowing it is there. This is what you did when your father burned your poetry book. As a child, you had no way of dealing with the amount of emotional pain you were feeling, so you not only buried the love of your poetry, but you also disconnected the memory for your own survival. In this way, forgetting is a process that protects you from the pain of an emotional wound until you are able to feel and release the pain the memory contains. Forgetting helps you for a certain period. But if the memory is not felt and experienced at a later date, then it may try to get your attention with depression, addictive behaviors, or the feeling that you are not living the life you have come here to live.

"The problem is, this deep wound never goes away and may appear later in life as some form of emotional dysfunction. Often people who have issues with anger or moodiness have some deep inner wound. The anger is not the problem. Anger functions like an orange light on the dashboard of our lives. It's trying to get our attention. Then you create another problem when you try to fix the anger or the depression without uncovering the deeper wound. This is like disconnecting the orange light from the dashboard. Many forms of addiction are created by deeply held emotional pain that the addiction numbs. This is why giving up an addiction is much harder than just using the intellect to stop whatever the addiction is. People with addictions often do not know what the deep wound is. They only know the deep pain or loneliness they feel, and the addiction numbs that pain.

"Years ago, I had a friend who was a chain smoker. She was also very tuned into her inner process. She once said to me that smoking was her best friend. It filled an empty void in her. She said, "If I did not smoke, I would probably die of the painful loneliness that lives deep within me." So, smoking was keeping her alive! I know this may sound odd, but people who do not have addiction issues can never truly know what people who do have addictions really go through.

"Many of the villagers struggled with addiction issues, and this was another reason the monks developed these powerful, deep emotional tools for healing. In particular, the use of color became a powerful healing tool that acted as a form of emotional X-ray. It was commonly used by the monks to help the villagers detect, release, and heal deeply held wounds.

"In the West, people tend to move away from pain. They often feel pain is the problem and do what they can to avoid it. The monks understood that pain is often created as a warning and for protection. Instead of numbing it or avoiding it, they sought the wisdom of the pain to help guide them to find the deeper healing, which meant release of the pain and the finding of the treasure that was held in the pain. This is what happened for you.

"Emotional pain often holds grief, as well, that is also is calling for release. As simple as this color process looks at first glance, it came from many years of deep, emotional inner work that the Shaolin monks did on themselves to truly know themselves."

I was struck by the wisdom of what Brock was sharing. "My next question is about my passion for poetry. I know a lot of people who have not truly found their passion in life. Does everybody have some form of creative passion within?"

Brock was quick to respond. "Absolutely. Look into the eyes of any baby. That sparkle and love you see is the unique gift and passion they bring into the world. However, the challenge is that it gets lost during their childhood, much like you lost yours.

"When the villagers learned how important it was to avoid emotionally hurting children, they asked the Shaolin monks to help guide their school system. The monks taught the villagers that the function of a school is not primarily education. This is the third priority. The first function or priority of a school should be that of discovering the unique gifts that each child brings into the world. It is important for children to know that their unique gifts are wanted and that they can express them. So often heavily structured educational systems bury the true gifts children bring to share with the world.

"The second priority of schools is to promote caring, trusting, and loving in children. The third priority then becomes education, which should be crafted around helping the child to become a whole and healthy adult. After the Shaolin monks transformed the education system, the children looked forward to going to school. They did not have things like attention deficit disorder, depression, bullying, or children committing suicide.

"I could go on and on about this," Brock said, "but we need to get back to your process. Maybe one day I will write a book about how children should be cared for. But for now, let's return to your question about finding your passion in life.

"A big misconception about finding your passion is that once you find it, you have to turn it into a living. That's not the case. Some people do that, but I know many people whose passion is a hobby and they work in other fields of employment. Take me, for example. I have never sold a woodcarving. I have given some away, but to put a monetary value on them and sell them would take something away from the process. I have one friend who has a passion for painting in oils. However, he works in the corporate world through the week and needs the income to sustain his family. He paints for a couple of hours one night a week and every other Sunday morning. So, his passion is alive and being nurtured, but it's woven around his regular work life. He enjoys his corporate career, and it is enriched by his passion being alive. So, people may or may not choose to let their passions be their main work in this world."

"That's good to hear," I said. "I did have a concern for how I would make a living as a poet. I am curious about how powerful the 'release of the father' process was for me. When you were representing him, there was one point when you had tears in your eyes, and it seemed as if they were his tears. How does that work?"

Brock took a sip of water. "When we are in relationship with a person through family connection or through friendship, we weave together their psychic fields of energy with our own. This is how we can achieve true intimacy. However, what few people know is that when we leave a relationship, or a person dies, often those psychic fields remain. This is what the grieving process of letting go is designed to release. However, in the West, there are very few rituals for releasing these old energy fields. When trauma is involved, the energy fields remain until they are released through processes very similar to the one that we enacted with your father. I allowed my energy field to tune into his field that you carried, which is why I felt the emotion. There are also parts of your father's psychic field that are still connected to him in spirit that needed to be released consciously, and this is why he wanted to speak and ask forgiveness. The process we did allowed you to release his field, and it allowed your father to reclaim the part of his spirit that was caught in the trauma."

"Wow!" I said. "I really felt the shift in my energy as he was released. I am wondering if things like depression can be caused by this sort of unreleased energy and losses that have not been properly grieved."

"Good insight. You are right on. The Shaolin monks said that knowing how to grieve is a form of medicine for emotional and physical health. Unexpressed grief is the cause of many health issues in the West. Anger is another symptom of a need for emotional healing and release."

I was feeling really good and thanked Brock for all that he had shared with me. He looked at his watch and mentioned there was a used-book sale at the local library going on and asked if I would I like to go see if they had any poetry books for sale.

"Hell, yeah!"

He said there was a diner near the library, and perhaps we could have some apple pie and vanilla ice cream as part of our healing ritual. We both laughed aloud and cleaned up to get ready to leave.

When we got out to the parking lot, Brock said that the library was about fifteen minutes away and suggested that we ride together. I liked that idea and hopped into his pickup truck. As he pulled away, he turned on the radio, and much to my disgust, the song "We Ain't Never Coming Back" was playing.

"Oh, no," I exclaimed. "Can you change the station?"

"Sure," he said, "but do you mind me asking why?" I explained the background to the song and how it pressed my buttons in the wrong way. "Got it," he said, and soon some lazy jazz music started to play.

He found a parking spot alongside the enormous tent erected on the green with tables of books underneath. Brock reminded me that I had just been through a major healing process and suggested I stay really relaxed and let him do the scouting for poetry books. I was feeling good but also a little tired, and I liked the idea of just tagging along with him.

The tent was roped off and had one entry and exit point, where people paid for their books. In front, a plump woman sat behind a table, collecting a four-dollar entrance fee, which would be taken off the price of any books we bought. Brock greeted her and asked where the poetry section would be found. She looked a bit puzzled and said there was no poetry section. Then Brock did something rather odd. He closed his eyes and sort of lifted his head as if he were listening to something nobody else could hear. After a few moments, he opened his eyes and said that he could sense that there were poetry books in the tent somewhere in need of a good home.

The woman gave him a *what are you on?* kind of look.

"May we go and look?" asked Brock.

She waved us in, saying, "Go knock your socks off, honey!"

Brock went quiet and started sensing the air again. Then he headed over to the far corner. He scanned some titles and then reached down and pulled out a book on poetry.

"Yay!" I said.

He went quiet again and pulled out another poetry book farther down the table. Now we had two. I was excited. This went on for twenty minutes, and we ended up with thirteen poetry books. I was elated.

When we headed back to plump woman, her eyes popped open. "Looks like you found some homeless poetry books," she said as she started to calculate the cost. They worked out to be around a dollar each. I could not believe our luck. She put them in plastic bag, and as we were leaving, she said to Brock with a smile, "Wouldn't like to come with me to the casino, would you? I think you've got the magic touch."

We all laughed, and Brock and I headed back to the truck to leave the books before walking to the diner. He asked me to close my eyes and pick one book that we would be reviewing over our apple pie.

We strolled to the diner a quick block away. Brock led us to a cozy booth. I opened my poetry book to read the list of poems and was interrupted by the slapping sound of two menus hitting the table. I turned to see a short waitress walking away. *That's a bit rude*, I thought. *No greeting or anything*. Brock left the menus where she had put them, and I started to read the titles aloud for us to choose one. The waitress returned with her order pad and a sour look on her face. She was heavily made up with black eyeliner that accentuated her glare. She was wearing a nauseating perfume and a scruffy name badge that said, "Mary." She gave a very curt nod to Brock as if to say, *What do you want?*

Politely, he asked for two pieces of apple pie with vanilla ice cream and two coffees.

Impatiently, she tapped the menu of main courses, suggesting we should be ordering dinner.

"Just the apple pie will be fine," said Brock.

What she did next really shocked me: she rolled her eyes, snatched up the menus, and walked to the counter. I was on the verge of calling her out for the rudeness. Brock could sense my annoyance and asked me to stay soft and let him lead. This was the first time I had been with Brock in public away from the coffee house, and I was curious to see how the way of the three loves played out in real life. *Will he confront her rudeness?* I wondered.

I started to read a poem, and then two plates of apple pie suddenly thudded down at the end of the table. Two cups of coffee followed with a crash of silverware, and she abruptly walked away. She did not even place the plates of pie in front of us. I was really annoyed. I looked at Brock, and he seemed to be studying the woman as she waited on other tables. Was he or was he not going to deal with her rudeness?

With the apple pie came one very small dab of vanilla ice cream. I wanted to ask the waitress for more but did not want to incur her rudeness again. As we were finishing our pie, she walked by, slapping the check on the table without even looking at us. Brock would never leave a tip for this sort of service. Or would he? I was curious to see what he was going to do.

He pulled a credit card from his wallet, and I thought this would be a good way to pay and avoid leaving a tip. Then he pulled out a ten-dollar bill, and I had to hold myself back from saying anything. He stood up, walked over to the cashier, and handed her the credit card. Then he handed the cashier the ten-dollar bill, and she counted ten dollars' worth of quarters into a dish. *Now what is he up to?* I wondered.

When he came back to the table, he placed the dish on the table and went very quiet. Then he picked up one of the quarters and placed it on the table. He picked up another quarter and placed it next to the first quarter. The way he was placing the quarters on the table reminded me of how the Tibetans did their sand painting of mandalas. They were created with focused, prayerful intention. What on Earth was Brock doing with those quarters?

Slowly, he created lines, curves, and circles with the quarters. Then I saw what he was doing. He was spelling out the name *Mary*. I felt my heart suddenly open. The beauty of what he was doing took my breath away. He carefully placed extra quarters around the *M* as if to make it bold. When the waitress came toward us, he very deftly covered the quarters with the poetry book so that she would not see them. The bill was about nine bucks, so a two-dollar tip would have been fair. But this was far more than a regular tip. I couldn't wait to see her face when she saw the coins spelling out her name. It would knock her haughty little socks off for sure. Just as he finished laying the last quarter, Brock whispered to me, "Please get ready to leave when I say."

He waited until the waitress was at the far end of the diner with her back to us and then he said, "Let's go!" and he headed out, not through the main entrance but through a little door at the back of the diner so she would not see us leave.

His orchestration of this whole event was very curious to me. Once outside, we walked straight to his pickup and jumped inside. He cranked up the engine and before he put it in gear, he turned to look at me and raised his eyebrows as if to invite a question.

"What the hell did you just do?" I asked.

He let out a little chuckle. "Well, the Shaolin monks said that the highest reflection of their way of three-loves process was in sharing acts of kindness. This was the true manifestation of love. The higher level, or what you would call in the West the PhD level, is when you share an invisible act of kindness. This means that you disappear and leave the act of kindness to be discovered. What I just did was simply an invisible act of kindness, where I did not hang around to see her response. Just doing the act of kindness was what I needed to wash away her rudeness."

I was stunned by this. He beamed one of his big, warm smiles at me and pushed the truck into drive. Just as he did this, there was an urgent tapping on his window. It was the waitress, and she had tears rolling down her cheeks.

She gestured for Brock to roll down the window.

Brock wound down the window, and she blurted, "Who are you? Do you have any idea what you just did?"

Brock flipped off the engine and sat there, quietly gazing at the waitress. She blew her nose in a tissue and then started to speak. "At five o'clock this morning, my beloved fourteen-year-old Labrador developed internal bleeding. I rushed him to the vet, and there was nothing that could be done to save him. I held him in my arms as the vet put him to sleep. I wanted to take the day off, but two other waitresses called out sick, and Bernie, the owner, was in shit street. So, I reluctantly agreed to work a shift. My tears have been frozen inside of me, and I was choking on them. As soon as I saw what you did with the quarters, my heart popped, and at last my tears were able to be released. I was in so much pain. The beauty of your act seemed to help my heart breathe again."

Brock remained silent, his eyes locked onto the waitress.

"I need to ask you a favor," she said.

"And that favor is?" Brock asked.

"I want you to come back for more apple pie, only please call me the day before, and I will personally bake the most amazing apple pie you have ever tasted," she said.

"On one condition," said Brock.

"And that is?" she asked.

"That we get two dabs of vanilla ice cream."

She laughed aloud and said, "Honey, you got three coming at ya."

We all roared with laughter. Then the waitress did something that took my breath away again. She reached into the cab and gently removed Brock's hand off the steering wheel and pulled it toward her face. Then she lowered her head very gently and placed a lingering kiss on the back of his hand. They both seemed to light up with a golden aura. She released his hand, smiled at him, and went back into the diner.

Brock slowly turned to me and said, "Ya know, ya just never know the trouble these acts of invisible kindness can get you into!"

We both laughed, and he started the truck again. When we pulled up outside his woodshop, he turned to me and said quietly, "No words. This has been a big day for you. Go home and rest to let everything integrate." He leaned toward me, and I leaned in toward him. The way his mouth was headed, I thought he was going to kiss me on the lips. Then at the last moment, he turned his head and kissed me on the cheek. I had the sense that he wanted to kiss me on the lips, but because of what I had just been through, he kissed me on the cheek instead.

I smiled and nodded at him as I closed his truck door. He smiled back.

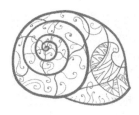

Chapter 47

An Eventful Day at the Clinic

I woke up before the alarm with a wonderful helium feeling throughout my body. There had been so many big shifts the day before. The return of my passion for poetry, healing my father wound, and of course, there was the "almost" kiss on the lips from Brock.

I had hit the radio alarm button the night before by mistake and instead of the usual buzzer to wake me, the radio alarm went off playing that awful song that my husband loved and I truly hated. I hit the off button with a vengeance. This brought me out of my little daydream. Then these questions appeared in my head: Why did David send those beautiful roses? What was I to make of that? What did I feel for him now? And how much of what I felt for him was simply from our old relationship before he walked out on me? My mind felt like a washing machine full of grubby thoughts all churning around in my head. Then I remembered that it was my chemo day at the clinic. Suddenly, the old familiar black ball of dread appeared in my stomach.

My light, happy mood soon slipped down into darkness, and thoughts about my cancer and having my breasts removed came in from right field and hit me sideways. Coffee shop! I need a visit with Goth Girl! That would set me straight. I reached for my phone and shot her a text.

Clinic day today. Any chance of 15 on my way in? ETA 7:30 a.m.

I hit the send button and headed to the shower.

The warm water made me feel a little better, but as I pulled my wig out of the cupboard, I caught sight of my bald head in the mirror, and I just fell apart. I threw myself onto my bed and cried my heart out. Just thinking about the day in the clinic gave me a nauseous feeling. It all began with Deborah, the receptionist from hell. Then there was Grumpy Nurse, who could never find my vein. I needed a very big latte and an even bigger hug from Goth Girl.

I arrived at the coffee shop at 7:30, and Goth Girl was sitting at the corner table with two very large lattes in front of her. As I walked toward her, I tried to put on a smile, but I knew that she would see right through it. We hugged, and as we sat down, she gazed intently at me with that psychic sort of reading-me look. I didn't know how this worked, but I knew that she had a way of seeing things that nobody else could see. But I was not threatened by being seen by her and knew how caring she could be. She went straight for the jugular. "Well, Wig Girl, you got some crap energy in you today, eh?"

I nodded in agreement as I sipped my latte.

"Clinic today and that bitch of a receptionist," she said. "Wasser name?"

"Deborah," I said quickly.

"Oh, and a grumpy-ass nurse." Goth Girl suggested we go over the seeing-beauty process using Deborah and Grumpy-Ass Nurse. I was in a flat mood and thought it best to pass. But Goth Girl was persistent. "You will only know if this stuff works if you use it, honey," she said supportively.

"Okay," I said. "Let's do it."

Goth Girl began. "To recap, you are going to see three aspects of physical beauty and three aspects of inner beauty, and you are going to imagine three acts of imaginary kindness you can do for each of these women. Right?"

I nodded in agreement.

She pulled out a napkin and slid a pen across the table toward me. "Remember, you deepen the effect of this process if you write it down."

I nodded acknowledgment, and I started to imagine three aspects of beauty for Deborah. I could see her beautiful nails, her beautiful nose, and beautiful hair. I was surprised at how this simple process seemed to soften the lump or dread inside. Then I imagined three aspects of her nature that were beautiful. I could see beauty in her administration skills. It was beautiful how she showed up for work every day. And I imagined that she had a beautiful sense of humor. Then came three imaginary acts of kindness. First, I saw myself bringing her a bar of chocolate—though I was tempted to imagine me eating half of it and just giving her the leftovers. But I shifted it to giving her the whole bar. Then I saw myself bringing her a single red rose in a small vase. The third act of kindness was the hardest: I imagined giving her a neck rub.

Goth Girl was quietly watching me as I wrote everything down. "How're you feeling now?" she asked.

I was surprised to hear myself say that I was feeling better and lighter.

Then Goth Girl handed me another napkin and said to do the same for Grumpy Nurse.

I saw her beautiful neck, her beautiful ears, and beautiful hands, even though they did not always find the vein. Then I saw her beautiful ability to show up every day. This was followed by imagining her caring nature that enabled her to spend five days a week looking after cancer patients. That one thought alone shot a warm bolt of energy into my heart. Guess I had never seen it that way before. For the third beautiful quality, I imagined that she was a very gentle person. For three acts of kindness, I saw myself bringing her a wooden heart that Brock had given to me. I would take her a large latte. And finally, I would give her hands a rub with lavender lotion. Once again, I felt a dramatic shift in my energy toward her. The black mass of energy was gone. I was actually feeling good.

"See, girl, I can tell by your face you just shifted that big-ass piece of darkness. Right?" Goth Girl said.

"Right!"

"Remember that by visualizing these things, you are also giving them energy, and you may feel called to actually enact some of them. If you do, try not to stop yourself, but trust the process. Remember, this is not to change them; it is to evolve you and your inner energy from negative to positive. This will keep your mind off the old negative, habitual patterns of thought that you have created around your clinic visits. It will also help to rewire the neural system in your brain so that this upbeat way of thinking becomes natural to you. And remember, this is medicine in the form of positive emotions that will make your immune system stronger. Tell me what else this will do," she said with her eyes locked onto me.

I beamed a smile at her and said, "Help me heal the cancer."

She slapped me high five and said, "Go get 'em, girl!" We shared a hug, and I headed out.

On the way to the clinic, I played through the seeing-beauty process with Deborah and Grumpy Nurse. I noticed the change in my energy as I drove into the clinic parking lot. Usually, I had a slow, growing sense of dread. But today I was feeling relaxed and in a fairly good mood. I was twenty minutes early for my appointment, so I decided to go over the things I had written on the two napkins. After ten minutes, I thought about going to the small hospital gift shop that was on the way to the clinic. I knew they sold single red roses in nice little vases. I remembered that this process was for me, so if I bought a rose for Deborah, I was really buying it for myself. Soon, I was walking out of the hospital gift store with a red rose. I could feel the law of attraction at work. I had been feeding this idea with energy, and now it was becoming manifest, quite effortlessly.

I was feeling very calm as I entered the waiting room. As usual, Deborah paid me no attention when I arrived at her desk. She kept her head buried in her computer screen. I noticed a small braid in her hair that was beautiful, and I noticed that she had beautiful nails. Without looking up at me, she confirmed my appointment. Then she gave me an impersonal glance as if to say, *You are done and can go now.* Usually, this really irritated me, but there was something about the rose I was carrying that seemed to keep my heart open toward her. Very gently, I placed the rose by the side of her computer, and without making eye contact, I quietly walked to the clinic.

First one down, I thought. I actually enjoyed fulfilling my first act-of-kindness mission. For the first time ever, I felt that my heart was open as I walked into the clinic. With Grumpy Nurse, I would simply focus on seeing her beauty and being grateful. I would not say anything or communicate in any way. I reminded myself that I was not trying to change her. I had no expectations other than to see the three physical aspects of her beauty, then the three personal aspects of her beauty. Then I would do the fun part of imagining three acts of kindness. My own energy was in a much better place than usual.

When I walked into the clinic area, Grumpy Nurse was attending to a chemo pump. She gave me a half glance as she pointed to an empty chemo chair. I was feeling a great peace inside and smiled as I nodded my response. Me smiling at Grumpy Nurse, now *that* was a first. As I made myself comfortable in the chemo chair, I thought Grumpy Nurse needed a new name. Florence popped into my mind, after Florence Nightingale, the famous nurse. That was it; her secret name, known only to me, was Florence.

This is fun, I thought. And then I remembered that this process was also keeping negative thoughts at bay. I watched Florence as she tended to other patients.

I noticed that she had beautiful hair, she wore beautiful sneakers, and there was a beautiful shape to her ears. I half closed my eyes, sank back in the chair, and started to do the spiral meditation with my tongue on the roof of my mouth. I was amazed at how this took my mind away from the usual judgmental and nasty thoughts I projected toward her.

As she approached with a bag of chemo and needles, she was looking quizzically at me.

"Good morning," I said cheerfully, surprised that I could be that nice to her. She placed the bag of chemo on the side table and set up the various tubes and needles. She kept giving me a sideways look and asked if I was okay.

I beamed a big smile at her and said I was great. And I really was. I had this inner peace going on and felt none of the anger and annoyance that usually oozed energetically out of me toward her.

Halfway through setting up my chemo, the alarm on the pump of an elderly woman went off. Florence knew that interrupting my set up by attending to another patient always annoyed me. Once, I complained to the doctor, and that really pissed her off. When I heard the pump alarm, I said, "Please attend to that. I am not in a rush."

She turned to me with a look of curiosity. What she did next completely blew me away. Instead of going to the beeping pump, she went to a heating cabinet and pulled out a heated pad. She came back to me and slipped it on my arm to raise my veins for the needle stick before she went to check on the other woman's pump. I was stunned. I had battled with her over this during my last visit. She had missed my veins two times, and I got angry and had to insist that she use a heated pad. She did it, but I could tell that she was fuming at me.

My relationship to Florence was like sand shifting under my feet. I felt as if I was in a bubble of peace. And all of this because of the seeing-beauty process. I was not wearing socks, but had I been, then they would have surely been blown off.

After ten minutes, Florence returned and prepped my arm. She was usually in a rush, and I think this caused the misses in finding a vein. Today, she seemed very slow and deliberate. I was shocked when she found the vein with the first stick.

Usually, Florence did not pay any attention to me during my four-to-five-hour infusion, but today she kept glancing over at me. Whenever she did, I said quietly, "Thank you, Florence" and would notice something of beauty about her. I really liked the deep inner peace I was feeling and did not look at any of the crummy magazines or soaps on TV the way I usually did.

Time passed very sweetly, and soon my chemo bag was empty, and the pump started to beep. Usually, I would be on the edge of my chair by then, giving dirty looks to Florence and urging her to hurry up. Now, I was just sitting there full of peace and being thankful for the way she was caring for other patients. When Florence came to me, I beamed her a big smile again and said nothing.

She had the same curious look on her face and kept gazing at me. This was new; she usually avoided any form of eye contact.

She pulled the needle out and placed the small cotton swab on my arm that signaled the end of my chemo. I reached into my pocket, pulled out the wooden heart Brock had given me, and placed it on her tray. "Thank you for your caring," I said.

She leaned into me and asked if I could spare a minute. She pointed to one of the small exam rooms.

Was something wrong? Was there bad news? This had never happened before, but I kept my energy positive and walked slowly to the small room. She followed me in, closed the door, and stood there facing me as tears came to her eyes. "What were you doing today that made you so friendly and centered? You have an aura of warmth around you. We usually dislike each other. What changed?"

I pondered how to answer. I remembered Goth Girl mentioning that it was best not to share in detail what I was doing.

The truth of the matter was that I had shifted my own attitude about her and about life in general. The bottom line was that I could now see beauty in her. All I could see before was negativity through my own distorted and judgmental lenses.

I decided to let truth guide me. I looked deeply into her eyes and said, "I realized today that you are a beautiful person, and I am grateful to have you as my nurse."

She froze, staring at me intently. Then she collapsed into my arms and sobbed on my shoulder. I was shocked. I had become like Goth Girl had been for me. This was truly an amazing moment. She sobbed for a few moments and then pulled back. She blew her nose in a tissue and started to talk. "I usually have a hard, protective screen of energy around me, which is the way I have learned to survive. The reason is that my husband is an alcoholic and is constantly shredding my self-esteem. We have two small boys, and I am frightened to leave him and raise the boys by myself. He makes me feel so unworthy, and I know this plays out in my nursing. But today, you seemed to see right through this, and I felt this beautiful energy coming from you that really touched my heart. And I know that I did not deserve it. I want to talk more about what you did today. I know this is very unprofessional, but I was wondering if we could meet for coffee and a chat sometime. I really want to know more about you and what you did today."

I was still in shock. "Ah, sure," I said. "It would be an honor. Do you know the small coffee shop out on route 7 by the Shell garage?"

"Yes," she said. "I drive past it on my way to work, but I have never been in there."

I pulled out one of my business cards and handed it to her. "Shoot me an email with some days and times, okay?"

"Sure thing," she said.

We hugged again, and I headed out. What a day in clinic this had been.

The last thing was to navigate past Deborah, and I planned to do it without being seen. Deborah's desk was on the left side of the wide, long reception area. There was always a lot of foot traffic, so all I had to do was walk on the other side toward the moving staircase that would take me to the lower-level parking area. Just before I got to the reception area, I paused to wait for some people to head in my direction. I wanted to keep them between Deborah and me as a form of shield. A small group of people appeared, and I slid in alongside for the fifty or so yards to the moving staircase.

We walked twenty, thirty, forty yards, and all was going well. Then with just five yards to the escalator, I heard someone behind me say my name.

I stopped, spun around, and there was Deborah—away from her desk and just a step or so away from me. Her eyes were full of tears. I was stunned. I gestured for her walk with me over to a small, quiet area of the reception room. When we got there, I could see that she was crying. I opened my arms, and she fell into them. I wrapped my arms around her and held her tightly. Her head was on my shoulder, and I could feel the moisture from her tears through my blouse. Then I had the flash: this was exactly what Goth Girl had done for me. I had collapsed into her arms just as Deborah had collapsed into mine. I held her gently as she quietly sobbed into my shoulder. After a minute or so, she pulled back with tears still rolling down her cheeks. I pulled some tissues from my bag and handed them to her.

"What did you do today?" she asked.

I replied, "I, um...ah, it was just an act of kindness, that's all."

"That's all?" she shot back. "You have no idea what you did today, do you?"

I shook my head.

"It was as if a battering ram came along and broke the door down to the emotional prison in which I had been trapped. You see, not many people know this, but I live in a rough area of town, and twelve months ago, I lost my only daughter to a drive-by shooting. She was seven. I have been barely hanging on for the last year. The pain in my heart is almost unbearable. Even though I know I am cold and unfriendly, coming into work is the only thing that has kept me from killing myself. My daughter had a favorite flower. It was the only flower people brought to her funeral. Her coffin was completely covered with this flower. And her special flower was a red rose."

I was crying as well, and we hugged again. Now my tears were soaking into her blouse. We pulled apart, and she said, "Jane, I need to know why you did what you did today. Whatever that is, I need to get some of it for my own life."

I was feeling a strong impulse to connect with Deborah outside the hospital, and I pulled out one of my cards and handed to her. "How about we connect on email and we can make a plan?" I said.

She held it close to her heart. "God bless you, honey," she said, and we shared another quick hug.

When I got to my car, I sat for a few minutes. I was stunned by the events of the day. I had put into practice the seeing-beauty process, and it had transformed not only me but also two people who had been causing me grief. Thanks to this process, I had become for these two women what Goth Girl and Mare had become for me.

For the first time since I began my treatment, I drove away from my day of chemo with a heart full of love.

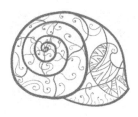

Chapter 48

A Pearl Necklace

I had a wonderful night's sleep and arrived in the office glowing from the day before. As I turned on my computer and took some sips of my dark roast, I reflected on my day in clinic and the experience of that amazing seeing-beauty process. My daydreaming was interrupted by an email from my doctor. More information about a double mastectomy. I felt a knot in my stomach. Then I felt annoyance with myself for being so displaced by my doctor's emails. A question floated into my mind. *Why don't I get a second opinion?*

I felt a flush of good energy and thought Goth Girl could help me with this. She had told me about her cancer specialist in New York, and I wondered if I could go and see her.

I dialed her number. She picked up quickly. I felt comforted hearing her voice say, "Hey, Wig Girl. Wonderful to hear from you! Wassup, girl?"

I told her about the emails my doctor was sending me about the double mastectomy, and Goth Girl got really annoyed. "Listen, let me put a call into my specialist in New York to see if she would be open to seeing you as a new patient. She is going to need all your current medical files sent to her. Lemme give her a call, and I will get back to you, K?"

"Great," I said and hung up. I felt a wave of optimism wash through me at the prospect of talking to a new doctor. Then I thought about my current doctor and wondered if she would share my medical files with another doctor.

I was tired of being emotionally pushed around by her and resolved to make the call as soon as I heard from Goth Girl.

The next email was from my husband. It began, *Darling Jane.* I felt the hairs on my neck shoot right up when I saw the word *darling.* He had used that word when he courted me and for the first month or so of our marriage. Then he seemed to lose it from his vocabulary. And here it was again. He had suddenly jumped into some new understanding about our relationship that I was not privy to. Initially, I felt annoyed by this. Then the word *darling* took me back to the happy memories of our courtship. Our chemistry had been so powerful, our lovemaking so full of passion. Those long weekends away when we would spend the whole day in bed. Having scrambled eggs for dinner. And once we had sex on the stairs of the hotel fire escape. We were wild and passionate. But was that love? I wondered. True love? Or was it some lust-filled Hallmark fantasy of love that I was eating like sugar? It annoyed me that I had not found peace with being single and living alone. I did not like having to pay all the bills, and then there was the early morning emptiness of having no one to wake up to.

I felt conflict inside around the word *darling.* Then I read his email.

Darling Jane, any chance we can have lunch today? There is a French restaurant five minutes from your office. It would mean the world to me. Yours lovingly, David.

I felt a tug on my heart strings, or were they lust strings? I was still feeling conflicted about the decision to hack into his private bank accounts. We had been together for twenty-four years. Surely, he wouldn't hide money from me. Or would he? What harm could one lunch do? I typed out my reply.

Hi, David. Sounds good for lunch. See you at 1:00 p.m. Jane.

The minute I hit send, I felt the doubts circling inside my head like buzzards. Was this real? Was he real now? Or was it just another emotional trap he was setting for me that would lead again to heartbreak. Perhaps he was a reformed lover. Could we go back to our log fires and lazy cups of morning dark roast after a night of glorious sex?

My daydreaming came to a halt when the phone rang. It was Goth Girl. She said that her specialist would be happy to review my files. "That was quick!" I said.

"It was just meant to be," she said. Her doctor had reviewing patient files and took her call right away. All I had to do was get my doctor's office to email or fax my records to her. The new doctor's contact info and a release form to sign was in an email that should arrive any minute. She said that my doctor may resist sending my records to a doctor out of state, but that it was now law that physicians had to share records. She encouraged me to kick a little ass if I needed to. "And remember to stand up when you talk to your doctor's office. Stand like a warrior," she said.

I knew that the medical system could be very intimidating, and I had a sense my regular doctor would give me some grief over this. I blew Goth Girl a kiss through the phone and then phoned my doctor's office with my request.

The receptionist got a little haughty about sending my records out of state to an unknown doctor. She put me on hold so that she could see if my doctor was available to speak with me. I heard a beep on the line, and I was surprised to hear my doctor's voice on the phone. Her voice sounded very serious. "Jane, you need to know that I always get the benefit of a second opinion from one of our other doctors in the office and there is very little for you to gain by confusing this with a third opinion."

I began to feel really small and feared that I may have upset my doctor. Then I heard Goth Girl's voice in my head saying to kick a little ass. These were my frickin' breasts, not hers. I imagined Goth Girl standing behind me. I slowly raised myself from my chair and stood like a warrior. I lowered the tone of my voice. "Thank you for your thoroughness," I said. "I want my records sent to the doctor whose contact information I will be emailing you in five minutes. How long will it take to do this?"

My doctor spoke again. "But Jane—"

I cut her off. "How long will it take?"

My doctor went silent. Then in a very cold tone, she said, "By end of day." And hung up.

"Bitch!" I said to myself as I hung up the phone. Then I gently touched my breasts. "It's okay, girls, we are going to get through this."

For the rest of the morning, I did my best to concentrate on grant research, but I kept thinking about David and where this lunch may or may not go. He had deserted me, after all! But he was seeing a therapist now. What does that mean? What is he really doing? He is back to calling me *darling*. What does this mean now? I had turned the washing machine of my mind on again, and round and round went my conflicted thoughts. The restaurant was five minutes away, and at 12:45 p.m. I went to the restroom to clean up. I splashed water on my face and then put on some light eye makeup and red lipstick.

Then a shrill voice in my head asked, *Why am I making myself pretty for him? Do I want to be back with him again?* It was all very confusing.

I walked around the block so that I would arrive a few minutes after one o'clock. David was waiting in his car in view of the restaurant entrance. When he saw me walking across the parking lot, he got out of his car and met me.

He opened his arms to greet me with a hug. He pulled me in tightly, but I let my arms hang loose by my sides. I did not want to communicate anything that might be misunderstood. He placed his arm lightly around my waist as we walked into the restaurant. He had reserved a nice, quiet, corner table. The maître d called him by his first name as if he knew him. This trick, I knew from his work in sales. He would get to the restaurant fifteen minutes ahead of the meeting time and drop a tip to the maître d in return for the old buddy/you-are-an-important-patron type of greeting designed to impress. Only this time, I knew the game he was playing. David was wearing a very smart dark-blue blazer, a light-blue striped shirt with tan pants well pressed. He really did clean up well.

He knew that wine at midday made me a little light-headed. Without consultation, a bottle of my favorite Chardonnay was delivered in a wine bucket to our table. He was playing his cards well. *What is he up to?* I wondered.

He made small talk as we munched on my favorite appetizer, garlic mushrooms. As the waiter cleared the plates, David did something that really caught me off guard. From his blazer pocket, he pulled a thin, velvet-covered jewelry box and placed it in front of me. I was shocked, then frightened, then curious.

"Please," he said, gesturing toward the jewelry box. "This is just a small way of saying sorry for walking out on you when you needed me most."

I felt my face go white, and a sudden chill shot through me. I had a sense that this was a frickin' emotional ambush. And I had just ridden right into it. I was now on my second glass of Chardonnay and without any sort of emotional defense. His dark-brown eyes were burning into me just like they did when he courted me. He was good, but was he real? I was really confused and just a little light-headed from the wine.

I flipped open the velvet case, and there was the most beautiful pearl necklace I'd ever seen. This really threw me a curve ball. For the last few years of our marriage, he had always promised me pearls, but to maintain a healthy business cash flow, he promised the pearls would arrive soon. But "soon" never came. And now, here they were. They were absolutely stunning, and the red velvet inside the case really set them off. I needed to reboot and excused myself, heading to the restroom. I splashed cold water on my face and looked deeply into my eyes. I felt untethered. Part joy and part fear. *Does he truly love me? Is this a new beginning? Or is he playing me?* I touched up my lipstick and headed back.

As I approached our table, I saw that he was checking his email. Damn, he knew that always pissed me off. But then there was the pearl necklace looking up at me.

Our main course arrived, and we continued our small talk. I kept feeling the urge to ask him about how his therapy was going, or to ask him to ask me how I was doing. I just wanted a sign that would tell me if he truly cared about me beyond the "what money can buy" signs. Our conversations were usually about him and his work, and that had always made me feel small and my life less important. The arrival of the pearl necklace had not changed the way that I felt smaller around him. The check came, and as waiter took his credit card away, David fired a question at me that hit me like a knife in the gut. He leaned toward me and said, "So, Jane, just checking. You still haven't filled the divorce papers yet, right?"

There was something in the way he asked that left me unnerved. The bubble he had been creating suddenly popped. What was it about the divorce that he feared? There was something amiss, but I couldn't quite put a finger on it.

I flashed a look at my watch to help bring me back to the reality that it was a workday lunch with a time consideration. He signed the credit card slip, and we stood. As we were leaving the restaurant, my phone rang, and a quick look at the caller ID showed me it was Goth Girl. I stopped in my tracks and took the call. He wandered a few yards ahead, waiting for me. She was calling to tell me there was a meeting with Tuku that evening. I told her I would be there and hung up.

As I walked to David, he asked suspiciously who had called me. I said it was my new friend, Goth Girl. He picked up on the name Goth Girl and asked, "Is she one of those crazy bitches who wears weird makeup?"

I felt annoyed with him for prying and had an impulse to defend Dar and our friendship. "What the hell is it to you?" I asked.

My anger surprised him, and he slipped back into Prince Charming. "Oh, sorry, sorry," he said lamely, becoming all smiles again. As we walked toward his car, he said, "Lovely lunch, darling! Hope we can do this again soon. Can I give you a lift to your office?"

I said that I needed the fresh air and wanted to walk. He gave me a peck on the cheek and headed to his car.

Back in the office, I made a cup of black tea to clear my mind. The pearls had really thrown me a curve ball. Perhaps we did belong together after all.

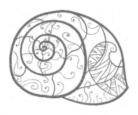

Chapter 49

Tuning into Loneliness

Back at work, I plowed through research data on potential donors. The highlight of the afternoon was a text from Goth Girl.

Remember: Tuku tonight. Golden ocean. Wear socks and be prepared to have them blown off!

I arrived at the coffee shop a little early around 6:40 p.m. As I was closing my car door, I noticed a police cruiser pull outside the coffee shop. Could there be trouble? Then I spotted Goth Girl sitting in the front seat. She rolled down the window and shouted, "Hey, Wig Girl, like my new taxi?"

I was in shock. Then I remembered that she was dating a New York cop named Tony. But New York was three hours away. Why she was in a police cruiser outside the coffee shop?

She jumped out and said, "Come meet my honey pie!"

As we were walking around to the driver's side of the cruiser, a rather handsome man emerged. He was around six feet tall with a slim, muscular build. Very sweet on the eyes, I had to say. Goth Girl introduced us, and we shook hands. He had a warm, strong hand and was rather sexy with his light-brown Mediterranean skin and deep, wanna-throw-yourself-into eyes. I was a little flummoxed and said, "Er, ah, a pleasure to meet you, Tony. I have heard great things about you." Then I said, "I thought you lived in New York."

Goth Girl jumped in, saying, "He changed jobs so that we can start living together!"

"Way cool!" I said.

Tony was very polite, and we shared some light conversation. Then his radio went off, and he was called away to an accident. As Goth Girl and I stood in the parking lot, she had a mischievous look on her face and said. "Bit of a cutie, eh? And without clothes, statue of David. Just heaven sent! He's gonna be my husband, you know!"

"Does he know that?"

"Not yet, but rest assured, at the right time, he will propose to me. Trust me, honey, I can already see it." She pulled out her "famous psychic" card and waved it in the air as she said, "I can see all things!" We both laughed and walked arm in arm into the coffee shop. Brock and Tuku had just finished setting up the room, and we hung out chatting as other people began to arrive.

By seven o'clock, all fifteen chairs were taken. Tuku welcomed everybody and began her talk. "Tonight, we are going to look at the term *grand design* and what this means to the way of the three loves. When the Shaolin monks developed this program, they had one aim in mind. I call this the grand design. Their aim was not simply about love and relationships, but it was about a way of living that makes this world a much more loving place for all. Real love to the Shaolin monks is when the primary function of your life is to share acts of kindness with yourself, with others, and for our planet. When this becomes your focus in life, then you become a self-generating force of love. It is this love that will transform your own life and the lives of all whom you touch. When we talked about the seeing-beauty process, acts of kindness were an important part of it. What we did with the seeing-beauty process was to build a vehicle. Now I am going to give you the ignition key with which you can turn it on. This is done with the unification of the three oceans that function as one, guided and inspired by the golden ocean and Divine Presence. The grand design is when your acts of kindness are made manifest in the world and become the focus of your life. This evening, we are going to talk about how to do this and how to manage the three oceans on a day-to-day basis."

I had the feeling that she was about to plug in or turn on the way of the three loves, much like they do with the tree-lighting ceremony for Christmas. She had been gently steering us to this place. Acts of kindness are about action and manifestation of love in the world. I was tired of people talking about love, singing about love, and complaining about love. To be real, love must be a word of action and doing.

"So, the three oceans become like a beautiful instrument you learn how to play," Tuku said. "At the core is Divine Presence. When I started to follow the way of the three loves, my challenge was how to maintain and use it like an instrument of self during my day-to-day challenges in life."

Dar put her hand up with a question. "Listening to myself was a real challenge until I discovered the way of the three loves. Could you talk more about this and the processes you use personally for communicating with yourself and the three oceans?"

Tuku beamed a big smile at her and thanked her for the question.

"Ah yes! Communicating with myself used to be a real problem for me as well," she said. "My blue ocean and rational mind had the loudest voice, and my white ocean of soul whispered very quietly. The golden ocean of Divine Presence made no sound at all. It communicates with feelings and intuition. In many ways, the way of the three loves could be called the way of the three voices because they communicate in different ways. Essentially, there are three voices within us.

"The voice of the intellect and ego, the voice of the soul, and the voice of Divine Presence. The secret is initially to know how and when to listen to each voice. Then the magic comes when they sing as a choir.

"When I seek a deeper communication and a listening with myself, I often use relaxing music and guided imagery to help me. I have a notebook on hand during the day to capture any insights or intuitions that come. There is also one by my bed. Sometimes I wake up in the night with important insights that will be gone in the morning if I do not write them down. The soul and Divine Presence are like twenty-four-hour diners. I had to learn how to honor this and truly listen around the clock.

"Another process that has helped me is journaling with my three oceans of three voices. I know this sounds a little odd at first, but it is a great way of achieving communication with these three aspects of self, the blue, white, and golden oceans. For example, I like to make tea, light a candle, and find twenty minutes or so when I will not be interrupted. No emails or phones. I select a voice or ocean I want to communicate with. I bring that color and part of me into awareness. I begin by writing with my dominant hand to ask a question or seek guidance. If I am in a low mood, I may ask a question seeking to know more about what the low mood has to share with me."

An elderly gent in the front row asked if she would talk about loneliness.

Tuku thanked him for the question and pondered for a few seconds before she began to reply. "I think loneliness is part of the human condition. I do not see it as something lacking, but as a sign that your life is calling for growth and evolution. In many ways, loneliness is like an orange light on the dashboard of my inner life. Rather than talk about my theory of loneliness, how about I share with you an actual story about loneliness from my own life?"

The old man nodded an enthusiastic yes.

"A few months ago," Tuku said, "I was in a very busy period with my work and had to work long hours. One day, I woke up and felt a sense of deep loneliness inside my heart. It was very distracting, and I could not focus on my work. It was not the usual form of loneliness that a chat with a good friend could fix. I decided to turn, face, and enter into the loneliness.

"When loneliness comes to visit, I first need to identify which ocean it is from. If I feel loneliness in the blue ocean or the rational mind and ego, it usually has to do with relationships in my life. It could be with a partner, a friend, or a family member. I look more deeply into the loneliness to track it, much like you do with the orange light on the dashboard. You need to track where the problem originates. Once I have located the origin of the loneliness, I can start to find resolution. It may be that I need to spend more time with friends, or it could have to do with a close personal relationship. This could have to do with releasing a partner, finding a partner, or making changes to the existing relationship. It is a sign that something is calling for change and attention. A close friend who lost his dog after fifteen years went through a period of grief and loneliness. After a year, he felt prompted to get a puppy. So, loneliness in the blue realm usually has to do with relationships in the world.

"If the loneliness I feel is in the white ocean, my world of soul, then it usually means that I have not been spending quality time with my inner self. I will take time to listen more deeply and reconnect to my inner self in a loving way. This may mean carving out some time to deeply relax, really listen, and be with my soul or inner self.

"The third form of loneliness I sometimes feel has to do with the golden ocean and my connection to Divine Presence. This usually means that I have not spent time being with and communicating with the Divine Presence within. If this happens, I will often go into nature or by the ocean for some quiet time. I may go to a monastery or a church in between services when there is nobody else there. I may need to read some spiritual material and look at my prayer life.

"So, you see, when feelings of loneliness come into my life, they have an intelligence and guidance that I need to listen to and be guided by. This is why

I do not numb loneliness or distract myself until it goes away. So, when the loneliness came a few weeks ago, I listened within and did not try to caffeinate it away or numb it by eating excessively. Twenty or so years ago, I struggled with being overweight because I was using food to numb the pain of the loneliness. I was working in the corporate world then, and some of my colleagues were addicted to smoking because of an inner loneliness that would not go away. We didn't have any resources or understanding as to how to access and be guided by our loneliness in those days.

"Anyway, back to my story. When I tuned into the loneliness, I was able to articulate where and how to respond to it. The loneliness I was feeling had to do with my white ocean and prompted me to spend time in nature. I trusted this impulse and went for a drive to a beautiful park overlooking a river thirty minutes from my home. I took a blanket and a notepad with me. By the time I got to the field, I was feeling lonely and sad. I laid out my blanket under a big oak tree and made myself comfortable. To help me communicate with my loneliness, I used the nondominant-hand journaling process. I used my dominant hand to write a question and then switched my pen to my nondominant hand to respond. Because the loneliness I was feeling was in my white ocean, I tuned into this for communication. As I started to write my first question, a few tears came to my eyes. I wrote with my dominant hand, "Why am I feeling so lonely?" When I moved my pen to my nondominant hand and tuned into my white ocean, I took a few deep breaths.

"The message I got back completely broke me open. I wrote, 'You have been neglecting me!' Tears started flooding down my cheeks. I guess I was having a mini meltdown. I knew enough to allow it to happen; I knew it would release the loneliness and sadness. As I tuned into this message, I became aware of how I had neglected my inner world of soul. My white ocean had become uncared for. My three oceans were out of balance. Work had taken over, and I had been mostly in my blue ocean of intellect and ego. I had lost connection to the inner world of my soul. The loneliness was a call to help me reconnect.

"Looking back at that experience, I would say that the feelings of loneliness came in order to get my attention. I did not override them. Instead, I let them lead me back to the beautiful inner world of my soul. It was there that I felt connected to myself again, and my feelings of loneliness went away. During this time of inner dialogue and listening, I also became aware of a couple of people in my life who were draining me. I needed to gently ease them out of my life. Even the awareness that I had to do this made my heart feel so much lighter.

"I was under the tree for just over an hour. I was feeling restored and took myself out for a nice breakfast. I took along my sketch pad, which always makes my soul happy. This is one example of how I dialogue with loneliness and use the communication process within to grow and take care of myself," Tuku said.

I also used this dialogue process to communicate with other parts of myself. It could be with my inner child or with a rather troublesome inner critic. She can be a real challenge. When I dialogued with the inner critic, she told me that I was carrying messages of being worthless from an old English teacher I had when I was nine. Once I found this out, I was able to release these negative messages, and my self-esteem was restored. Because of this, my inner critic became unemployed and moved away."

The group laughed.

"In this way," Tuku said, "several of my negative character traits have yielded valuable information that has helped me to heal and grow. Once I respond to and heal the underlying negative character trait, the loneliness or moodiness usually leaves. Learning how to communicate with myself has been the key to finding my true passion in life and for finding and maintaining true and lasting love."

I felt as if Tuku had just given me a flashlight for looking inside to find out what needed attention. I loved the process of communication she used and couldn't wait to try it out for myself.

Tuku said, "I think it is important to mention that there are different forms of loneliness. The three most common are found in the three oceans, but there is another form of loneliness that can be emotionally painful. This is a different process, and I would like to invite Dar to share her perspective and personal story with you. This form of loneliness is a deeper call to enter into and evolve the inner pain that has been carried for a long time."

Goth Girl stood and seemed keen to share. "I often use the journaling process for exploring my inner world of emotions," she said, "but there was a time when this process was unable to help. Words and the intellect could not go into a deeper place of me that was holding pain and loneliness. Tuku used a special guided meditation to take me deep down inside to face the pain. My usual response to emotional pain was to numb it and hope that it went away. Tuku guided me to surrender into the pain and to fully experience it.

"Initially, I resisted this," Goth Girl said. "I was frightened of feeling emotional pain. I know this is common in our society. My loneliness and pain were buried deep inside of me, and the guided meditation took me down into the pain. It felt as if I was slipping down into a dark abyss within myself. The pain of the loneliness became very intense, and I kept surrendering into it. I could not see or reach the sides of the abyss. All I could see below me was darkness that seemed to go on forever. Tuku helped me to surrender and free-fall into this dark, bottomless pit inside me. As I went further and further down, I suddenly came to a place where I seemed to break through the darkness into another realm that was filled with light. It was a place of incredible peace and love. I became aware that this beautiful realm represented a part of me that had been lost or buried many years ago. It was buried under the pain and loneliness.

"The loneliness acted as a sort of SOS light that eventually got my attention when I was ready to reclaim this part of me," she said. "The pain inside had always been there. I had just come to a time in my life when I was ready to reclaim it and face the emotional pain.

"What I did not realize at the time was that going into the pain took great strength and courage. Facing the pain actually increased my strength and courage. It seems paradoxical, I know. It was this strength and courage that I needed to reclaim the treasure buried inside. So, the process of working with the pain gave me what I needed to be able to reclaim that part of me. It is one of the most amazing healing processes I have ever experienced. And to think that for all those years, I ran away from any form of emotional pain. Gee, if only I had known Tuku!" Goth Girl smiled and turned to Tuku for a hug.

Tuku thanked Goth Girl for sharing.

"The pain that Dar was dealing with was not about brokenness or dysfunction. It was a deeply wise part of her that helped her to reclaim and release the wounded part that she buried as a child. Facing the pain gave her the strength she needed to reclaim that special part of her. This is a wonderful story that communicates that pain is not always what we think it is. This process is similar to what shamans do with their soul-retrieval work."

As I reflected on Goth Girl's story, I began to understand the age-old concept that suffering can be a means to spiritual growth. I was seeing how the word *suffering* was not the destination but a place of transition and transformation. In facing suffering, there was a strength to be gained that could enrich life beyond suffering. My whole relationship around suffering was shifting under my feet.

For many years, I had been formed by the Disney approach to a "happily-ever-after" version of life. I thought that pain and suffering were signs of failure. I was wrong. I now realize that even though I'll always try to avoid pain and suffering, if they show up, then I have powerful opportunities for healing by facing them.

Tuku suggested we take a ten-minute stretch break, and I headed out to the parking lot with Goth Girl.

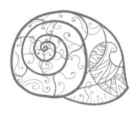

Chapter 50

Acts of Kindness

Tuku was chatting with Brock when we returned. We all took our seats, and Tuku said, "Now I would like to look at acts of kindness. They come in all shapes and sizes. There are regular acts of kindness, which make you feel good. These are like a master's degree. Then there are invisible acts of kindness, which are the equivalent of a PhD."

Everybody in the group laughed.

"The aim is not for you to simply achieve balance between the three oceans and three states of gratitude, peace, and being loved," she said. "That would be good, but you would limit their power to bring you happiness. The purpose in achieving harmony among your three oceans is that together, they will merge and produce beautiful acts of kindness. In doing this, you will be making the world a better place, and when your time to leave this planet arrives, you will pass onward with a full and satisfied heart. And if you get the chance to spend a few moments reviewing your life before you die, you will realize that the only things that really matter are whether you made a difference and whether you brought love to this world.

"If you have spent your life sharing acts of kindness, then chances are your soul will travel on from this life expanded and full of love. This is what happens to the Shaolin monks when they die. Their core teaching is that the journey of life is about sharing love through acts of kindness in and with the world. They teach that love is like a tree of fruit. It provides fruit through acts of kindness that feed people. It produces new trees through being inspirational examples of doing acts of kindness. So, when you share an act of kindness, you offer two things to the world: love in action and inspiration through your example. This is how we can change the world, one act of kindness at a time.

"The beautiful thing about acts of kindness is that they generate more acts of kindness. So, you could say that acts of kindness become a self-generating force of love. If someone shares an act of kindness with you, you have a natural tendency to want to do an act of kindness back. As I said, acts of kindness come in all shapes and sizes. Sharing a heartfelt smile or compliment. Sending someone a little note on the back of a napkin to say how much you appreciate the other person will transform two lives, yours and the recipient's. There are no limits to the acts of kindness you can offer. Helping people in trouble and even donating money to a non-profit are wonderful acts of kindness.

"One thing to remember is that acts of kindness should not be done to change, influence, or manipulate people. Acts of kindness are done by you for your own evolution and happiness. That said, you will find that your acts of kindness may affect beautiful responses in people. These will be even more well received because they are not expected.

"One other thing to remember is that your thoughts affect your health. Every cell in your body is tuned into the emotions you are feeling. So, acts of kindness become a sort of medicine as well. In simple terms, they will make you happy and healthy.

"The energy that is created and shared by the act of kindness is love in action. Anonymous acts of kindness are also real fun, as are imaginary ones. They help to release you from old patterns of bartering for love and being needy for love. They will help to create new patterns of positive, nurturing thought. Because the golden ocean represents and connects to the Divine Presence, acts of kindness that originate from the golden ocean have incredible power to spread love and healing in this world. The Shaolin monks taught me that two of the greatest acts of kindness are to truly listen to another and to truly listen to yourself."

A middle-aged, smartly dressed woman put her hand up. She said that she was undergoing treatment for cancer, and she was always receiving, but it was hard to give back with acts of kindness. People kept wanting to help her and do things for her. She had a freezer full of dinners that neighbors had prepared for her. They would often ask her how she liked what they had prepared, so she felt obliged to eat their meals. What she really wanted to do was cook and feed her family. She said these were beautiful acts of kindness, but it felt as if she was breathing in all the time and not breathing out by being able to easily do acts of kindness for others.

Tuku thanked her for the comment. "For the villagers who were battling cancer, the Shaolin monks set up what they called 'creative work centers' within the hospital. These were areas where patients could go to make things to be given to other people. They also sold some of these items in the hospital shop to raise funds to support the program. The Shaolin monks knew the therapeutic value of being able to do something for others. The most popular program was a woodworking program, where adult cancer patients made wooden toys for children with cancer. Instead of cancer patients sitting around waiting and waiting and waiting as chemo slowly dripped into them, they were given the chance to build and create works of art that would bring joy to children. The medical staff was amazed at how energized the cancer patients became. This promoted sociability among the patients, and there was a lot of laughter and shared joy whenever they came to create in this way. Compare this to the chemo clinic and people sitting alone hour after hour, staring into space or at soap operas and mindless TV shopping programs. Can you see the difference?" Tuku paused for a sip of water.

"The Shaolin monks made a point not to call this a therapeutic program. They were called 'workstations,' and cancer patients felt real again in having meaningful and purposeful work to do. As you can imagine, this affected every cell in their bodies, and ultimately, their immune systems became stronger, and they healed much quicker. Woodworking was the most popular and therapeutic program because it empowers so many aspects of a human being. Using tools and building with wood engages the inner will force that is deep within the soul. This is like an energy that radiates out through every cell in the body. So often cancer patients are inactive, and these essential inner forces atrophy and diminish.

"Human beings are designed to create and manifest lasting beauty. Just working with wood sends wholesome energy to the immune system. The motivation to create a strong and lasting form of beauty is a deep part of the human psyche.

"The completed wood project becomes like a mirror that reflects back the health and beauty of the person who created it. Building with wood produces a creative energy that is likened to when you jumpstart a dead battery. There is powerful charge of creative and psychic energy that floods your body and spirit. The monks' woodworking program elevated the patients' moods, and they always went home happy and feeling as if they'd made a difference.

"The permanency of the wooden project is also a wonderful metaphor for long- term health and beauty, which communicates this message on a cellular level.

"The doctors used to write prescriptions for woodworking as part of the treatment protocol for cancer. Men and women loved building with wood and felt great joy because they were bringing joy to children. There is no medicine that fills the heart with joy the way the woodworking program did. A common comment to the Shaolin monks was that building with wood seemed to make cancer patients taller when they left the hospital. It was increased self-worth, pride, and making a difference that made them taller."

I was really struck by what Tuku was sharing. Woodworking as medicine for the body and spirit made so much sense.

An elderly man in the front row put his hand up with a question. "I like the idea of feeling loved by Divine Presence and the golden ocean. How do you achieve this?"

Tuku smiled and thanked him for the question. "In terms of how you achieve being loved by the Divine Presence, it is not something you can achieve. You can only prepare yourself with humility, gratitude, and reverence. In terms of how it works, imagine a rosebud. Have you ever tried to open a rose bud by peeling back the petals? You will only damage its fragile form. Imagine then the effect of warm sun on a rosebud. Joyfully, the bud opens and blooms.

"It is the same with Divine Presence. You can bring yourself to that place of silent reverence and simply let it shine on you. The greater the humility and silence, the greater will you bloom."

The old man said, "Amen to that!" and everybody laughed.

I was becoming distracted, as thoughts about my doctor started to pop into my mind. I was wondering if she had she sent my patient file to the new doctor. Her reluctance was a source of annoyance to me, and she had made me feel guilty for asking. Tuku said that we had a couple more things to discuss about the importance of truth and saying "no" with love. She suggested a ten-minute stretch break. I headed to a restroom for a pee and to check my email to see if my doctor had, in fact, sent my file.

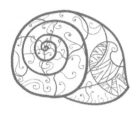

Chapter 51

More Than a Tattoo

I hit the "new email" button and found a long email from my doctor. She really ripped into me for seeking a third opinion and not trusting her judgment. She also emphasized how long she had been caring for me and that she was personally disappointed because in seeking another opinion, she felt that I was in questioning her ability as a doctor. Her email really beat me up emotionally. I just wanted to have a good cry. I considered going home but knew that if I did, Goth Girl would follow me, and she would miss Tuku's talk. I decided to return to the group, but I sat near the door, so I could leave if it all became too much.

As I walked back to the group, I began to feel anger toward my doctor. How dare she write me such an upsetting letter, especially when I was battling cancer! I was really boiling with anger by the time I got to my seat. I knew I was a firework about to go off and wanted to keep a low profile. Goth Girl was sitting on the far side of the group, and I could feel her eyes upon me. I could not hide anything from her. I slowly turned toward her, and I could see her studying me with a concerned look on her face.

Tuku was sitting in the front of the group. To try to distract myself from my anger, I looked for beauty in her. I noticed that she was wearing a beautiful maroon skirt and matching blouse. Her outfit seemed to accentuate the beautiful curves of her body. And my curves? Angry thoughts about my doctor surged back inside my head. My own curves were under threat from a knife! I felt scared and alone.

Tuku welcomed everybody back. "Now I would like to talk about the importance of speaking your truth to help you create clear lenses through which you may shine your golden ocean out into the world. We are also going to look at the importance of using the word *no* when it comes to living your truth."

I thought about my doctor and how I would be truthful with her. First, I would give her a big mouthful and put her straight about wanting to hack off my breasts so quickly. I could not get her out of my head, and my thoughts were running around like hungry rats in a pantry. All I really wanted to do was throw a chair at somebody.

Tuku began by explaining how she'd learned how to say *no* with as much love as she said *yes*. It was good to hear this, because I was the original say-yes girl, and then I would kick myself afterward. She said that saying *no* is saying *yes* to yourself.

I was finding it hard to focus on what Tuku was saying. I could feel the anger coursing through me. I was angry at the man in front of me for being tall. I was angry at myself for being so weak. I was angry at David for buying me pearls and then asking about the divorce. I was angry at my doctor for the fear I was feeling about losing my breasts. Tuku started to talk again. I lowered my head and eyes to the floor, taking deep breaths. I knew that Goth Girl was watching me. Then I reached down into my bag and pulled out my car keys. I couldn't do this. I flashed a glance at Goth Girl and tried to flip my head in a way that communicated I had to leave.

I was waiting for a natural pause in Tuku's talk so that I could quietly leave. I could feel my face getting red, and the fuse of anger was dangerously near the gunpowder within. Any minute now, I was going to blow.

Then Tuku said my name, and suddenly, the attention of the group was on me. I looked up and saw she was looking right at me. I knew she could sense something was going on within me. Then she dropped the gauntlet. "Jane, I welcome your truth!"

My truth? I thought. *Oh, my goodness, if you know what's good for you, you had best leave me and my truth alone.* I sat there feeling the rage boiling in me. I flashed a quick look at Goth Girl. She knew something was really off with me. Then she gave me a light nod of her head as if saying, "Let your truth have a voice."

My anger and rage were past the point of no return. I stood slowly.

Tuku also stood. We were like two gunslingers meeting at high noon. Only one would leave alive.

Tuku spoke again. "Jane, please share your truth."

My anger was now in my throat, and my words mixed with rage poured out of me. "My fricking truth is that they want to cut off my breasts. I have breast cancer, and I am really angry. I am angry with cancer. I am angry with my doctor. I am angry with me. I am angry at everything."

I could feel the veins in my neck bulging. I waved my car keys in the air. "I should go, right?" I shouted.

Everybody in the group looked stunned and a little nervous. I was expecting Tuku to rebuke me in some way or ask me to leave. She just stood there with her eyes on me. Then I noticed tears rolling down her face. She was not crying in the usual sense. I had a sense she was feeling the pain that was under my anger. She spoke quietly. "Your truth is beautiful, Jane. Is there more you would like to share?"

I was shocked. I had just given her an almighty mouthful, and she was asking for more! The rage in me eased a little, and I started to slow my breathing down. I still felt anger and stood there glaring at Tuku.

"May we go further into the truth, Jane?" she asked.

"What the hell do you mean?" I barked at her.

She spoke quietly. "You are not your breasts, Jane. You are more than your breasts."

That was it. She'd really hit my rage button, and I screamed at her with spittle shooting out of my mouth and over the big guy in front of me. "What the hell do you know about cancer? What the hell do you know about having your breasts removed? Look at you and your nice breasts! Stand in my shoes, honey, and you may not want to say I am not my breasts! And what the hell does 'I am more than my breasts' mean anyway?"

This had become ugly. I had no way of backing down. My anger was volcanic, emotional lava erupting out of me. Tuku and the group were deathly silent. Tuku did not move. She just held me in her gaze. Then she spoke again. "Jane, please come and stand in front of me."

Wasn't she frightened that I may take a swing at her? As I started to move toward her, she said, "Take some deep breaths, Jane."

I took several deep breaths and was now standing at arm's length from her, looking right into her tear-filled eyes.

She spoke again. "Together, Jane, may we go deeper into the truth?"

I was still feisty. "Sure! My anger is my truth, understand?" I said defiantly. I had a sense she was going to give me a little lecture about anger, and I was going to cut her off at the pass if she did. I was in no mood for some dumb-ass words of comfort. But what she did next completely blew me into a thousand pieces.

Tuku untucked her blouse from her skirt. She took a deep breath and moved her hands behind her and up under her loose blouse and unhooked her bra. Then she lowered her hands to grip the bottom edges of her blouse. In one smooth upward motion, she pulled the blouse and bra over her head, and I could see in the bra two artificial silicone breasts. My breath froze. What I saw next rocked, changed, and completely transformed my world. Rising from the waistband of her skirt was a tattoo of a beautiful tree with branches that spread out all over her chest, extending along her arms. On her upper chest, there were no nipples but two four-inch scars where her breasts had once been. Each of the scars was inside a long graceful branch of the tree tattoo.

Her chest was completely flat. All my anger suddenly vanished as my heart broke open.

"Come close," Tuku said.

I moved a little closer and took a deep breath. She reached down and gently took my hands in hers. Ever so slowly she raised them up and placed my fingers on the two scars where her nipples had been. Tears were now flooding down my cheeks. She removed her hands, leaving my hands resting gently on the two scars.

She lifted her hands to cradle my face. "What do you feel, Jane?"

I had no words. I just stood in front of her, sobbing, with my hands gently resting on her chest.

"Welcome to the truth," she said. "Stay here awhile. Let it open and open and open your heart."

I wasn't sure if my heart was opening, expanding, exploding, or breaking. I only know that I was held in the purest form of love I had ever known. Our eyes were locked onto each other's. The whole room seemed to disappear, and we were transported into a huge bubble of light.

Her hands were gently holding and caressing my face as she began to talk. "Jane, know this. I love my body as it is. The light of my soul resides in my body. I am not my body. I am a radiant and beautiful eternal spirit living in my body. You are a radiant and beautiful eternal spirit living in your body. My body is a gift on loan for my journey through this life on Earth. Your body is a gift on loan for your journey through this life. You and I are eternal souls. Nothing can ever take this away from you or from me.

"When I was diagnosed with breast cancer fifteen years ago, I was working in a manufacturing company in the Far East. There were very few options for women with breast cancer at that time, and they removed both of my breasts. I fell into a deep despair."

She lifted her hands away from my face and showed me her wrists. I was shocked to see the scars from what looked like knife cuts.

"Yes, I tried to commit suicide," she said. "I did not think I could live a full life without my breasts. I was desperate. A social worker friend of mine arranged for me to go and stay with the Shaolin monks for three months. This was when I started to study the way of the three loves. They took me under their wing and transformed me, my life, and my relationship to my body. My whole world turned upside down.

"When I lost my breasts, I realized how caged in I had been by the sexual expectations and projections of our culture. Up to that point, my identity had been formed around having an attractive body with beautiful breasts. I dated men whom I knew were attracted to my body. Many of them were looking for women who could satisfy their visual and sexual needs. I was a prisoner living in this self-inflicted prison. When I lost my breasts, I also lost a distorted relationship to my body and my breasts. When my breasts went, so did my prison, and I began to experience true freedom.

"The Shaolin monks and the way of the three loves helped me to find the love that existed in me all along. My initial reaction to my breast cancer was from my blue ocean of ego and intellect. The monks helped me to experience my life from the white and golden oceans—a soul with a Divine Presence. They helped me to come home to my soul and the Divine Presence that both lives within me and loves me.

"When you first stood up and raged at me, I knew that you were in your blue ocean of ego and intellect, where anger and rage live. Fifteen years ago, I was a victim of my breast cancer. I thought it was done *to* me. As I began to see that it could be used *for* me, I found incredible people and love pouring into my life. I do want to say that I think it is important to do everything possible to keep your breasts. However, please know that if you do lose one or both of them, your life may well be richer than it ever was before. The compass for your life is in the golden ocean where Divine Presence resides."

Then I felt a warm hand on my back. I turned to see Goth Girl standing behind me. Tears were pouring down her cheeks. I took a quick glance around the room, and everybody had beautiful tears in their eyes. They did not seem to be crying in the usual way. They seemed to be crying angel tears of love and caring. It was the most beautiful outpouring of love I had ever experienced. Tuku leaned toward me and gently planted a kiss on my forehead. I felt a bolt of warm energy surge down into my heart. Then she whispered, "We are complete for now, Jane. Go in peace and love."

She said for us to take a ten-minute stretch break, and she went to the back room to get dressed. Goth Girl walked with me outside for some air.

"What the hell just happened in there?" I asked.

"You went for a sail on the three oceans," Goth Girl said, laughing.

"I feel as if some form of birth just took place. I love this feeling!"

Goth Girl smiled. "That's what it feels like when your three oceans become balanced and in harmony."

I went quiet. Something had shifted my relationship to my breasts. Before today, I felt as if my breasts were full of dark energy and were sick. I now had a sense that they were full of light. They were not my weakest part but my strongest and most beautiful part. Before the doctors discovered the cancer, my breasts had been fighting the cancer all alone. They had done valiantly, and now it was time to love them more and do all that I could to make them stronger. I had the sense that the cancer was dark energy, and I wanted to cleanse it from my body. I was wondering what Goth Girl thought about surgery and asked her if she was open to share this part of her inner journey.

"Hell, yeah!" she shot back. "This is how I see it. The primary question for me now is not whether I do or do not have my breasts removed. My question has to do with whether I am living fully alive. Or am I living small and in fear? I used to think that eating kale and doing yoga alone would cure me. I believed that there was Divine Presence in them both and in all other holistic remedies. Then I realized that Divine Presence may also be in the hands of the surgeon. I realized that I had to listen deeply for my own truth and be strong in how I use the word *no*. Same for you, honey. Go deep into this for yourself, and you will know. Just remember, whether you do or do not have them removed will not determine how powerfully you will live and love going forward. Kale, yoga, and/or surgery will only help you to love more and care more. Ultimately, it is all about acts of kindness, right?"

In these few words, she had suddenly released me from my knee-jerk reaction to surgery. For some, it would be the right choice; for others, it may not be. The right choice for each is to decide from that higher place inside. What decision you choose will be the right one. This realization brought immediate peace to my heart and a sense of inner freedom. Now, my truth was about getting another opinion from a new doctor. Whether I did or did not choose to go the surgery route would be decided from my inner place of Divine Presence and not from my fear-based ego and intellect.

Goth Girl gave me a nod to communicate that it was time to go back in.

We took our seats, and I could sense a wonderful energy in the room. Tuku was fully dressed and sitting in front of us, radiating a warm glow. She began speaking. "First, I want to thank Jane for walking along the path of truth with me. What you all just witnessed is the power of the three oceans to transform your lives into something bigger and more powerful than you could ever imagine they could be. And it could be that cancer is the provocateur to a new and bigger way of loving and living.

"I don't think we need many more words this evening. May I suggest you find a little quiet time over the next few days to ponder what happened this evening." She gave us all a blessing, and the evening ended.

As I was walking out to the parking lot, Brock came over and reached out for a hug. As he wrapped his long, strong arms around me, the aroma of pine and his body scent seemed to wash over and into me, making me feel dangerously sensuous. I felt my legs go a little wobbly, and I became light-headed in a really good way.

He picked up on this and released me slowly from the hug. "I have a new name for you," he said, looking deeply into my eyes. "I am going to call you Warrior Woman from now on."

It felt like a baptism of sorts. What is it about his energy that does this to me? I wondered. Goth Girl was looking at me, and I knew that she knew there was something beautiful and sensuous bubbling between Brock and me.

For my drive home, I chose not to play the radio. I just wanted to stay with this expanded feeling. I now understood that I am a beautiful soul whether or not I have breasts. It was as if my soul just got birthed into life. This is who I truly am and who I have always been! And it rocks! It was a glorious feeling.

Sleep found me sweetly and quickly.

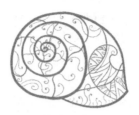

Chapter 52

The Hacking Begins

I woke up feeling on top of the world. There was some new research I wanted to get a jump-start on, and I arrived at the office thirty minutes early. As I turned on my computer, my cell phone rang. I did not recognize the number on caller ID, so I screened the call. A deep male voice with a Southern drawl said, "Hi, this is Hank calling for Jane."

I immediately hit the speak button. "Hi, Hank; this is Jane. First, may I apologize for my rather rude behavior the other day. It's a long story I do not want to bore you with, but I was having a really bad day."

"Water under the bridge, ma'am," he drawled.

"What are your thoughts going forward?" I asked.

He said that we needed to get a jump on this right away. I agreed for him to come over that evening. I felt a knot in my stomach. I knew it had to be done, but I also felt great conflict, given the way David and I seemed to be connecting again. As I put down the phone, I felt relief at the prospect of putting to rest the suspicions around my husband being a bad boy with our finances. At least with his innocence proved, we could continue to explore the possibility of our getting back together again. The red roses and the pearl necklace must be good signs.

As for Brock, there was a definite sense of connection with him. But I did not know much about his background or even if he was in a relationship, though Dar said he was not. Flirting with Brock was fun, but I had to consider my long-term security.

I plowed through my research and headed home just after 5:00 p.m. I arrived home around 5:20 and took a quick shower. I put on a loose-fitting tracksuit, boiled water for tea, and sprinkled some cookies on a plate for Hank. *What a name he has*, I thought. *Hank the Hacker*. I had a sense that David was clean with nothing to hide, and this hacking exercise would get my brother, Bob, off my case.

At seven sharp, the doorbell rang. I swung the door open and invited Hank in, directing him to the dining room table.

He greeted me with an "Evening, ma'am" and sauntered past me carrying his two black, FBI laptop cases. *Definitely no James Bond*, I thought. If looks were anything to go by, I still had doubts that he knew one end of a flash drive from his backside. As he started to set up his laptops, I offered him tea.

"Well, thank you, ma'am," he said. "Black with a touch of sugar. I am kind of partial to sweet things."

I held back the urge to laugh. He had a sense of humor, if nothing else. I slid the tea and the plate of cookies near him. "Thank you most kindly, ma'am," he said in his lazy Southern drawl.

"You can call me Jane," I said.

"Happy to. Can you please boot up your laptop for me, ma'am...er, Jane?"

When I returned with my laptop, the sight of the two FBI laptops made me feel uncertain. I pushed my laptop toward him with trepidation. "Will David know I am hacking him?" I asked nervously.

He gave me a slow smile. "Nothing to worry about. Stealth is my middle name."

Even though he was a little odd, there was something likeable about his gentle, easy manner. His fingers started flying across the keyboard with dizzying speed. Without looking up, he said, "Two minutes, and we will be ready to go. Jane, can you give me a little background as to what we are looking for and why?"

I suddenly felt vulnerable and a little embarrassed that I was essentially spying on my husband. He sat quietly waiting for me to gather my thoughts. I gave him a quick rundown of the pending divorce and how Bob suggested we track our invisible savings.

"Got it," he said very casually. I had the sense he had done this many times before.

I saw him look at the roses in the living room. I wanted him to know that this was probably a wild goose chase, and I popped upstairs to get the pearls. He was typing away on his laptops when I returned. I flipped open the velvet case and lay the necklace by the side of his laptop. Trying not to sound nervous, I said, "The roses and these pearls came from David, my husband. Just want you to know you may not find anything out of the ordinary."

He stopped typing and turned his head sort of sideways and raised one eyebrow as if studying me. Then he lifted his nose up in the air and pretended to be sniffing something. "Just because you can't smell a rat don't mean there ain't no rat. Some rats know how to use soap, you know!" At that point, we both cracked up.

"Okay, okay, okay," I said. "Point taken."

He pushed a zip drive into my computer and started to download files as I sipped my tea nervously.

"I think it best to mention that my husband is very web-security savvy, and he has every security system you can imagine in place. Don't be disappointed if you're unsuccessful," I said. I think it was the word *unsuccessful* that made him sit bolt upright in his chair.

His easygoing, ex-hippie persona seemed to fall away, and he narrowed his eyes as he peered at me in silence. Then he spoke again with cold steel in his voice. "Honey, I can tell you what President Vladimir Putin had for breakfast and how many bowel movements he has in a day!"

My jaw dropped, and now I was sitting bolt upright. He held me in his steely gaze for a few moments, and now I could see this other strong, tenacious side of him.

Then he started laughing and fell back in his chair, spitting cookie crumbs onto my nicely vacuumed rug. I started laughing as well and I said, "You got me on that one."

"Oh no," he said, "don't think I was joking." There was something about Hank the Hacker that I really liked. He obviously had some serious layers of professional expertise, but he had also integrated them into a super nice guy with a great sense of humor.

"Do you have a wireless printer?" he asked.

"Sure," I said. "It is upstairs, though."

"Please bring it down. Bob wants a paper trail. If you have any rewards statements from credit cards, please bring them too."

I ran off to get the printer and statements. *Rewards? What on Earth is he going to do with them? I thought he was going after important stuff.* When I returned, I placed the printer near his laptops and plugged it in. "I need to get my access code for the wireless service," I said.

"No need," he said, and he started typing on my laptop. I hadn't given him my security code to get in and was surprised to see him typing away in my personal email system. Then the printer kicked on, and two pieces of paper shot out.

In a rather demanding voice, I asked, "Okay, how did you just do that? I have a three-password-access security system on my laptop. Nobody, repeat, *nobody* should be able to get into it!"

His fingers ran over my keyboard. Without moving his head, he flashed his eyes up at me and broke into a grin, showing a partly chewed cookie in his mouth.

No French kisses for this guy.

He reached for the rewards statements that I had placed near him.

"But I thought you were going after the big financial info," I said.

He looked up at me. "Well, I have to say your husband has done a good job protecting his financials. He has really done his homework. He has built an electronic fortress that has sealed windows, a heavily bolted front door, and barbed wire all around it, with attack-and-kill dogs patrolling the perimeter."

"Does that mean we cannot get into it?" I asked.

"Not at all," he shot back. "There ain't nothing that can stop me. Only thing is, if I go in the front door, he may be able to see my footsteps, even though he will not know whose footsteps they are. That may scare him. So, I am going in through the servant's entrance, where I will be invisible. In other words, I can get in through the rewards statements because everything has an electronic connection."

I sat quietly, sipping my tea, as he rattled his fingers across the two black laptops. "Please don't be disappointed if my husband is squeaky clean. We don't know for sure if he is playing any games. This is more Bob's instincts than my not trusting him."

Hacker Hank gave me another sideways glance and said quietly, "Peace of mind is what I want for you, honey. That's all."

He picked up the rewards statements and started to study them.

"Why are these rewards in your name? Where are the rewards that come from his credit card spending?" he asked.

"Well," I began a little shamefully, "he wanted the credit cards in my name so that he could use them without transactions showing up on his accounts directly. Untraceable by the IRS, is what he told me."

Hank widened his eyes as if in disbelief over what I had just told him.

"I am a very trusting person, you know," I said rather weakly, trying to justify this odd credit card arrangement.

Then he said, "You have a bucket load of free air miles here. Where did they come from?"

I knew the answer to that question. "They come from his monthly business trips, which take him all over the world. To Europe, the Far East, even to South America. He has been accruing air miles for the last two years. That's why there are so many of them. He kept saying he would take me with him, but he never did."

Hank said he was going to do an "analysis of origin" search on the air miles.

I began to feel nervous. After a few minutes, he hit the printer button, and three pages shot out. Hank pulled them out of the printer and handed them to me with a serious look.

The first date on the sheet was two years ago, when David started his world travels. For the first year, there were twelve postings for Tucson, Arizona. One for each month. Then I looked at the next year's statement, and it had twelve more postings, all to Tucson, Arizona. I felt a cold shiver from head to toe. I picked up the recent statement for the last five months. Same thing, Tucson Arizona listed five times. I felt a knot forming in my stomach. My eyes darted to Hank for an explanation.

He gazed at me expressionless.

Then a deep sense of dread stirred at the bottom of my stomach, and I went pale.

"Sorry," he said. "I've seen this before. Your husband has been going to Tucson for the last twenty-nine months."

"No, No, No!" I said. "There must be some mistake!" I could hear terror in my voice.

"'Fraid so," he said. "Wanna go deeper?"

"What do you mean by deeper?" I shot back.

"Oh, this is just the surface. Now the journey really begins."

I was feeling nauseous. Hank could see I was moving into shock. "Take some big breaths," he said as he studied me closely.

I was feeling cold all over. My throat was tight, and it was hard to speak. I squeaked out a faint, "Go deeper."

His fingers started again like a machine gun going over the keys.

The printer kicked on again. I grabbed the paper it produced. It was a credit card statement, and I scanned it with fear-filled eyes. My name was on the statement, but I knew from the last four digits that it was the card that David used. All I could see were regular business expenditures. I handed it to Hank. He glanced at it and said that it was called a "masking account."

"What the hell is that?"

"Well, this is set up to mask the true expenditures that are incurred in a second, subaccount. There could be one or several sub or feeder credit card accounts under this masking account. These are controlled by a very clever software app called Masquerade. This app is illegal in this country. It takes the feeder account information and formulates it into proportioned numbers that fit under the various IRS limits for business expenditures. This way, it will not trigger an audit from the IRS. Basically, there are fixed amounts that can be written off as overhead and business expenses. The Masquerade program adjusts the figures given to it with a set of logarithms based on the IRS trigger levels. The IRS hates this program but is unable to detect it. It is often used by people who are going into bankruptcy to hide money and, of course, by husbands who are up to no good. It is a kick-ass good program and one that your husband has obviously learned how to use well. What I am going to do now is track the Masquerade program to the sub credit card accounts your husband has created. There may be one or more of these."

With that, Hank the Hacker put his head down and started punching the keyboards on both laptops. I was still in shock. There must be some simple reason for Tucson, Arizona, to keep showing up. A computer error, maybe?

After five minutes, the printer started to whir again. It spat out four sheets, and I grabbed them. There was a new credit card number on the top of the statement. Under it was a lump sum posted to the masking account number. Then there was a list of merchant payments. It seems I had been making regular purchases in Tucson. My sense of nausea started to grow as I read Tucson Hilton, Tucson Happiness Hair Salon, Tucson Lingerie Shop. Tucson Flower Shop.

I tossed the statements on the table, threw myself onto the sofa, burying my head in the pillows, and started to cry. Hank sat quietly behind his computers as I sobbed my heart. I felt invaded, stupid, hurt, cheated, and completely broken as waves of pain-filled tears washed through me. After a few minutes, I felt Hank gently place a hand on my back. In a soft, caring tone, he whispered, "Name what you are feeling with the in breath. Pause and feel it. On the out breath, release it." He kept saying, "Name, feel, and release. Name, feel, and release. Name, feel, and release."

I felt an incredible pain in my heart. It was as if someone had just stuck me with a dagger. My first impulse was to close my heart down to stop myself from feeling. I thought the pain would be too great. But the name, feel, and release process seemed to be releasing the pain that was filling me.

I kept naming, feeling, and breathing. On and on it went. My chest began to feel lighter and freer, and the pain eased. Hank released his hand, and I sat upright. I was still a little dazed but much better than before. Hank sat quietly in the easy chair, watching me.

"Where the hell did you learn to do that?" I asked.

He replied, "An old wood-carver buddy of mine taught me."

"What?" I exclaimed. "You are not talking about a guy called Brock, are you?"

His eyes suddenly opened wide. "You know Brock?"

"Holy crap!" I said. "I don't believe it. So, you know about the three oceans and all?"

He replied, "Know about them? They saved my emotional life!"

"How so?"

He picked up his empty teacup and said, "We still have more to do, but I am happy to share about me later."

Then I noticed that when I threw myself down on the couch, I must have dislodged my wig, and it was sitting sideways, revealing my half-bald head. Hank was studying me. I knew that he knew that I had cancer. He spoke first. "I think we should take a few minutes to talk. How about a fresh cup of tea?"

Without looking directly at him, I took his cup and headed to the kitchen. As the kettle was boiling, I took time to straighten Henry and secure him with some fixing gel.

With our cups of tea, we sat in the comfort of two easy chairs. I felt it best to remain silent and wait for him to talk. He took some sips of his tea. "Well, Jane, I think I should tell you that when I saw the baldness, I knew exactly what it meant. Ya see, my mother, God bless her, is upstairs looking down on me. She developed a very rare form of bone cancer when I was ten. She battled it for seven years and went through various chemotherapy protocols, and she lost her hair many times. I was seventeen when she passed away. I was with her up to the end. For this reason, I have a special place in my heart for people who are battling cancer. I just wanted to tell you that and say that it will only make me more determined to help you resolve this issue with your husband."

I thanked him for his honesty and welcomed anything he could offer to skin my rat of a husband. "So how did you meet Brock?" I asked.

"We both volunteer at a food kitchen. He is one amazing dude," he said, looking at his watch. "We gotta keep this ball in the air, Jane. Okay to get going again?"

I was feeling better and somehow relieved that he knew about my cancer. I was starting to trust this guy and felt better not having to hide it. "What's next?" I asked.

"Pee break for me, and then we start digging," he said.

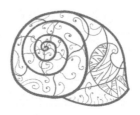

Chapter 53

More Than I Thought

I mentioned to Hank Bob thought there may be a lump sum stashed away somewhere that had come from my husband's earnings. As Hank typed away on his laptops, he said that he had just found a bank link to one of the other sub credit-card accounts David had been using. "Clever guy, this husband of yours," he said.

"*Ex*-husband!" I shot back.

"Found it," he said. "He has been paying one of his sub credit-card accounts from a bank in Tucson. But this is only a fronting bank, so he only keeps the money in there that he needs to maintain his various credit card accounts." He hit the printer button, and two more sheets popped out. He handed one to me and kept one for himself. It was a bank statement for a bank in Tucson with my husband's name on it. I was hoping to see a large amount of money deposited, but there was only around $5,000. "So, no hidden pile of cash, eh?" I said, rather disappointed.

"Not here," Hank said. "He has to have an offshore setup." He started rattling away at the laptops again.

Then he called me over to look at something he had pulled up on his screen. It was a statement from a bank in Chicago for an account I had never seen before.

"This is another fronting account. What I am looking for is probably underneath this one. I can track it by his transfer records, which are kept private by his bank in Tucson. He pays large bank fees for this service, which ultimately protects everything he wants to hide, especially from the IRS. I helped design the firewall the bank uses," he said with a smug smirk. "Just gotta decode some encrypted passwords, and we should be good to go." He kept typing.

"Ah-ha!" he said. "Another masking account. Gee, this dude is good. But not good enough." Two more documents shot out of the printer. I took one and handed one to him. This was another statement from a bank in Chicago with next to nothing in the account.

Hank scrutinized the statement and then said, "Got it! Now I can see the hidden link to the offshore account. This is how he sends in money to keep the credit-card payments on track. Three more minutes, and I should have what you want."

I sipped my tea.

After some furious typing, he sat back in his chair and put his hands behind his head with his elbows spread like wings. He was looking rather satisfied with himself. "So, Jane, do you have any idea as to the amount Bob or you are looking for in terms of squirreled-away cash?"

"I have no idea," I said. "Perhaps twenty or thirty thousand dollars?"

Hank smiled and hit the printer button. I moved quickly to the printer and eagerly pulled out the first sheet. It was yet another bank statement, and it was for Irving Bank in Bermuda. I looked at the balance and was shocked to see $830,000. My mouth dropped open.

"Guess you had no idea, eh?" he said.

I felt excited and frightened. "But he is controlling this money. Is there any way I can get any of it back?"

"Let me check the bank's operating mandate." He pulled up some legal-looking documents and started to read them. Then he said, "We're good to go because it was your salary check they registered, so you are the primary signer on the account. I don't want to say too much too soon, but I can say that so far, it's looking good."

He kept rattling away at the keys. "Thought so," he said. "Seems like he is buying a home in Tucson with someone else. Here are the agent-fee withdrawals. The name of the Realtor is Davis and Clark. There is a bank transfer withdrawal order pending, which will close this account in Bermuda. Seems that there is a sixty-day notice period that is being served, which explains why he does not want to trigger the divorce. You see, all offshore banks are linked to the national divorce register to make sure their clients are not going through divorce. This is to prevent husbands from doing what your husband is trying to do and hide the money from you. If your husband's name appeared on the national divorce register, then the bank in Bermuda would freeze the account until it received clearance from a divorce court. Once this transfer goes through, the money will vanish and will not be traceable."

I was in shock. The roses, the dinner, and the pearls were all a ploy for time. "Makes me want to throw up," I said.

"We have to move quickly, Jane," Hank said. "Pull up your online banking account."

I promptly did as he requested.

Then he told me to hit the "open new account" tab and set up a new bank account under my name only. Because my husband and I were customers of long standing, we had the ambassador privileges for opening new accounts. Only problem was, to have it opened immediately online, I needed a special code from a notary who was registered in the bank's system. "We're stumped!" I said and explained the problem.

Hank responded, "They set this notary application process up several years ago to help people who had lost a spouse manage their money without going to probate. The good news is..." He paused as he reached into his bag and pulled out a small, black, velvet bag and waved it in the air.

"So, what's in there?" I asked. "A white rabbit?"

He smiled and pulled out a notary's stamp. "I am registered with every bank in the country through my work with the FBI. All I have to do is email my ID into the bank, using my special email address, and you are good to go."

I was in shock.

Then he asked me how many accounts we currently had with this bank. I said we only had one. He grunted and hit the print button. I grabbed the sheet from the printer and saw that it was from our bank, but from another account. I could see the large deposits and the large transfers to the bank in Chicago. "What the hell is this?" I asked.

"They call it a sleeper account," he explained. "It is a facility the bank created for people who work the stock market. It allows you instant access to funds that are transferred instantaneously to any bank, including foreign banks. It was designed for stock traders, but it is also used by crap bags like your husband for squirreling away cash. Your husband has been using this sleeper account to hide and transfer his earnings, which is your money."

He started to read some legal jargon. Next thing, he jumped up and punched his fist into the air. "Yes! Yes! Yes!"

"Yes what?" I asked.

"The account David set up in the offshore bank in Bermuda has a retro deposit facility that allows funds to be returned to the bank of origin instantaneously upon request. Once again, this was set up for people who worked the stock market, so they could respond quickly to market opportunities. Your husband chose this particular account so that he would always have quick access to move and hide the money.

"Your husband is just a little too smart for his own good." Hank had a mischievous grin on his face. He started punching the keys again. "Ooooh!" he exclaimed. "Seems your husband is buying a home with a Cathy Jones, 47 Wayside Avenue, Tucson, Arizona.

"What? The bitch!" I screamed.

"Whoa!" Hank said. "Look at your energy. How are you feeling?"

I said I felt angry and bitter toward this woman who had stolen my husband.

He asked, "How do you know that she knows that he is married?"

That stopped me in my tracks. "Well, I don't!"

Hank asked if Brock had shared the sunflower story and how, by only seeing the surface layer, we did not see the truth. I was aware of how much poisonous energy I was creating by assuming this Cathy Jones was guilty. In truth, I did not know. I could see that I was on an emotional roller coaster, and it was really chewing me up inside. I sat back and closed my eyes to process the events through the lens of the sunflower story. A good way to test a philosophy is to see what happened when the shit hits the fan. And a tractor-trailer load of shit had just hit my fan. As I began to process the events through this lens, I could feel inner shifts, and a warm peace returned to me.

I knew Hank was concerned for me. After several minutes, I opened my eyes and felt tremendous peace. Just minutes before, I had felt anger and rage, but now, there was just a great feeling of peace. "Holy crap!" I said. "Now I see how this process works. What's next?"

He started hitting keys on the laptop again. "Ah-ha!" he said. "I have a cell phone number for Cathy Jones. She used it with the Realtor. Wanna call her?"

I suddenly felt threatened. But I was aware that I was seeing only my own projections about Cathy Jones and perhaps there was more to this than I had surmised. I went silent for a few moments. Then I nodded in agreement. I would call Cathy Jones.

Hank picked up the phone and handed it to me. "Eight o'clock here, six o'clock in Tucson. Truth and courage, Jane!" Hank said as he pushed a piece of paper with her number on it toward me.

I gave him a narrow-eyed look as if to say, *You really are a pain in the ass, you know!*

He smiled and reminded me to stand like a warrior when I called. As instructed, I stood up tall like a warrior, sucked in a deep breath, and punched in her number. Hank picked up the extension to listen in.

The phone started ringing. I was expecting an answering machine. Then a woman picked up, and I was shocked to hear her say, "Hello, David, darling. It's your honey bunny here!"

I swallowed hard and almost smashed the phone on the table in anger. Then Hank started tapping his heart as a sign that I had to stay in the golden ocean. I sucked in another deep breath and said in a strong but kind tone, "Hello, Cathy. My name is Jane, and I wondered if you have a few minutes to talk."

"Who are you?" she asked.

"I am Jane, David's wife of twenty-four years."

I heard a loud gasp. Then came, "No, no, no! There must be some mistake here. David is not married! He lives with his mother, who is seriously ill with cancer and has just weeks to live!"

In a gentle tone of voice, I said, "Sorry, Cathy. That is one big lie. He has betrayed both of us!"

I heard sobbing on the line. Then came, "I am so, so sorry. I am so, so sorry!" and the sobbing continued.

I was surprised to hear myself say, "Breathe, feel, and release, Cathy. Breathe, feel, and release."

The sobbing went on for a few minutes, and then she said. "Oh, Jane, I feel awful. I just had no idea. He said his mother was seriously ill and I should never call this number for fear of disturbing her. He called me from time to time when, as he said, his mother was sleeping. I feel so bad for both of us. How did I ever get sucked into this lie? I feel confused and don't know what to do."

Hacker Hank gestured with his arm that he wanted to join the conversation. I said to Cathy, "Listen, I have a friend who can help us with this. I am going to ask him to jump into this conversation, okay?"

"Sure," she said.

"Hi, Cathy, my name is Hank, and I am a friend of Jane's. Sorry to meet you under these disturbing circumstances, but I am a bit of a tech guy and want to help you and Jane resolve the property purchase you are involved in with David."

She gasped. "Oh yes! But how do you know about that?"

He replied, "As I said, ma'am, I am a tech guy. I'm helping Jane to straighten things out and I would be happy to work with you to get your money back."

"Oh, could you?" she replied.

"Sure can," he said. "Let me put you on speaker so I can check some things out on the internet while I have you on the line."

Hank went back to his laptop and started punching the keys. Then he started talking on the speaker phone. "Seems the new home is in both your names. You each put five thousand dollars down as a deposit with the cash balance arriving in two weeks when you will close on the property. Sound right, Cathy?"

She seemed a little shocked. "Well, er, yes. But how do you know all this?"

Hank chuckled. "Well, I ain't just any old kind of hacker, you know. Now, let me check some things out about your contract with the Realtor." He hit more keys. "Good news!" he said. "You both transferred your deposits into the Realtor's account. I can easily transfer it back out, but the full balance will go direct to your account. In your contract, there is a 20 percent penalty for early withdrawal, so you will see eight thousand dollars arriving first thing to-morrow. What I suggest is that you open a new checking account with a new bank and transfer everything in this old account to the new account, then close this account. I suggest you do this ASAP, as he is going to know about this in forty-eight hours.

"Then I suggest you send David's portion of the deposit—three thousand dollars—to Jane once you get your new checks. How does that sound?"

"I would rather split the eight thousand and send Jane four thousand," Cathy said. "Given the circumstances, I feel this is the fair way to go. I will take care of this first thing in the morning before I go to work."

"Nice suggestion," Hank said. "I will email you the mailing address."

"I...ah...don't know how to thank you both for helping me resolve this." Cathy sounded very emotional. "You saved me from one mega-sized asshole! Again Jane, I am so, so sorry that I got suckered into this, and thank you for being so gracious."

I asked Cathy if we might talk in a couple of weeks.

"That would mean a great deal to me, Jane," Cathy responded, and we hung up.

Hank was sitting back in his chair with his arms up and hands behind his head again. "Almost there," he said. "We just gotta move a big chunk of dough around for you." Hank pushed his teacup toward me, and I headed to the kitchen to put the kettle on.

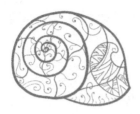

Chapter 54

Transferring a Big Chunk of Change

As I returned with cups of tea and a fresh plate of cookies, Hank was busy on his laptop. Without taking his eyes of the computer screen, he took a cookie and pushed the whole thing into his mouth at once. Then he took a sip of tea, all without looking up. "Got it!" he announced. "Because your name is on your regular bank account, I can transfer everything from the Bermuda account in one lump right into your new account. Just make sure that your new bank account has automatic notification to the IRS. The IRS will automatically take 40 percent of this amount as standard procedure. You will see a credit of $830,000 in your new account with a debit entry of $332,000 paid to the IRS, and a balance of $498,000.

"I am going to set the time for this transaction at end of day today. This means that he will receive notification six hours after the banks open tomorrow. This will give us time to enact a final ritual of parting for you."

"Final ritual of parting? What is that?" I asked.

He beamed a big smile at me and said, "This is the fun part. You so deserve this, Jane. But we have one more thing to do. I call it the final act."

"What is that?" I asked.

"This is your chance to orchestrate your final meeting with David when you can cut the cheater down to size," he replied.

"How do I do that?"

"How do *we* do that," he corrected. He started to type again. Then he stopped and said, "I see that his BMW is leased in your name. Let me check the lease company. Ah! Good news. I know the manager of this leasing company. This is a slam dunk. And then there is your husband's phone; I see this is in your name as well. This is really cool."

"Oh yeah?" I asked. "What exactly are you up to?"

"You'll see," he said spitting a few crumbs in my direction.

He took another sip of tea and started to talk in a slow, calculated way. "Okay, it begins with the transfer from the offshore bank at end of day today. I need Bob to file the divorce papers tomorrow promptly at 9:00 a.m. They will appear on the register at 10:00 a.m. David will have the bank's early notification app that will notify him at 10:30 a.m. At 10:31 a.m., he will call you in panic," Hank said. "You need to sound very innocent and surprised to hear that Bob filed the divorce papers. How far is his office from your home?"

"About twenty minutes," I replied.

"You will offer to resolve this right away and ask him to come by at eleven," Hank said. "I'm going to email my friend at the car-lease company and have a tow truck here at 11:05. I'll tell them that you won't be making any more payments, and they will be appreciative of the heads-up. It will save them the usual legal fees when people default on their payments. They'll be very cooperative with us. You need to terminate his phone service at 11:10 a.m. tomorrow as well. You can go online to do that."

I liked the thought of David losing his BMW, but how he would get back to his office? Then I thought of the blue bicycle that I'd bought for him that he was too haughty to ride. Now was the time. I would leave it outside the garage the following morning. It felt a little spiteful, but the idea of lowering the saddle to make him look awkward just seemed the right and fair thing to do. The visual I saw of him in my imagination cycling with his knees up around his chin made me smile.

Hank packed up his computers and said he would be here at 9:00 a.m. the next day for the party. He grabbed a cookie and headed out.

I felt exhausted and crashed on the couch. As I reflected on the last couple of hours, I began to think about Brock. My heart began to quicken. My heart was truly connected to his. I thought about his scent, his touch, his eyes lingering on me. I thought about his kiss on my cheek and his moist lips, which would soon meet mine.

I imagined inviting him to my home and cooking an amazing candlelit dinner for him. My offering myself to him would coincide with his desire to take me. I began to feel a warm stir of energy down in my groin.

Then I thought, *Underwear!* Mine was mostly the old, functional, granny type. It was time for an excursion to the new lingerie store downtown, Aphrodite's Allure. I guessed I could get some nice, flimsy little things for $498,000.

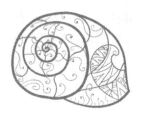

Chapter 55

A Sweet Good-bye

I woke up with mixed feelings. A part of me was looking forward to taking down my crap ass of a husband. Yet a part of me was also a little nervous. This type of aggressive behavior was not something I was used to. But the sweet taste of revenge was now on my lips, and it was really juicy. Then my thoughts shifted to Brock. My husband had been a smoke screen, preventing me from seeing all that Brock had come to mean to me. Brock made my heart race. His touch stirred sensuous forces deep within me that I thought were lost to me forever. And his eyes, they were like oceans I wanted to launch my all into.

Now I was ready to claim the love that I knew existed between us. Only the final act of destroying David awaited. And today was the day. I sprang from bed like a Navy SEAL on a mission. At 8:45 a.m., I put a pot of coffee on for Hank. Then I went to the garage to lower the saddle on the blue bike and left it outside so David could easily see it. At 9:00 a.m., there was a knock on the door. I swung it open and Hacker Hank was standing there in a slim-fitting checked shirt that gave his six-foot-three-inch frame a very powerful presence.

"Morning, Jane! A question for you," he said. "Do you have a dog?"

He had seen the numerous dog poops on the lawn and had not seen the dog that was responsible. I smiled and told him my lovely, eighty-three-year-old neighbor, Doris, and Duke.

Hank smiled as he walked in and started to set up his laptops. I went to the kitchen to pour the coffee, and within minutes I heard him rattling away on his keyboards, making the final tweaks to our game plan. As I walked in with his coffee, he asked me to get the offshore bank statements ready, along with the letter from Cathy Jones. I flipped on my laptop and found an email from Bob.

Hey, Sis. Confirming I am set to file divorce papers electronically at 9:00 a.m. your time as requested. Hugs and love, Bob.

The game plan was coming together well. Then another email arrived from the BMW leasing company. It confirmed that the collection of the vehicle would take place at my residence at 11:05 a.m., as requested. I was beginning to feel excited.

Hank wanted to review how it was to play out. When David arrived, I was to go out the front door and stand on the porch, looking down at the path where David would be standing. I was to ask him to stay on the path and not approach me on the front porch. "I want you looking down at this piece of crap when you execute our game plan. Okay?" said Hank.

"Okay with me," I said.

At 9:10 a.m., Bob sent an email confirming that the divorce papers had been filed. Operation Kick David's Ass was underway. We had some time to kill until 10:30, so I made some eggs and toast. I placed my phone in front of me, ready for the call that was due to arrive just past 10:30.

At 10:35, my phone rang, making me jump. Caller ID told me it was David. I let it ring and ring, then picked up. "Hello, darling!" I said.

David's voice was urgent. "Jane, the divorce papers have been filed. What's going on?"

"Oh really?" I said with a pretend innocence. "Must have been my attorney. Let me check with him and get back to you."

"You have to stop this!" David barked.

"Of course, darling," I said. "Would you like to come over so that we can resolve this together?"

"Yes!" he said

"Would eleven work for you?"

"Yes!" came the reply, and he abruptly hung up.

I felt my heart racing in a good way. Hank gave me a sideways smile and said, "Oh, I like the *darling* bit! Very smooth!" We both laughed.

At a couple of minutes before the hour, I walked out the front porch with my papers in hand. At eleven o'clock, David's large, white, BMW sped around the corner and screeched to a halt outside the house. David leaped out of the car and started running up the front path. He was dressed in smart tan slacks and a crisp white shirt with the sleeves rolled up. As he came close to the porch, I pointed my finger at him and in a strong voice told him to stop there. He stopped abruptly and said, "What are you doing?"

I said, "Darling, I have a question for you."

"What?" he asked impatiently.

With a steel tone in my voice, I said, "So, darling, I am curious, where did all of my frequent flyer miles come from?"

He held me in a questioning gaze as he pondered the question. "From my trips to my clients all around the country," he said impatiently. "I told you that months ago!"

"So, which one of your clients lives in Tucson?" I asked.

He was now staring at me through narrowed eyes. He paused to think before he answered. "Well, ah, that is a Mr. Biggs."

"So, as part of your financial consulting service, do you have to purchase lingerie and flowers for him?" I asked.

An angry frown appeared on his forehead. He paused for a few seconds again before answering. "What makes you think I have been buying lingerie and flowers?" he asked suspiciously.

I pulled out the credit card report that itemized his purchases. "On this credit-card purchase report, it says that you bought lingerie in Tucson. Well?"

He seemed to be caught off guard. "Er, oh that? Oh yeah, now I remember. Mr. Bigg is going through some marriage challenges with his wife, and he asked to pick up some things for him on my way from the airport."

Was this guy slippery or what?

Then David regrouped and barked at me. "Where the hell did you get that credit card report from?"

With a pretend innocence in my voice, I said, "Oh honey, you know I am the curious type, right? So, darling," I said, completely ignoring his question, "tell me why your air-miles statement shows that you have been going to Tuscan once a month for the past two years."

Anger flashed across his face. "Where the hell did you get that from?"

"Well, darling, you know I have a curious streak in me. Oink, oink oink!"

He looked at me puzzled and asked what the oink, oink, oink meant.

With steel and strength in my voice, I replied, "You are a lying pig, and I am speaking to you in your language!"

His face suddenly became very dark, and his eyes flashed rage at me. In the distance, I heard the tow truck. Right on time, it pulled up in front of David's BMW. He spun around quickly to see what was going on. A short, stocky man got out and started to pull out the tow wire. When David realized his car was going to be towed, he sprinted toward the tow truck, cursing and swearing. Then the passenger door of the tow truck opened, and out came a huge character with tattoos on his neck and forearms. He must have been six foot five, and he looked as if he'd just come from a wrestling ring. He was chewing on a toothpick. I was looking at a mountain of a man built of muscle and sinew. He stood menacingly with his legs apart and his hands on his hips. When David saw him, he screeched to a halt. The tattooed man said to him, "Is there a problem here, little man? I use sticks like you for toothpicks!" Then he spat his toothpick in David's direction.

David turned to look at me, and his face was burning red with anger. As he started to walk back toward me, I could sense rage emanating from every cell in his body.

Ever since I met David, I'd had the sense that a dark, angry, violent side to him lurked somewhere in his shadowy inner terrain. I saw it once when, in a flash of rage, he slammed a kitchen cabinet door, smashing it to pieces. Then there was the time when he caught Duke pooping on the lawn. He flew into rage and came very close to kicking the dog. I ask you, wanting to kick a poor old three-legged dog? Then he phoned the police and reported Doris. This showed me that he also had a vengeful side to his nature. His polished professional persona had mostly covered it up, but now huge cracks were appearing, and a very nasty, spiteful, little man was emerging. As he walked toward me, I saw him clench his fists into balls.

I felt a flash of cold fear. Had I pushed him too far? Would he unleash his poisonous, violent rage at me? I had nowhere to run, and I could not match his strength. My breathing became shallow, and I felt a chill all over. I remembered this story about the time he got into a fistfight at school. He told me proudly how he had permanently marked the face of the other boy with his fingernails. He was violent, nasty, and headed toward me. I imagined the headlines in the paper: Wife Beaten Almost to Death. Face Permanently Disfigured. I was in fear for my life.

"Stop! Stop! Stop!" I shouted nervously.

He kept coming. He was just a couple of paces away when I heard the front door open, and out walked a very muscular six-foot-three-inch tall Hank with his shirt wide open, revealing a very hairy chest. David stopped dead in his tracks. In his lazy Southern drawl, Hank very coolly said, "Hey, Jane. Just wanted to let you know I made the bed."

David's jaw dropped open in shock, and he froze like a statue. I picked up immediately on Hank's lead. I turned and said in a light, flirty tone, "Oh, thank you, honey. I'll put some eggs on shortly."

The appearance of Hank had suddenly put steel back into my spine, and with a stern look, I said to David, "Game is up, douchebag!"

David was silent for a moment, then he let loose angrily. "Okay, okay. So, I have a honey in Tucson. That is where my true happiness now exists. I am out of here to start my new life in Tucson."

I pulled out my purse and said, "Would you like some spending money?"

"Screw you," he barked at me. "I gotta nice little pot of cash stashed away that you can't get your sticky hands on."

"Oh," I said as I pulled out the statement from the bank in Bermuda. "Would the name Irving Bank in Bermuda mean anything to you?"

"What?" he screamed at me. "What have you been up to?"

I leaned forward and offered him the statement showing a zero balance. He snatched it out of my hand and scanned it quickly. Then he shouted, "You can't do this! Half of this is mine!"

"*Was* yours, darling!" I said. "Lying and cheating are expensive hobbies, you know! Oh, and, for your peace of mind, for the time being, the money is in an account that has an IRS reporting link. I don't need to remind you that this means that the IRS will not audit me, but it might audit you. Between you and me, darling, I don't think prison clothing would hang well on you!"

Hank turned away, trying to contain his laughter.

David stood frozen as he pondered what I was saying. When the penny dropped, he barked at me. "Take it, take it. See what I care. I have a sweetheart waiting for me, the true love of my life, so it's happily ever after for me. Ha ha ha. Last laugh is on you!"

Then I said, "Oh, did I mention that I have a new friend called Cathy Jones? We had a lovely chat, and it seems that she mistakenly thought that your mother was in hospice care. And for some reason, she did not know about me, your wife."

"What?" he screamed. "You stay away from her, you hear?"

With a cold steel in my voice, I said, "Too late, asshole. Your game of deceit and lying is up!"

David stood there pale, dazed, and staring into space. Slowly, he pulled out his phone to call a cab. He tried to find a ring tone and then realized his phone was dead.

"Got a problem with your phone, honey?" I asked. He quickly understood that I had cut his service, and he angrily tossed the phone into a bush.

He turned toward me, looking very much like a pathetic and broken man. "So, how do I get back to the office?" he asked.

I gestured toward the blue bicycle. He rolled his eyes as a fresh wave of angst washed over his face. He was looking at me as he turned and toward the bicycle. He did not see the very large, fresh, slippery poop Duke had left earlier that morning. His right foot shot out from under him, and he landed on his butt, slap bang in the poop. In his attempt to break his fall, he thrust his left arm out, and it found another poop left by Duke. Now he had poop all over his pants, hands, arm, and shirt.

I heard Hank collapse with laughter behind me. David stood up very slowly, looking disgusted and shamed. I glared at him from under my lowered eyebrows and pointed to the blue bicycle by the garage door. Hank was still rolling around on the porch behind me, guffawing. The two guys in the tow truck had been watching, and now they, too, were laughing.

David stomped across the lawn toward the blue bicycle. He angrily jerked it away from the garage door and swung his poop-covered leg over the saddle. The lowered seat was the perfect touch. He looked like a lost little boy as he rode away hunched over the handlebars, his knees coming up to his chest as he pedaled. And that was the last time I saw him. He was riding off like a petulant little kid in search of his mother. A more glorious sight had never met my eyes!

I turned to Hacker Hank, who was still rolling around on the porch, holding his side.

Then, a big bubble burst inside me, and I fell to my knees and joined him, guffawing with laughter. This went on for several minutes, then I heard my phone ring. The caller ID told me it was my brother. I took the call.

"You okay, Sis?" came his concerned question.

In between bursts of laughter, I said, "I have never felt better. This guy Hank is one hell of a cool-ass guy!" I put the phone on speaker and lifted it into the air so that my brother could hear Hank's laughter.

"Way to go!" Bob said. "Shoot me an email later and let me know what went down, okay?"

"Sure, big brother. Oh, and one more thing. I love you!"

Hank and I headed into the house to put on a fresh pot of coffee.

As we reflected on the morning's adventure, I thought about the words of Winston Churchill: "This is a day that will live in infamy!"

Oh yeah, baby...what a day of infamy it was! Hank packed up his laptops. Then I remembered about the name, feel, and release process.

"When can we chat about the name, feel, and release process?" I asked.

He thought for a while and said, "In two days, I am heading out of town for a week. We can either get together tomorrow at 7:00 a.m. in the coffee shop or when I come back."

"Tomorrow works just fine for me!" I quickly replied.

"Great. See you at 7:00 a.m.," he said, and he gave me a hug as he headed out.

As I sat cradling my warm coffee mug, my thoughts went to Brock. It was time to make my move. I needed to cook him the best dinner of his life and show him just who this passionate, red-hot mamma really was. Then I thought of his lips, the scent of pine mingling with his body perfume. My thoughts went mischievously to my bedroom. It needed a good clean, a supply of candles, and some satin sheets. And how about my lingerie? Yikes! Red light on that one! Since David left, I had been wearing old granny knickers. I needed something flimsy in black lace. Then I remembered the lingerie store that had recently opened downtown called Aphrodite's Allure. Suddenly, I had a use for some of that $498,000.

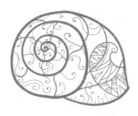

Chapter 56

The Name, Feel, and Release Process

As I sat cradling my coffee mug, I felt a sense of sadness deep inside me. This surprised me. Removing David from my life the day before seemed to go really well. But I was feeling sad that our relationship had turned out the way it did. I was also deeply hurt by his betrayal. As I lay in bed, I started to do the name, feel, and release process.

It really seemed to lift the heaviness in my chest. I was surprised at how quickly I was able to lighten my mood. The thought of seeing Hank for early morning coffee cheered me up, and I enthusiastically hopped into the shower. With warm water running down my naked body, I thought about Brock, and a naughty visual of Brock sharing this shower with me popped into my thoughts.

I arrived at the coffee shop a few minutes before seven. As I walked in, I noticed Hank at the corner table, pounding away on his laptop. He glanced up and gave me a wave, gesturing for me to get a coffee and join him. I walked to the counter, and Mare was there with a big smile and large latte waiting for me. "You are too much!" I said.

She blew me a kiss and said, "Love ya, sweetie!"

When I arrived at his table, Hank had put his laptop away and was sitting very peacefully, looking out the window. As I eased my steaming latte onto the table and took a seat, he smiled at me. "Frickin' awesome day yesterday!" he said. "I laughed all the way home!"

"Yeah!" I said. "And I am so, so grateful for all that you have done for me."

"Hey, that big ugly brother of yours owes me now!" he said, and we both laughed.

Then he asked me how I was doing. I told him about waking up feeling sad and low, and how my outlook had shifted with the name, feel, and release process.

"To be expected," he said. "You ended your twenty-four-year marriage yesterday after a betrayal. That is one of the hardest ways for a relationship to end. It has a way of negating the good bits, and there must have been many. The deep emotions you stirred yesterday will reverberate in you for some time to come."

I reiterated how much the name, feel, and release process helped me and told Hank that I wanted to learn more.

After taking a long sip of his coffee, he said, "Well, we have another name for this process, which is 'bye-bye blues.' Brock gave it this name because the people he taught it to kept saying how it helped them shift the blues. He is the real teacher of this process, but I am happy to share with you what I know, and he can fill in any gaps. As I understand it, the Shaolin monks developed the process to help the villagers with sudden emotional trauma and shock. As with a physical wound, there is a need for quick action that helps to support and empower the longer healing process. When we experience a form of emotional trauma, as you did the other day, we are deluged with pain that could be overwhelming. If this pain is not cleared, it forms into a mass of congealed energy that is hard to release. This is why people can carry emotional hurts all through their lives, never releasing them. Sometimes, they manifest into physical illnesses.

"As you learned yesterday, the key to emotional pain is to release it, but first it needs to be felt. People find it hard to release emotional pain because they naturally resist feeling it. But by linking it to the breath, a very natural and controlled healing and releasing process unfolds. This process can be used for any form of emotional pain and can be used as a regular tool for emotional maintenance. In the same way we keep our bodies clean, this is a wonderful tool for keeping our emotional bodies clean. The beauty of the process it that you do not always have to know the actual cause of the hurtful emotion. Sometimes, long-held emotions bubble up to the surface, and it is hard to determine the origin of the pain. This process is like a magical bar of soap for the emotions. I often use it in the morning, when some emotional pain may have bubbled up during the night.

"The other day, I took you through a quick version. How about I go over the full process for you now?"

"That would be great," I said.

He took another long sip of his coffee. "There are four parts to the process, which is done over one full breath. There are pauses on the inhale and exhale, hence four parts. The first part is to name the feeling during the in breath. This provides a sort directive for your awareness to locate the emotion in you. Once you have named the emotion, then you need to feel it, which gets it ready for release. Feeling the emotion is done when you pause after the inhale. Once you have felt the emotion, it can be released with a long out breath through an open mouth. I often imagine a stream of black smoke pouring out of me and vanishing into the air. After you have exhaled the sadness, you then pause with empty lungs and visualize golden light inside of yourself. These are the four parts, and each should take between five and seven seconds. It is best to practice the breath by itself first, so you create the natural pattern of deep breathing and breath retention. Once you have balanced the in and out breaths with pauses, you can easily apply the process to the breath. You can do this for any emotion you want to shift.

"Just to recap, you name the emotion, feel the emotion, and release the emotion. You fill yourself with golden light," Hank said. "You can use this process for any form of emotional release. I used it last year when my dog passed away. I was really heartbroken, and I would wake up each morning grieving with a very heavy heart. The first thing I did before getting out of bed was to take three or four of these emotionally cleansing breaths. The problem with grief—or any form of emotional hurt—is that unless we have a way to gently release the emotions, they congeal and stick with us, turning into depression and moodiness. I used to resist feeling emotional pain because I was frightened that it would overwhelm me. With this process, I can feel my emotional pain in bite-size pieces and release it gradually.

"There are three core emotions that I cleanse myself of most days," Hank said. "These are sadness, loneliness, and pain. I can feel and release these emotions without having to know their origin.

"I am interested in keeping up with daily news, but sometimes it can leave me feeling sad and upset. So, before I go to bed, I like to do a couple of these cleansing release breaths. This also works well for anger that can turn into toxic energy if we carry it for extended periods of time. The process helps to release the emotional charge of anger, which is helpful in finding resolution.

"Being a very sensitive person means that I often feel the empathetic pain of others. Once again, this process helps me to release it." Hacker Hank took a sip of his coffee and asked if I had any questions.

I was feeling good about the bye-bye blues process and thanked him for his time.

He looked at his watch and said he had to run. We stood and hugged, and he headed out. I sat quietly with my back to the counter, looking out the window and pondering the bye-bye blues process—yet another amazing tool I could use on my quest for love and healing. I took a few quiet moments and then headed to the office.

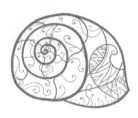

Chapter 57

My New Doctor

I arrived at the office early and before starting work, I checked my personal email.

There was one from the new doctor in New York. I was suddenly thrust back into the world of cancer. I felt excited and nervous as I opened her email.

Dear Jane.

I have reviewed your medical information and would like to talk with you. Please call my office at your earliest convenience.

Dr. Julie.

Without hesitation, I dialed her number. The receptionist picked up. She was very chirpy and put me through to Dr. Julie's secretary. "Hello, Jane," she said in an upbeat manner. "I know Dr. Julie wants to speak with you. She has just gone into a team meeting. Let me see if she can take your call."

She put on some elevator music. Then came a clicking sound, and a warm, relaxed voice, said, "Hi, Jane. This is Dr. Julie. Thank you for calling so quickly. I wanted to speak with you because I have reviewed your files and wanted to run an idea by you. First, I should mention that I have shown your file to two of my colleagues here in the clinic who are also breast cancer specialists, and they fully endorse what I am about to share with you.

"We have a new treatment protocol here that is only available in five centers around the country. Your doctor probably knows about it, but she does not have access to it yet. Your cancer is stage two, and we have been treating stage-four cancer patients who have responded well to it. I have a sense that your cancer would also respond well to this treatment. I wanted to invite you in for an interview so that we can explore the possibility of you becoming a part of this treatment protocol. How does this sound to you?"

Without hesitation, I said, "Tell me when and where."

"Oh good!" said Dr. Julie. "Short notice, but I have just had a cancelation for a ten o'clock appointment tomorrow morning. Would this be an option?"

"Tell me where and what I need to bring," I shot back.

"Oh wonderful, Jane. I have your up-to-date medical records. We will need about ninety minutes of your time. My nurses will work with you for around thirty minutes, taking blood and doing some tests. I will plan to spend around sixty minutes with you, looking at your lifestyle and psychological profile in depth, to make sure this new treatment protocol is a good fit for both of us. The address for our clinic is included in the email I sent to you. If you need any help in finding us, please call my assistant Rosemary."

"Sounds fabulous to me!" I said. "I am so grateful that you are doing this for me."

"Dar has told me wonderful things about you," Dr. Julie said, "and she is very dear to me. I consider it an honor to be working with you."

I thanked her again, and we hung up.

I felt a buzz of good energy from head to toe. It was as if a bright light of hope just got turned on. I had an immediate sensation that I was important, and not just my cancer. I shot a text to Goth Girl to update her and thank her. Next was an email to my boss requesting the day off.

For the rest of the day, I had difficulty focusing on my work. Thoughts about my new doctor and my impending trip to New York kept whizzing around in my head. Eventually, five o'clock came, and I headed home. I decided that Henry deserved a nice shampoo and blow dry for our day in New York.

I slept well and arrived at the train station several minutes early. It gave me a few moments to run the three ocean spirals to center myself. First was the blue ocean of gratitude. Then came the white ocean of deep peace. And third was the golden ocean of being loved by Divine Presence. I was glowing as I boarded the train for New York. I found a nice window seat and snuggled down with my music for the seventy-five-minute train ride.

After a ten-minute cab ride, I arrived at a tall and dignified-looking gray stone building. In the lobby, I found the name of my new doctor on the third floor, suite 7. As I stood waiting for the elevator, I was feeling excited but also a little nervous. A lot of questions were rumbling around in my head. Would I qualify for this new protocol? Would I like my new doctor? Would this save my breasts? Would this cure me? I checked my watch and noticed that I was thirty minutes early for my appointment. What to do? I decided to show up early and spend time in the waiting room.

As I walked into the waiting room, I was immediately struck by the soft peach-and-aqua color scheme. It felt more like a spa than a doctor's office. The receptionist was very cheerful and seemed pleased to see me. "Hi, Jane, lovely to meet you," she said. "My name is Sarah. Great that you are so early. This means that we can get a jump on your paperwork." She handed me an aqua-colored clipboard with three sheets that needed my signature. "I have most of your medical information. These forms are about file sharing and patient confidentiality. Like something to drink, Jane? We some wonderful teas and organic coffees."

This genuine gesture of kindness really touched my heart, and I felt tears forming at the backs of my eyes. I turned to look at Sarah full on as she was gazing at me. "Do you have any idea how that one gesture of offering me a warm drink has just transformed my fear into trust?"

Sarah looked at me and smiled. Then she leaned forward conspiratorially and whispered, "Dar told us that you are working with Tuku and the way of the three loves. She is one cool lady. She's come into our clinic several times over the last six months to run programs for our staff, so don't be surprised if you are inundated with acts of kindness." As she said this, she stood up and walked out from behind her desk to give me a hug. It was like being in the coffee shop. I felt immediately loved and welcomed. And this was a doctor's office! Acts of kindness and medicine seemed so natural together.

I took a seat in a chair upholstered in a beautiful floral tapestry and started to complete the paperwork. After a few minutes, a young nurse walked over. "Hi, Jane," she said. "My name is Barbara. I will be your nurse today. I'm pleased to meet you." She reached out her arms for a hug.

I stood a little clumsily and took the warm hug. Once again, I was struck by how a simple hug could completely transform the role of nurse into healer and not just a chemo-hookup lady. "I'll be back for you in about ten minutes. Please relax and let Sarah know if you need anything."

"Will do," I said and sat down.

I was struck by how the energy of the waiting room was so peaceful. There was a scent of rose in the air, and I spotted a small diffuser in the corner spreading this beautiful aroma throughout the room. Just sitting there made me feel better, and I completely forgot that I had cancer. I finished the paperwork and handed it to Sarah. I was still fifteen minutes early and watched as several patients came in for their appointments. The same warm and gracious greeting was given to them all.

After five minutes, Barbara came back and invited me into one of the treatment rooms. I knew she was about to take some blood, and I began to tense up. She tuned in right away. "Okay to use a warming pad on your arm, Jane?" she asked.

I was shocked. "Oh, absolutely" I said.

The first thing I noticed was that none of the needles or implements were visible. There were flower-patterned pieces of fabric covering them from view. I remembered my old clinic and how just seeing the needle made me tense up. Sarah came to sit by my right side and prep my arm. As she was talking, she directed my attention to the left, toward a painting on the wall of a country scene that reminded me of the south of France. She started to gently massage my arm as she talked about the artist who painted it. Then she asked me to pay attention to the light and guess what time of day the picture had been painted. I started looking much more closely at the shadows and the color of the sky and tried to work out what time of day it was painted. Before I was able to give her an answer, she said, "All done, honey," and moved her tray way.

"What?" I exclaimed. "You just took blood without me even knowing it? Where did you learn to do that?"

She beamed a smile at me and said, "Our friend Tuku. She helped us create a series of sequenced processes. I disengaged your awareness of your arm as I was discreetly redirecting your attention. That's why I massaged your arm—so you were used to being touched. My timing of the question about the light was sequenced to when I inserted the needle. Pretty cool, eh?"

I was in glorious shock. "I simply don't have words. I didn't even see the needle. All I could see were beautiful pieces of fabric."

Barbara responded quickly. "What goes in through our eyes has a direct effect on our emotions. So just seeing a needle will create the energy of fear and contraction, which will diminish your immune system. Whereas seeing beautiful, pastel-colored fabric creates the energy of warmth and relaxation.

Tuku taught us nurses to see ourselves as healing artists and to see each patient as a painting. The brush strokes are our acts of kindness and caring. Staff morale in this clinic is through the roof."

Barbara spent another fifteen minutes doing a few more tests and going over the new treatment protocols. Then she ushered me into Dr. Julie's office and a very comfortable armchair. "She will be with you in a few moments," Barbara said, and she gave me a hug before leaving.

Dr. Julie's office was more like a living room than a doctor's office. There was no desk piled with patient files. Instead, it was furnished with a rather stylish table, a nice lamp, and a vase of flowers. Near it was a smaller table and next to this, a filing cabinet.

The focal point of the room was a suite of lounge furniture around a nice coffee table. The rug was deep pile and matched the pretty drapes. I almost had to pinch myself to make sure it was a doctor's office. After a few minutes, in walked a very smartly dressed woman in heels and light makeup.

She beamed a big smile at me and said, "Hi, Jane! Welcome. My name is Dr. Julie, but please call me Julie." Like the other staff, she greeted me with a hug, and soon we were sitting facing each other in the comfortable armchairs.

"So, Jane," she began. "Is everything okay so far for you?"

"More than okay," I said. "Everything is top notch, and the staff is so caring."

"We have Tuku to thank for that," she said. "Before she came to work with us, we were the usual sort of medical clinic—very functional for working on the body of a patient, but no sensitivity to the spirit of the patient. Tuku really opened our eyes. She helped us to reinvent ourselves based purely on patient kindness and care. As you can see, even my office is different from the regular kind of doctor's office. She took us back to the roots of how to care for a person's body, mind, and spirit. I was amazed at how the staff responded. Morale shot up along with patient satisfaction. But the most important result of all was our success in treating women with breast cancer. In comparison studies with similar centers around the country, we came out far ahead. This is why our small clinic was given the new treatment protocol along with four of the biggest hospitals in the country.

"My aim today is to look generally at the quality of your life so that I can see the bigger emotional picture. The reason for this is simple: your immune system is the key to your healing and staying well. By optimizing it, we are also optimizing the potential for our treatments to succeed. From a medical perspective, I know that you are good match for the program. But I would like to learn about your emotional life and what your passions are. We do not work with the old model of having cancer patients sitting around in chairs, staring at other cancer patients and trying to make conversation. This is a real emotional damper. We have started to use the model developed by the Shaolin monks for cancer patients by giving them a way to do acts of kindness for others. We believe that a healthy person should be able to give and receive in life. This is especially important for cancer patients, as they are under so much stress and their physical appearance is often diminished.

"In a way, we have turned acts of kindness into a sort of medicine that helps the body to fight cancer and prevent it from returning. This does not take great physical effort. It may be a simple gesture, such as writing a card that generates beautiful energy for the person writing it and the person receiving it. Then we have other projects like making bracelets. You can also build and create wooden toys. The woodworking program is the most popular one we offer and really strengthens a person's will to live. The physical aspect of creativity is something given to us at birth, but often it atrophies through lack of use. We combine it with a sense of purpose, and the effect on our patients has been remarkable. It has made their lives happier and given them a new and empowered sense of purpose.

"One of the questions I have for you has to do with your work. I see that you are a grant writer. May I ask, are you passionate about what you do?"

I shook my head slowly to say no. I explained that I was going through marriage problems and was kind of asleep at the wheel workwise.

"Are you content with this?" she asked.

"No."

"Then it may be time you did something about it. Being a cancer patient does not mean you have to take second-best in anything, especially your work, where you spend so much of your time." She took out a prescription pad and started writing. I thought she was writing a prescription for medicine. Then she handed me the prescription, which read, "Spend one hour with Dar talking about finding passion and purpose in my work life."

I was shocked. A doctor who actually cared about my inner life. Now this was something different.

"Jane, your body is comprised of billions of cells that are all communicating with each other," Julie said. "They listen and respond to the positive and negative messages you send them. It's like the coach on a football team. A motivated coach inspires players. And a negative coach? There is a force deep within the human psyche I call the 'will to live.' Through the everyday challenges and stresses of living, this force becomes diminished. The will to live directly affects every cell in your body with 'get healthy' or 'don't bother' messages.

"Because of the extra stresses that cancer patients must endure, their will to live is further diminished. There are two keys to feeding and strengthening the will to live. These are passion and purpose. Ironically, cancer patients often go into a form of energetic withdrawal from life, and their will to live is diminished. I know that cancer treatment can be very physically draining, but I am talking about the psyche, which is like an inner fire. The fire is roused just by thinking about something that stirs purpose and passion. When this is engaged, the negative forces of thought and worry are overridden and are not able to further diminish the will to live."

She reached for her prescription pad again and started writing. I waited and wondered. She smiled as she handed me the new prescription. It read, "Build and paint five wooden race cars for hospitalized children. See Brock for the kits and how to donate the cars."

Just reading the prescription stirred something inside of me. I could build and paint five race cars that would enrich the lives of children with cancer. I felt a wonderful flood of positive emotional energy.

I said, "I can feel how this works. I think it makes great sense. I will be in touch with Dar and Brock ASAP."

"Wonderful!" she said. "When you do this, you will feel tremendous power that brings warmth and happiness to your heart. And woodworking is the best activity to empower your will to live. This is because you expend physical force to manipulate the tools to create a sturdy project that will stand the test of time. The permanency of the wood acts as a metaphor to empower the human spirit. Plus, it is a lot of fun and will boost your self-esteem. Any questions?"

I did have a question, not about the prescriptions but about why my doctor was pushing to remove my breasts.

Julie pondered the question. "Jane, different doctors have different perspectives about how a patient should proceed with cancer care. For some, it is right to remove one or both breasts. For others, it may be right to pursue other treatment options. From my own perspective, a patient should become as well informed as she can and make a decision based on all the facts and what her gut tells her. That way, whether you do or do not have a breast or breasts removed, the decision is the right one.

"It is a very personal decision, and both options have many success stories. How does that sound?"

"I think what you just said makes absolute sense. I feel good about our decision to run with this new treatment protocol."

Julie said we were done for this session. I had to come back once a month for six months for monitoring, and we would have a chance to chat again. She gave me a big hug, and I headed out to catch a train home. I was lucky to get another window seat. I selected some good music and settled in for the ride. I started to think about purpose and passion in my life. These were definitely weak in me. Then I thought of the kids with cancer for whom I could build wooden race cars and felt a wonderful flush of enthusiastic energy course through me. Just thinking about this made me feel so much better. I liked the idea of using my hands to create something beautiful with wood.

I sent a text to Goth Girl, sharing the prescription Dr. Julie had written for me to spend an hour with her. I relaxed back in my seat and gazing at the passing scenery as I pondered my amazing time in New York.

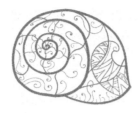

Chapter 58

Purpose and Passion

I arrived home around three in the afternoon and ran a hot bath. I heard the ping of a text arrive and saw that it was from Dar.

Great. One hour of power, it is. Coffee shop tomorrow at 7??

I typed a quick response.

See u there. Hugs. WG.

After a good soak, I spent a lazy evening with a glass or two of Chardonnay, some organic chicken soup, and the Movie Channel.

I slept well and woke up looking forward to my hour of power, as Goth Girl had called it. As I swung into the parking lot, I noticed that she was already sitting at our corner table. Mare had a hug and a large latte ready for me. Goth Girl beamed a big smile at me as I walked toward the table. Next was our customary rib-crunching hug, and then I took a seat across from her. She had placed a file on the table, and I wondered what was inside. I gave her a quick rundown on my wonderful day in New York and how supercool I thought Dr. Julie was.

"So, girl, on the hunt for your purpose and passion, eh?" she asked.

"Got that right," I said.

She opened the file and pulled out a sheet of paper showing the nine spirals. "As they do with medicine, we are going to do a CT scan of your life to see what treasures and clues we can find. We will be looking for three things:

what you loved to do as a child, your unborn hopes and dreams, and what has shown up in your life.

"There are nine circles in the spiral on the sheet of paper. We are going to divide your age by nine, so each circle will represent a certain period in your life. You told me you were forty-five, so each of these circles represents five years. Take your time and reflect back as far as you can and think of the things you loved to do as a child."

This was easy for me. I told Dar that I could remember from around three years of age that I loved poetry. Then at six, it was stolen from me. I started to enjoy words and writing, and my parents guided me in that direction. I also used to create pictures with markers. I remember how I liked to draw pictures of my father in his army uniform. Goth Girl started to make notes on the two inner spirals representing the first ten years of my life. "From ten onward now," she said.

As I reflected, the theme of writing was very strong for me. I won awards at school and began to see that this was what I would do for a living. "My father was in the army, so we moved around a lot. I was used to seeing a lot of people in uniform, and Dad and I would often watch war movies together. It seemed a funny thing to do, but I loved my father and loved sharing things with him. My passion for writing led me into grant writing when I was around twenty-two. This is where I have been ever since, and I feel trapped," I said.

She kept making notes on the spiral sheet. "How about your unborn and secret dreams?"

I took a sip of my latte and reflected. "Being a writer was really up there. But there was also a period when I thought that I would be an army nurse. I felt very comfortable around uniforms and knew that soldiers were often wounded. I never wanted to join the army, but I wanted to help soldiers in some way. I had this dream until I got married and was pushed into the grant-writing job. I used to dream of being a famous writer. I could see myself writing books that would become movies. I also liked the idea of helping people, but I didn't know how these two could come together, so I kind of gave up on the helping-people piece."

Goth Girl continued to make notes. Then she asked, "So, what has shown up in your life either by chance or coincidence?"

I reflected over my life, thinking about the times I'd helped people, such as my elderly neighbor, Doris. I also felt an urge to reach out to some of the other cancer patients in the clinic to offer them comfort. Workwise, grant writing was something I had a talent for, but I had no emotional connection to the work. Then my boss and the special project for homeless vets he had earmarked for me popped into my mind. I never understood why he thought I was the right person for it.

"Interesting!" Goth Girl said as she continued to make notes. "Nice CT scan," she said as she turned the spiral toward me so that I could see it.

"What do you make of it?" I asked.

"It is not what I make of it, but what you make of it that matters," she replied as she handed me a red marker. She asked me to put red marks where I felt energy or passion.

It was really interesting to look at my life in the form of a snapshot. Poetry and writing as a child got red dots. Then came my dad and the army. I put a red dot when I began grant writing, but later on, there were no red dots. Then I put a red dot for when I helped my neighbor, Doris. It was an interesting process.

Goth Girl handed me a gray marker and asked me to make marks for where I felt blocked or dead energy. I put a lot of gray dots for the last twenty years of my work as a grant writer. Then I put a big gray circle around the homeless veterans' project my boss had offered me.

Goth Girl picked up on this right away. "See what you did? You didn't block this out; you just drew a circle around it. Can we zoom in on this?"

"How do I do that?" I asked.

She pulled out a blank sheet of paper and drew a big circle with the gray marker. She asked me to draw a sort of zoom picture of what was inside. Then she laid out a box of colored markers and said I could use words, shapes, and colors.

It was a fascinating process. First, I picked up a green marker and made a happy face. This represented my dad. Then I picked up a black marker and made a black circle inside the gray circle.

"What does the black circle mean?" she asked.

I closed my eyes and tuned into the feeling. "It represents the feeling of entrapment that I feel working for the grant-writing agency. I have no freedom there."

Then I picked up a blue marker and drew squiggles. These represented how I felt about writing grants in the early days. But the squiggles were short because I stopped enjoying it. Then I picked up a red marker and drew a small heart. As I did this, I realized that a part of me once did love this work. But it was really small. As I pondered this, I felt a surge of anger and picked up the black marker and drew a thick square box around the gray outer circle. I started to cry as I realized that this represented my husband and how he had wanted me to do that work because of the salary and benefits. He was only interested in my salary and had no interest in what I was doing.

This really surprised me. I was aware of his pressure for me to earn a salary. But I had no idea how it had imprisoned me and stolen my joy. My tears felt full of sadness. Goth Girl handed me a tissue for a good blow of my nose. Then she asked me if anything at work had shown up that held good energy. I pondered her question and wrote "homeless vets" but then I put a dark gray box around the words.

"Interesting," she said.

The word vet in connection to your father was red and passionate. But here the word vet linked to homeless has turned into a negative feeling.

She ripped a blank sheet of paper in half and wrote *homeless* on one sheet and *vets* on the other. She placed the sheet bearing the word *vets* in front of me and asked me to draw a zoomed-in picture of what I felt.

I was shocked when I picked up the green marker and drew a happy face. Then I picked up the red marker and drew a heart around it. I felt a movement in my heart, and a warm burst of energy came out.

Then she placed the piece of paper with *homeless* on it in front of me. I immediately felt my hackles rise, and anger started to course through me. She asked me to represent this with a drawing or a shape. I went straight for the black marker again and drew another black box that I filled in with black.

I stared at the black box. Goth Girl encouraged me to gaze gently at it and enter into what meaning the word *homeless* held for me. As she did this, she placed the spiral of my life in front of me and invited me to travel back to see where the origin of this memory could be found. As I started to travel back in my memory, there was nothing of note until I got to around the age of sixteen. Then a very dark and scary memory seemed to emerge like a sea monster from a dark lagoon inside of me. The memory was of a school friend who was on her way home from the movies one night with her boyfriend. They were walking past a park, and two homeless men attacked them. They beat up her boyfriend, sending him to the hospital, and they raped her. It was a terrible time. The homeless men were arrested and sent to jail. The town purged the streets of all the homeless men, and we were taught in school not to have anything to do with them. Since that experience, the word *homeless* creates in me a knee-jerk reaction of repulsion and fear. As an adult some twenty-nine years later, I realized that I was still a victim of this deep trauma.

I felt as if some essential part of the puzzle had just been unlocked. I looked at Goth Girl and said, "Where the hell did you learn this process? I feel as if in less than one hour, you just unlocked a door that has been imprisoning my passion and purpose all my life."

She smiled and replied, "It was our Mr. Brock who taught me this. I know he seems all quiet and humble on the outside, but this guy is steeped with gems like this. Some years ago, he studied curative education in Europe, when he was working with severely handicapped children. This is called the 'biography of color process' and is one that they use to communicate with profoundly handicapped children. He has adapted it for working with adults.

"By using color and shapes, you move away from the rational mind and can access deeper aspects of your psyche. This is the process he used on me when I was lost and needed to find my direction in life. It really put me on track and gave me tools that I continue to use to this day. Cool, eh?"

"What's next?" I asked.

"It's a process he calls 'entering into the arms of serendipity.' This is when we move toward what seems to be calling us. The key is to be open and let serendipity unfold naturally," she said.

"What would you suggest we do?"

She pondered this as she sipped her latte. Looking up with a sparkle in her eye, she said, "Well, honey, I'm thinking we should go downtown to the bus station next to the homeless shelter and have us a nice old cup of coffee and see what happens. Only thing is, we gotta shift this *homeless* word for you. We will be hanging with people we are going to call 'people with no homes,' got it? No more 'homeless' for you, because this is a major emotional trigger point."

"Sounds cool to me. When?"

"I am thinking tomorrow would be good. Let's meet at the bus depot at 9:00 a.m. by stop 42. Sound like a plan?" she asked.

"Roger that," I said and gathered the papers as I stood for a farewell hug.

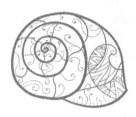

Chapter 59

The Bus Depot

I woke thinking about what I should wear to the bus station. I was going to be around homeless people, who, as Goth Girl had suggested, I had to see as people without homes. The last thing I wanted was to attract their attention. I decided on some old blue jeans and a dark-blue, loose-fitting sweater. I wanted to be prepared for anything, so I slipped a small canister of Mace into my bag, just in case.

I arrived fifteen minutes before the scheduled time to scope out the bus station and tune in to the energy. I noticed there was a coffee shop near the ticket counter and thought this would be a good place for us to hang out. I poked my head inside; it looked fairly clean. There were several empty booths where we could sit and observe. Or we could sit at one of the beat-up tables near the food truck outside. Grubby-looking people who I guessed were "people without homes" roamed the area. I was feeling very uneasy.

I wandered toward bus stop 42, where I was to meet Goth Girl. The place was like a zoo. Buses whizzed by, spewing nasty fumes. An endless stream of agitated and frenzied people hurried to and fro. At five minutes to nine, a bus sped into the station and screeched to a halt at stop 42. The doors slid open, and Goth Girl emerged in a striking, all-black outfit. She looked as if she'd just stepped out of a science fiction movie with her snow-white complexion, heavily made-up eyes, and scarlet lipstick. She looked both scary and stunning. I saw men eying her. We shared a quick hug, and I led her toward the coffee shop.

"Oh, no," she said. "We'll sit over there." As she gestured toward the food truck, a wave of panic shot through me. She couldn't be serious. But away she went, walking with a quietly determined air.

I noticed one empty table next to the narrow corridor where people lined up at the food truck. As we moved closer, I sensed eyes shifting to look at me. I slipped my hand into my bag and gripped the Mace. I felt like a gunslinger from the Wild West ready to draw and shoot at the slightest provocation. Goth Girl led us to the table. My skin was crawling. The smell of body odor and stale cigarette smoke hung in the air. One guy in a hooded sweatshirt was gazing at me. I flashed him an angry don't-screw-with-me look, and he turned away. Goth Girl gestured for me to sit. "Coffee, right?" she asked as she headed to the food truck.

Was she expecting me to drink anything from that dirty truck? This was getting worse by the moment. As I took my seat, I nervously pulled my bag close to my chest. I noticed men sitting at other tables stealing furtive glances at me. This was not going well. I felt like a goldfish in a bowl. Each time a bus came or left, a fresh burst of blue diesel fumes washed over me. My resolve to see this through was crumbling fast. I could sense the hooded guy eyeballing me again. I clutched the Mace in my bag and gave him another nasty look. He sheepishly looked away again. *Frickin' creep!* I thought.

Goth girl returned, carrying two small, Styrofoam cups of what I guessed was coffee. She placed them on the table and took a seat. She was quiet. I was feeling like a prickly cactus and angry at her for bringing me into this frickin' awful place. I narrowed my eyes and looked back defiantly.

After a moment of this stare down, she said, "Well, talk to me, honey. Tell me what is going on behind that pretty little face of yours."

Now she was deliberately pressing my buttons. The polluted air was making my lungs feel tight, and I could hardly breathe. As for what I was feeling, it was a combination of fear, embarrassment, revulsion, and annoyance at her. She waited quietly for my response. My defenses were bristling, and I was on red alert. "So what bus is serendipity arriving on?"

She burst out laughing. It was a good line, and I reluctantly let a small smile slip out. I felt like a fly caught in a spider's web. I was super pissed and really unhappy with what was going down.

"May we look at some layers?" she asked.

I should have known this was coming. I am being ogled by some hooded creep, and all she wants to talk about is damn layers? "Knock yourself out, honey," I said.

She smiled at my response. "Talk to me about what you are perceiving."

She didn't have to ask twice. "What I am perceiving is really simple. There is a creepy, hooded guy over there who keeps eyeballing me. What I am perceiving is my grip on my Mace spray, and I am locked and loaded and ready to fire at will." I could feel my anger flaring.

Goth Girl said, "You seem to have an issue with that guy in the hoodie."

I barked out my response. "Got that right. He keeps eyeballing me. Frickin' creep!"

She smiled at me. "Remember the story about the guy in a cream suit on the train and his perceptions of the father who disturbed his peace?"

I nodded yes but wondered why that was relevant.

"How do you know your perceptions about that hooded guy are correct?"

The question pissed me off. Whose side was she on? I wondered. Then she did something that shocked me. She stood up, went over to the hooded guy, and sat next to him. I thought for a moment that she was going to admonish him and tell him to stop eyeballing me. She talked to him for a few moments, and then they both stood up and walked over to the food truck. What the hell was she doing? I wondered. I watched as Goth Girl pointed to the breakfast-sandwich menu, and the stumpy little guy in the food truck handed the creepy hooded guy a ball of foil, which I guessed was a breakfast sandwich. Next came a very large cup of coffee. Goth Girl handed over some money, and I wondered why the hell she was buying him breakfast after what he had done to me.

I was even more shocked when they walked toward our table. I averted my eyes, pretending not to see them. Goth Girl pulled back a chair for the creepy hooded guy, and as he sat down, a wave of stale body odor filled the air. This guy needed a bath. His hood was pulled over his face, and I could not see his eyes. He pulled hungrily at the foil and took a big bite of the sandwich, which he seemed to swallow without chewing. Goth Girl sat quietly, watching him. I sat in shock and disgust. In between bites of the sandwich, he would suck down mouthfuls of coffee with a loud slurping sound. Egg yolk oozed over his dirty fingers. No manners! What a pig! And a smelly one at that.

The chomping and slurping went on for a few minutes. His hood was still pulled over his head, so I could not see his face. I wanted him to finish quickly so he would leave. As he crunched up the empty foil, I noticed his big, powerful hands. Surely, he could find some meaningful work to do with those. Instead of getting up to leave, he started to rummage around in his pockets. Then he pulled out a pack of cigarettes. A loud voice in my head said, *This is really not happening, right?*

He fished out a cigarette and rather shakily lifted it to his mouth. His hands were shaking so badly he could not get a flame on the cigarette. Then Goth Girl shocked me by reaching out and cradling his hands in hers. His shaking stopped, and together they lifted the flame to his cigarette. I noticed that some of the egg yolk was now on her hands. Soon, puffs of blue smoke billowed out from under the hood and hung around me like a cloud. Everything inside of me wanted to get up and angrily walk away. Yet a part of me sensed that something bigger was going on here. Goth Girl was up to something, and I was curious as to how it would unfold. I continued to sit through the puffs of blue smoke as I pictured throwing all my smoke-infested clothes in the washing machine as soon as I got home. After a few long sucks on his cigarette, he casually flipped the lit cigarette butt into his empty coffee cup.

Goth Girl turned to me then. "So, Jane, I want you to meet John," she said. "John has agreed to share his story with you."

I almost fell off my dirty little chair. My eyes widened in disbelief at Goth Girl. I pursed my lips tightly and lowered my eyes as I tried to decide whether to walk away. I slowly reached into my bag and gripped the Mace. Reassured that I could hit creepy hooded guy right between the eyes if he tried anything, I resolved to stay and see it through.

Still with the grubby hood covering his face, Creepy Hooded Guy, now called John, picked up a paper napkin and blew his very congested nose a couple of times. This was awful. I sucked in a deep breath and deepened my resolve not to run away. We all sat in silence for a moment. Then John slowly pulled back his hood. With my body facing Goth Girl, I turned my head slowly to look at him. The first thing I saw was the dirty baseball cap he was wearing backward. His face was covered in a layer of grimy dirt, and he had a scruffy stubble over his lower face. He kept his eyes lowered to the table, and I could not see them. Goth Girl reached out very tenderly and touched his hand again. "Take your time, John. Share when you are ready," she said in a warm, caring voice.

Then I noticed it: a long, deep-pink scar that started just below his ear and traveled up the side of his head. It looked nasty. I felt a sharp prick in my heart as if a needle just stabbed me. I sensed that this would play into whatever it was that Goth Girl was trying to achieve. I tried to look relaxed and interested. I picked up my warm cup of piss water that was masquerading as coffee and took a couple of sips. It was hard to believe that it tasted worse than it looked.

John slowly raised his head and stared into space between Goth Girl and me. For the first time, I saw his eyes. They were a beautiful shade of blue, and I was struck by the innocence and vulnerability I could sense in them. His dirty face made him look older and seemed at variance with the youthful eyes.

"My name is Johnny," he said. "I live in the shelter outside the bus station. When I was twelve years old, my mother died. She was the only person who ever really loved me for myself. My dad was a vet. PTSD and all that crap. He was an angry, bad-ass guy. When I was eighteen, I had some buddies who were going into the army, and to get away from my dad, I signed up. I am proud of my country, and the army gave me a purpose in life. I was one fit and strong dude, and they put me in a crack marine special-ops unit. Then I married my childhood sweetheart. And soon, two beautiful twin girls came along.

"Life was good. When I was twenty-one, I did a one-year tour in Afghanistan. Then, three years later, I did my second tour in Iraq with my best buddy, Joey. We were out on patrol one afternoon...."

John seemed to choke up. Goth Girl gently touched his arm and told him to take a few breaths. He lowered his eyes to the table and went quiet for a moment. Then he lifted his gaze to the same place in between Goth Girl and me and continued. "Well, we were on patrol, and we got our asses blown sky high with a land mine. It blew Joey to pieces and left half of my frickin' brain in the Iraqi dirt."

I flashed my eyes to the pink scar behind his ear and felt a shiver all over me.

"I came home with this PTSD thing. Some days, my head is like an empty tin can. Some days, it's hard to move my legs. They just go numb. I was so lost, angry, and frightened. The drugs they gave me just numbed me for a while but did nothing to really help me. The talk therapy they did with me just seemed to stir up bad shit. I was, and am, one angry bastard.

"I just could not focus on anything. My anger got out of hand. I was no good for the kids to be around, so my wife went to live with her mother. This was a real frickin' heartbreak for me, and I just spiraled down and down." Then he gestured to the homeless shelter outside the bus depot and with sadness in his voice, he said that it was now his home.

I looked at Goth Girl. Her loving gaze was locked on John. She seemed to be holding him in some form of energetic, loving field of energy. I had seen Tuku do that. The energy was palpable. I was in a state of shock. John's words had broken something open in me, and I was doing everything I could to hold back my tears. It felt like some sort of bomb had gone off inside my heart, and I was losing the ice barrier that I had created around it for protection. I had never talked to a homeless vet before. I had the sense that he had only shared the tip of the iceberg, yet I was completely blown away by his story. I felt the urge to reach out and hold him. To thank him for what he had given for our country—for the freedom his wounds had given me. I glanced at the scar and felt the urge to touch it lovingly. I wanted to heal it. I wanted to take away his pain. I wanted to take away his suffering. He had put his life on the line for my freedom. And what had I really done with my life? All I did was sit on my fat ass, writing bullshit grants. Here was a real person, more real than I could imagine being. My heart was breaking one painful crack at a time. I felt a deep desire to do something to help him and other vets like him.

Then a light went off in my head. For three months, I had been ducking a homeless-vet project at work. My purpose and passion had just shown up in the form of a wounded guy in a hoodie. John was quiet. Then Goth Girl asked softly if she could ask him a question.

His eyes were now lowered to the table between us. "Sure," he said.

Her question surprised and embarrassed me. "Johnny, may I ask why you were looking at Jane?"

I shot an annoyed look at her. She kept her face toward John and slowly turned her eyes to meet mine. Then she quietly raised one eyebrow as if to say, *Get ready, honey. The payload is headed your way.* We both turned our eyes back to John.

He paused to ponder the question, then started to talk.

As he began to speak, for the first time he raised and turned his head to look at me. When our eyes met, everything about his dirty, smelly presence disappeared. His soft blue eyes seemed to hold me in some form of spell. "My mom was my source of unconditional love. She was always there for me. Always told me how special I was. Always loved the hell out of me. When she died, her love died too. I have this special memory of her. I was ten, and I'd just won the school wrestling competition. She came to the award ceremony wearing dark blue jeans and a plain, dark-blue, loose-fitting sweater, just like you. Her hair was your color too. When I looked at you, it made me think of my mom. When I look at you, her love seems to come alive in me again. I am sorry, ma'am; really sorry. I know it was wrong of me to stare and all. But you remind me of my mom, and that warms my very cold and lonely heart."

Then I completely lost it. It was as if my heart finally cracked into two pieces, and a torrent of tears flooded down my cheeks. I reached out with both hands for his hands. Our eyes were now locked in a teary embrace. "Thank you, thank you, thank you for what you just shared. I am so, so moved by you and your story. I feel honored that you saw your mother's love in me."

He was now crying too, and I noticed that his tears had washed away the grime, revealing thin strips of pink flesh on his cheeks. Goth Girl offered us tissues. Then I realized I had been gripping his hands tightly. His hands were big and strong, just like those of a wrestler. I released them, and we both took tissues from Goth Girl and began to wipe away our tears.

We were all silent. Then I thought of my father. I felt a thump in my chest, and a huge ball of sadness suddenly broke loose inside of me. I started to sob again. Goth Girl and John both reached out at the same time, each taking one of my hands in theirs. Wave after wave of tears crashed through me. My whole body was shaking. I had lost it. This went on for a few minutes until I slowly regained control of my senses. John said in a gentle whisper, "Sorry if my story did this to you."

I thought for a while and then replied, "I'm not crying because of your story. I am crying because of the way I wrongly judged you and for how wretched a person I am." I was in meltdown mode and emotionally broken open. But I could feel how much caring and support these two incongruous people were lavishing upon me. As we sat quietly in a sort of daze, I was aware of a figure walking toward us. It was the stubby little man from the food truck. He was carrying a tray of fresh coffee for us. As he lowered the tray onto the table, he said, "Excuse me, but I gotta sense you all may be ready for this." I noticed his thick powerful wrists and a tattoo that ran the length of his muscular forearm.

"This is Stan," John said. "He's a vet, like me. One of the best!"

Stan extended his fist toward John, and John raised his fist, and their hands met in a bump, a gentle kiss of acknowledgment. That gesture of the bond between them touched me. I wanted to do that. I wanted to share that bond. I wanted to reach out and touch my fist to Stan's and have my fist touched by his fist. Their sense of brotherhood was palpable. As Stan walked away, I noticed that John was looking at the food truck. Goth Girl picked up on that and said, "I am guessing it may be time for another sandwich, right?"

He smiled at her, and they both got up. As John walked over to the food truck, Goth Girl whispered a question to me. "So, what showed up today? How does it make you feel?"

I knew right away what she meant. I took out my phone and speed-dialed my boss, Mark.

"Hey, Jane," Mark said. "Nice surprise. You okay?"

"Never been better," I responded quickly. "I'll explain more when I see you. I want the homeless-vet shelter project. All of it! Please set up a meeting next week with the board. Pull me off the other projects. I want this to be my focus. I wanna kick some ass for these guys and gals in the shelter!"

"Great!" Mark sounded shocked. "This is wonderful news. What caused the shift?"

"I'll explain when I see you," I said. "Thanks, Mark." I hung up. Then I speed-dialed my hairdresser friend, Dorothy, to call in a favor. In her spare time, she ran a non-profit shelter for cats. It had a small budget and could never afford to hire me officially through the agency, so I wrote grants for it under the table on weekends. I pulled in a lot of cash for Dorothy's shelter, and she always asked me if there was anything she could do for me.

The phone rang twice, and Dorothy picked up. "Hey, Jane. Great to see your name on my caller ID. Wassup, girl?"

"I am calling in a favor," I said. "I got this super nice homeless guy that needs some of your TLC and a damn good haircut. Gotta warn you, he also needs a shower."

Dorothy responded enthusiastically. "Been waiting to have a way to say thank you. I have a shower in the back and will get him clean and sparkly for you."

"And that Anthony guy on your board who owns a clothing store?" I said. "Would you mind asking him if he could set my buddy up with three new outfits? Jeans and a casual shirt, a dark suit for interviews, and a sports outfit for the gym. Oh, and ask Anthony to get a seven-day gym pass for my buddy, will you?"

"Sure thing, honey. We owe you big time, and all of this is easy to do," she said. "We have both been itching to do something for you."

"What are you up to today?" I asked.

"I worked last Saturday, and this is my admin day at home," she said. "My girls are running the salon."

"Great," I said. "Any chance you can come down to the central bus station and pick my buddy up to take him to your salon?"

"Sure. When works best for you?" she replied.

I checked my watch and said, "How about in half an hour?"

"I am there, baby cakes! Front or back entrance?" she asked.

"In the front by the food truck. You know it?" I asked.

"Sure do. I have a white car," she said.

"Perfecto! See you soon," I said and hung up. As John and Goth Girl waited at the counter, I sat back and pondered the passion and purpose I was feeling. Something that was already in my life had just come alive. I was on fire for the project that had been stalking me for over three months. I gazed at John's back. Even though he was wearing baggy clothes, they did not hide the fact that he had a powerful body. I guessed his height was around six feet, and his strong neck had a broad taper that ran into muscular shoulders. That somebody like him had to live in a shelter made me feel very sad.

As they walked back to our table, John was carrying a rather large bag of food and looking relaxed. Goth Girl had seen me on the phone and asked me who I'd called. I knew that she knew that I'd called my boss.

"I am on fire for the homeless-shelter project," I said, beaming a big smile at her. I could sense Johnny was watching me closely. Then I turned to him and told him about my work and how I wanted to help him and his homeless-vet buddies. I could see he was moved. I asked him what sort of work he felt drawn toward. He lifted one of his powerful hands and said he loved to build things with wood. I thought of Brock immediately and asked if I could introduce him.

His eyes became soft and glistened, as if tears were close. What he did next shocked me. He reached into his pocket and pulled out his pack of cigarettes. In one slow movement of his powerful hand, he crushed the pack and threw it into a nearby waste bin. Then he opened his jacket and started tugging at the lining. Goth Girl and I traded puzzled glances when John popped a couple of threads and pulled the lining open. Then he reached inside and pulled out a Ziploc bag of white powder. I was shocked. It was obviously some form of dope or crack. Pulling the bag open, he turned and poured the contents into the trash can.

Goth Girl lifted one eyebrow and asked him if he was open to sharing why he had just thrown away his cigarettes and drugs.

"Sure," he said. "You see, the smokes and dope helped me keep this big, dark, painful thing inside of me numb. Without 'em, the pain of this dark thing would take over. What Jane just gave me was hope, and there is like a beautiful light inside me now. She believes in me, and that has changed everything."

A lump came to my throat, and a sense of wanting to look after him came alive in me. I felt protective, as if he were my little brother. Goth Girl shifted her gaze to me. She knew that big emotions were stirring in me and waited in silence for me to share. Very softly, she said, "Be in your truth, Jane."

Well, that opened me up, and I blurted my feelings of brotherly caring for John. Funnily enough, I did not feel uncomfortable saying it aloud and looking directly at him.

Tears had formed in his eyes, and he said, "I just don't believe this." His tear-filled eyes shifted upward. It was as if he was looking up to heaven.

I flashed a look at Goth Girl, wondering if he was having some form of religious experience.

Then he said, "Thanks, Joey. You came through. You came through!" He lowered his eyes, and tears rolled down his cheeks. Goth Girl gently touched his arm and invited him to share. John picked up a napkin and gave his nose a big, loud blow. He turned to look at Goth Girl, whose hand was still on his arm. "Ya see, the night before my best buddy, Joey, and I got blown up, we had a few beers under the stars. Joe had this big sister that he loved and adored. He used to tell stories about how they looked out for each other. I was an only child and loved to hear these stories about his sister. I did not have a sister, but I had a chocolate Lab called Dibbs. His mom was allergic to dogs, so he could never have a dog. So, as we were sipping our beers, we were sharing stories about his big sister and my dog, Dibbs.

"After we had popped quite a few beers that night, we got to talking sort of sentimentally like. We knew were in some heavy-duty enemy territory, and danger was all around. It was a high-risk combat zone, and we had no idea if we would make it out alive. I am not sure where this came from, but I said to him that if I got to heaven first, I would pull some strings and send him a chocolate Lab. We got a bit teary at that point. Then he turned to me, and with tears in his eyes, he said that if he got to heaven first, he would pull some strings and send me a big sister."

At that point, all three of us simultaneously reached out our hands and formed a triangle of love as tears and laughter flowed. The laughter came from a place of joy that was overflowing.

Goth Girl gave both our hands a squeeze and said, "Ever heard the word *adoption*?" My eyes flashed onto John's eyes, which were locked on mine. "I'm game," I said.

"Hell, yeah!" John said. "I'm game too."

Quick as a flash, Goth Girl pulled out two wooden hearts that I guessed she got from Brock. "Open your right hands," she said. We did. She placed a wooden heart in each of our palms and then closed our fingers around them. She gestured for us to move our hands up to our own hearts. Looking at Johnny, she asked him to speak his intention to adopt me as his big sister.

In a quiet, strong voice, he said, "I, John Carson, do take Jane to be my adopted big sister."

We were all flooding tears. Then I said, "I, Jane Harris, take John Carson to be my adopted little brother."

Goth Girl then guided us to exchange our wooden hearts. As we did that, I felt as if a golden cord had been tied between John and me. It was glorious. It was like a homecoming.

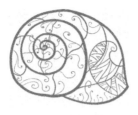

Chapter 60

A Menacing Bunch

Boisterous men's voices broke into our precious time together. I spun around to see four men walking toward us from the shelter. They were talking loudly, and I could tell they had been drinking. They were all big men, but what caught my eye was a *really* big man who must have been well over six feet tall and weighed at least 250 pounds. He was powerfully built. My mind flashed to a BBC series I'd watched a few years ago. In it, there was a large rugby player who was described affectionately as a brick crapper. Being a writer and lover of words, this term stuck with me. The really big man reminded me of Brick Crapper. His loud voice carried, and the other men seemed to flock around him. Brick Crapper was the obvious alpha male in this sorry bunch.

They seemed to be headed toward us, and then it dawned on me that they were headed to the food truck and would be going right past me. I was sitting with my back to the narrow corridor between the chairs and tables. My dirty little chair was bolted to the pavement, so I could not move it. As the menacing group came nearer, I pulled myself forward and took a sip of my lousy coffee to pretend I was not looking at them.

As they walked by, I felt a sharp thud on my right side, and my coffee spilled all over my hand. I turned quickly to see who had bumped me. Brick Crapper was standing over me, glaring menacingly down a broken nose at me. His eyes bulged out from under a dirty baseball cap. This guy was scary. "Get the hell out of my way, bitch!" he barked at me.

I spun my head back to the table and felt a flash of fear course though my body.

What happened next shocked me. Like a missile taking off, John launched himself from his chair toward Brick Crapper and drove his left elbow forcefully under the man's chin. Brick Crapper stumbled backward, until his head hit a concrete pillar with a sickening thud. John had him locked up against the pillar with his elbow under his chin and his right hand menacingly clamped around his throat. His thumb and fingers were buried deep within the neck of the Brick Crapper guy. Brick Crapper's eyes bulged with rage, and his face was red with anger. I was scared that he might lash out at John.

But John's right hand held something deep within Brick Crapper's neck that seemed to freeze him. John's eyes were narrow, and he held him in a piercing laser gaze. The two men were locked in a hate-filled stare down. The three other guys were in shock and standing like statues. Other people in the area scattered. Then I saw Brick Crapper's hand moving slowly in the direction of his jacket pocket. What if he had a knife? One quick thrust, and John could be dead. I felt the urge to call out, but what would happen if I distracted John? I was frozen stiff with fear.

Just as Brick Crapper's hand was about to enter his pocket, John said, "Don't even think about it!"

Brick Crapper lowered his hand and let it fall limp at his side.

With barely a movement in his face, John said, "I guess you got two options, douchebag. You can say you are sorry, or I can break your filthy neck."

That enraged Brick Crapper, and his already bulging eyes bulged even more. His red face got redder. I was scared for John.

He slowly tightened his right hand that was buried into Brick Crapper's throat. Suddenly, the bigger man's eyes seemed to shrink back in their sockets, and his face lost its color. At the same time, I could sense the alpha energy seeping out of him and into Johnny. Meekly, Brick Crapper said, "Sorry."

John tipped his head toward me as the person to whom he needed to apologize, and he very slowly released his grip around Brick Crapper's neck. But he remained coiled, and his gaze did not falter. I could see the deep-red welt marks left by his fingers on the man's neck.

Brick Crapper meekly stepped toward me, and looking down at me, he said, "Sorry."

I nodded in response. Then John coughed. We both spun to look at him. With the greatest of economy, John pointed to his knees and then to the ground.

Holy crap! Brick Crapper has to get on his knees to apologize, I thought.

Slowly, Brick Crapper lowered his big frame until his knees were on the pavement. Now he was looking up into my eyes. He said the word again. "Sorry."

John coughed again. We looked, and John gave a little nod, suggesting that Brick Crapper remove his hat. Slowly, Brick Crapper pulled off his grubby baseball hat, revealing a greasy mass of dark-brown hair. Now he was looking very meek. "Sorry, ma'am," he said.

"Apology accepted," I said.

Brick Crapper looked at John, as if asking for permission to get up. John nodded, and Brick Crapper rose and walked meekly away. I was dumb struck. Johnny had controlled Brick Crapper with a series of small gestures as if he were a marionette. John then spun to look at the other three men, who were standing dumb struck. He gave them a piercing look that seemed to say, "Any of you want a piece of this?" All three of them turned, lowered their heads, and walked away.

John came back to his seat still wearing the fierce, steely look on his face. As soon as he sat down, he smiled. For the first time, I saw his strong chin and his youthful, handsome good looks. With a mischievous grin, he said, "Didn't I tell you that your new brother comes as part of a bundled package?"

I gave him a questioning look. "I come with the 'ain't nobody ever gonna mess with my big sister' package."

I felt warm energy touch my heart, and we all burst into laughter.

As the laughter died down, Goth Girl reached into her handbag and pulled out what looked like a new flip phone. She looked at me and said, "Phone number?" I told her my number, and she entered it. My phone rang. Then she gave the flip phone to Johnny and said, "There ya go. You are connected now."

I'd noticed that a guy in a wheelchair over by the food truck was looking at us. John followed my line of sight and waved his hand in the air, beckoning the man over. "My lucky day," he said. "You get to meet Billy." In a few moments, Billy was at our table, and John rose and gave him long, tight hug. I sensed the affection and respect the two men shared. John introduced us, and we shook hands. Billy was very charismatic. He had lost both legs, but his upper body was powerfully built like John's. It was obvious that he was another vet.

Then we heard a honk, and Dorothy's car pulled up. She was waiting in the bus loading area, so we had to move quickly. I took John over and introduced him as my younger brother. Dorothy's mouth dropped open; she had never heard of me having a younger brother. I gave John a hug, and he jumped into the car.

He wound the window down, and I instructed him to tell Dorothy the story of how we had just become brother and sister. "Call me later," I said as they sped out of the bus station.

When I returned to our table, Goth Girl was in conversation with Billy, who was explaining that he had been posted with John in Iraq. "That's where I lost these suckers," he said, pointing to his missing lower limbs. "Saved my life, he did, that Johnny boy."

I felt a lump come to my throat.

Goth Girl asked if he would be open to sharing the story. Just then, Stan, the guy from the food truck, arrived with a big cup of coffee for Billy. They touched knuckles as a sign of mutual respect. I knew that this gesture of greeting was a brotherly vet thing, and a part of me yearned to belong to this brotherhood.

Billy took a long sip and said, "Johnny and I came home two years ago in pretty bad shape. Me with my legs gone, and him with half his brains blown away. We also had crazy-ass PTSD. We created this 9:00 a.m. daily check-in process to support each other. PTSD can be pretty brutal, and having a bud on the end of the line can be a lifesaver. For the first year, we did not miss a day of calls. Then one day just before Christmas, the mail man brought me a letter from the VA declining a benefit I had been waiting for. My wife had a very low-paying job, and I was banking on this to buy a Christmas tree and presents for our kids. When the letter arrived, it really hit me hard. I just lost it. Everything crashed, and I knew that I could not go on. My wife was at work, and the kids were in school. I was in a death-wish state. I took the phone off the hook and got my service revolver from under my bed. I loaded it with one bullet, and I was sitting at my kitchen table with the gun up against my forehead at ten minutes after nine. I pulled back the safety catch and said a prayer asking God to forgive me for what I was about to do. Then I heard Johnny shout through the mail slot in the door, 'Don't you dare do it, you asshole!' Next thing I knew, he shouldered in my front door and wrestled the gun off me. We fell on the floor and held each other as we sobbed our hearts out for the longest time. I was just seconds away from blowing my brains out.

"I told him about the letter, and he pulled this crumpled check from his pocket. It was made out to him, and he signed it over to me. Then he loaded me in his truck and took me out to buy a Christmas tree and presents for the kids. We spent every last dime of that check. I never wondered for one moment what that check was for. Not only did he save my life, but he gave Christmas to me and my family. We continued our morning check-ins, and I leveled out. It wasn't until three months later that I found out from another vet buddy of mine where this check had come from. Ya see, Johnny had this nice little apartment and was beginning to get his life back together after his surgery. Turns out, the check was his rent payment from the VA. Because he could not pay the rent that month, he got put out on the street, which is why he lives in the shelter. The VA system is kind of screwed up, and they thought he had blown it on booze. Johnny is a proud man, and he would not go begging to the VA. That's why he ended up living in the shelter.

"But he never told me that," Billy said. "He doesn't know that I know the story. Pure salt of the Earth is that Johnny." Billy looked at his watch and said he had a doctor's appointment to go to. He gave us both hugs and headed out.

Goth Girl and I were both in tears. The thought that Johnny was homeless hung heavily with me. As I pondered options for helping him, I thought of an old college buddy who lived on the outskirts of town. His wife had walked out on him, and he was living by himself in a four-bedroom home and struggling with loneliness. I called him and gave him the scoop.

"I didn't know you had a younger brother," he said.

I said it was a long story best told over coffee.

"For your brother, no problem," he said. "When does he want to come over?"

"How about tonight?"

"Er...ah...well, sure, I guess. Just need to make up the bed," he said.

"Love you," I said. "Expect him late afternoon."

I put a call in to Dorothy, and she agreed to drop off John after his cleanup.

Goth Girl was watching me set this up. "Seems you've got some passion going here," she said, smiling.

"Passion is red hot!" I replied. "I've got this fire going inside to help homeless vets. Thank you for popping me open and helping me to see what was there all along."

Goth Girl smiled and said we were done for the day. We hugged, and I headed home, glowing from the events of a day that would live in my heart for all times.

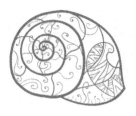

Chapter 61

The Golden Breath?

I woke up feeling energized, as if I was beginning a whole new life. I couldn't wait to get to the office to start my work with homeless vets. To celebrate this new adventure, I planned a quick visit to the coffee shop to pick up a latte. As I walked in, Mare greeted me with the usual beaming smile, followed by a big hug. As I was waiting for her to make my latte, I noticed Tuku tucked away in the booth in the far corner of the coffee shop. In front of her were books and a notebook. She was quietly gazing out of the window and seemed to be in some form of angelic trance. It was mesmerizing. She always had a peaceful inner glow, but this was different. It was hard to capture with words. There was an aura of golden light around her that I had never seen before.

Mare returned with my latte and followed my line of vision to Tuku. Then she said, "Beautiful to watch, isn't it?" I turned to Mare and asked what Tuku was doing. Mare closed her eyes for a few seconds, as if going inside. Slowly she opened her eyes and said, "She is doing the 'golden breath.'"

"What's that?" I asked. Mare said that it was not for her to share; only Tuku could explain the golden breath. I turned to look at Tuku again. Her aura was magnetic. I wanted to go over and say hello, but I also felt great reverence for her privacy.

I thanked Mare and headed out to the office. During the drive, I kept thinking about the term *golden breath*. It was an alluring concept, and I could not stop wondering about the golden aura that came from Tuku.

As soon as my computer booted up, I shot an email to Goth Girl.

Hey, GG. So, what is the scoop on the 'golden breath' process?

She was quick to reply.

> Hey, WG. Golden breath is not something I can explain. But final session with Tuku is tomorrow night, and the subject is the Golden Breath. Are you tuned in or what? Guess you need to be there, right?

I emailed back,

Got that right! Seven o'clock?

> Roger and out. See you then, she replied.

The next email was from Mark, my boss, requesting a planning meeting for the homeless-vets project. It was beginning! My purpose and passion were locked and loaded, and what felt like a whole new life was about to begin.

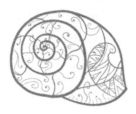

Chapter 62

Sea Creatures of the Mind

I arrived at the coffee shop at 6:45 p.m. Brock and Goth Girl were in the back room talking to Tuku, and I chatted with a very nice elderly gent, who was a retired professor of literature.

At 7:00 p.m., Tuku welcomed us and explained that this was the final evening in her series of presentations. The agenda for the evening consisted of two parts. The first part of the evening would be spent looking at how to work effectively with thoughts. The second part would be about the golden breath. I felt an immediate stir of curiosity and anticipation. Tuku opened the meeting by reviewing the common challenges of managing thoughts. This was a big problem for the villagers, she said, and the Shaolin monks came up with a fun process that was drawn from the ocean theme. I had always struggled to control my thoughts and was looking forward to what she had to share.

Tuku took a sip of tea and started. "The mind and thoughts are like the ocean. They are constantly in motion. Meditation can soothe and slow down thoughts, but it cannot stop them. The Shaolin monks developed what they called the "aquarium process" for gaining control over the natural movement of thoughts. The monks likened thoughts to fish swimming around in the blue ocean. As there are all sorts of thoughts, they used their imaginations to create fishes and sea creatures to represent them. This process gave each thought an identity and form that could be managed and directed. Some thoughts are loud and tenacious in grabbing our attention. An example would be thoughts of cancer, money worries, and broken relationships, to name just a few. Then there are the happy thoughts like vacations, time with friends, and joyful events. As I am sure you all know, it is often the loud and tenacious thoughts that tend to get the most air space in our heads. In my case, it was hard to stop thinking about cancer. This was a loud and tenacious thought that became harassing, dominant, hard to get out of my head, and kept me awake at night. Negative thoughts such as these can also lead to excessive stress and ultimately diminish your immune system.

"The Shaolin monks taught the villagers to use their imagination to create images of fishes and sea creatures that represented each of their negative and challenging thoughts. With the thought represented as a fish or sea creature, it was natural for it to be in motion, and the next part of the process is to see it swimming from left to right, away from you. It is important to remember that you are not trying to stop or get rid of thoughts.

"As most of you know, the more you try to *not* think a thought, the more it keeps showing up. This process acknowledges the thought and gives it an identity that you can control. With distressing or worrying thoughts you can create a fun visual with the colors of your choice. For example, when I was dealing with worrying thoughts about my breast cancer, I saw it as a brown shark with pink pinstripes. I gave it the made-up name *Dirga*. Whenever it popped into my mind, I acknowledged it and saw it moving from left to right as it swam past. I found that giving it a name like Dirga displaced the impact of the word *cancer*, and I felt a new sense of power over the word.

"I also had happy thoughts. For example, I had planned a vacation to a beautiful mountain resort that made me happy whenever I thought of it. For this vacation, I visualized a sparkly pink dolphin that I called Molly. Whenever Dirga came swimming by, I would visualize Molly swimming behind. If Dirga hovered, I would imagine Molly nudging Dirga to keep going. Giving this sort of identity to thought forms made them much more manageable and fun. I did this for large and small thoughts. The more I practiced, the more they all seemed to be swimming in the same direction. As a result, my mind became much more peaceful, and I had a real sense of control. So, I went from being controlled by my thoughts to being *in control* of my thoughts.

"The key for me was not trying to stop or eliminate challenging thoughts. I know that this process sounds almost too good to be true. But trust me, the Shaolin monks spent years developing these processes. What they taught the villagers was the essence of powerful psychological tools developed through deep inner work that were cultured into simple and fun-to-do processes. As with all processes, you need to allow yourself time to learn and practice them," Tuku said, taking a sip of water.

"I want to repeat that the aim of this process is not to eliminate or numb your thoughts," she continued. "Thoughts often have messages and important information for you. This process is designed to provide you with a tool for managing and relating to your thoughts. In particular, it will help with the more challenging thoughts of worry around the word *cancer*.

"This process provided me with a way to order and direct my thoughts. One of the things that really helped me with the more challenging thoughts was to set a time of day when I would communicate with them. It was like making a date. For example, if I had a worry about losing my job due to my cancer, I would set a time of day when my energy was strong to sit down and commune with it, using the nondominant handwriting process. I was often surprised with the insights that communication with challenging thoughts provided. For instance, I had sad thoughts about the loss of my mother. When I did the nondominant handwriting process, the sadness communicated to me that I needed to slow down and grieve her loss. I had been running fast and did not take the time I needed to deal with the loss. It was the reoccurring thoughts about my mother and the sad feelings that guided me to do the work of fully grieving her. After I did this, the sad thoughts about her went away, and my thoughts about her were happy ones.

"I felt gratitude for what a wonderful mother she had been and how lucky I was to have had her as a mother," Tuku said.

"When I was initially diagnosed with cancer, I was deluged with negative, worrying thoughts. It seemed that all my fishes were dark and troublesome. I had no hopes and dreams. Cancer is not just a physical illness. It has a psychological presence that directly affects your physical health. The Shaolin monks taught me that healing cancer is not just about removing it from your body. This is obviously the priority. But the other level of healing is to remove the fear of cancer. Even just the fear of getting cancer, or the fear of cancer returning is a form of invisible cancer that can feed the physical manifestation of cancer.

"The Shaolin monks taught that the way to eliminate the fear of cancer is not to try to remove the fear of cancer. This attention actually *feeds* it with energy. The way to remove the fear of cancer is to live, love, and thrive more.

The two key words are purpose and passion. The key action is doing acts of kindness. In this way, the treatment for cancer and the prevention of cancer are the same. The monks' message was simple: choose to live with purpose and passion on your own terms.

"I have taught the 'aquarium process' to a number of people. I did this with a friend who had been cheated in business by a partner. The partner syphoned off the company profits behind the other's back, which led to bankruptcy. My friend carried enormous rage and anger toward the cheating partner, and it began to have a debilitating effect on her health. She imagined the face of the partner on a fat, flabby, gray fish, and it helped her to release the energy of anger. She also communicated with the fish and gained valuable insights into how to move beyond the anger and rage. If she had not done this, the anger and rage would have destroyed her life. By using her imagination, my friend was able to heal and learn valuable lessons that helped her develop her own, more successful company.

"I personally like using the imagery of fish and sea creatures, but you should listen within for what works best for you. Another friend of mine had a cheating husband, and whenever he popped into her thoughts, she gave him the image of a scrawny rat swimming past her. The key is to use images that work for you and your imagination. The more fun it is, the easier and more effective it will be.

"One final thing," Tuku said. "Thoughts and worries only exist in the blue ocean. They cannot exist in the white ocean of the soul or the golden ocean of Divine Presence. To minimize the tyranny of negative thoughts, it helps to spend time in the white and golden ocean within."

Tuku invited questions. The elderly, retired gent I had been speaking with put his hand up. What he said shocked me. "I have just been diagnosed with prostate cancer. My head is full of worry and fear. I like all your processes and use them from time to time. But there are certain situations during treatments when I can't even keep focused for three breaths. Do you have any suggestions as to what I might do?"

Tuku thanked him for his question and asked him how many breaths he could focus for.

"Honestly, all I could manage is one full breath," he said.

She smiled and said, "Good. I know of a one-breath meditation that Brock developed called the credit-card meditation. It consists of one breath."

What on Earth was a one-breath credit-card meditation?

The elderly man looked a little confused as well.

Then Tuku asked Brock if he would be open to sharing this process with the group.

Brock sat next to Tuku. It was good to see him in plain view at the front of the group. I felt a strong energetic connection right away. He was wearing a nice, white, cotton shirt with a light-blue check. My eyes went straight to the curly chest hair that seemed to be trying to escape from his unbuttoned shirt collar.

Flashing into my mind came a naughty visual of me ripping his shirt off, throwing him to the floor, and climbing on top of him. I had to forcibly shift my attention to what he was saying. Perhaps this was a premonition of what was to come when I invited him for dinner. I felt a nice little stir of teasing energy down in my groin. A rather loud voice in my head shouted, *Focus, focus, focus!* And I brought my attention back to the room.

Brock thanked Tuku for inviting him to share. "The credit-card, one-breath meditation I am about to share with you came out of a visit to the bagel store. First, I would like to share with you the story of how this was created.

"Early one morning," he said, "I popped into my favorite bagel store for a bagel and a good read. The manager of the store is a friend, and he was running the counter. 'Brock,' he said, looking rather tired and stressed. 'Can you recommend a book on meditation?'

"I have many books on meditation I could have recommended, but I was unclear as to what he was really asking. So, I asked him what he wanted to achieve with meditation. He shrugged his shoulders and said he wanted to relax more. Knowing that he had a newborn baby and a three-year-old at home, I asked him how much time he had each day to devote to meditation. He shrugged and said, 'I don't really know.' This meant to me that he did not have any spare time to devote to a regular meditation practice.

"When the time came to pay for my bagel and coffee, I handed him my credit card, which he inserted in the credit-card machine. At that point, we both went silent as we waited for the card to be read. It was a glorious little window of silence and stillness that lasted for the length of one full breath. Then he pulled out the card and resumed his busy pace. I watched him do this with all his customers.

"As I was munching on my bagel, I pondered the question of how to use one full breath for a meditation, because this was all the time he had.

"From my musings I came up with the credit-card, one-breath meditation and wrote it on a piece of paper. After I finished my bagel, I gave him the sheet of paper and spent one minute explaining it before heading out. I went about my day and didn't think about the credit-card, one-breath meditation I had shared with him.

"A week later, as I was headed for another visit to the bagel store, I pondered the credit-card meditation and wondered if it had made any sense to him. I entered the bagel store aware that he might look at me as if I were nuts.

"When he saw me, he immediately came out from behind the counter and pulled me to a quiet corner. Then he shared with me why he had asked me for a book on meditation. He had been having serious relationship problems with his wife and was on the point of leaving her and their two children. He said that the credit-card, one-breath meditation really helped him slow his thoughts down and become focused, which helped him to see how much he was about to lose. They had both made the decision to work things out.

"I was shocked. After he shared his story, I ordered my regular coffee and a bagel. As I went to hand him my credit card, he waved it away and said, 'This one's on me.' So that's the origin of the credit-card, one-breath meditation process I am about to share with you. This meditation is taken from the golden breath process and that of feeling loved by the divine," Brock said.

"I am going to explain the credit-card meditation process first. Then we can all do it together. There are four parts to the one full breath. Breath in. Breath in retention. Breath out. Breath out retention. Breath in and breath in retention is one half. Breath out and breath out retention is the second half.

"There are two sets of words that go with the two halves. The first set is 'I am.' It is said quietly as an inner voice during breath in and breath retention. The second set is 'loved.' It is said quietly as an inner voice during exhalation and exhale retention. The flow of the breath is one slow breath in and hold it for a few seconds. During this time, you say, 'I am.' Then you breathe out slowly and hold the breath out for a few seconds as you say 'loved.' This is the first phase of the credit-card breath.

"Once you become comfortable with phase one, you have the option of moving on to phase two. For phase two, as you breathe in and hold the breath, you imagine golden light pouring down from above through the crown of your head and filling up your heart. As you breathe out, imagine the golden breath is expanding your heart like a balloon and there is a beautiful bubble all around you. Imagine that the outside of the bubble is six inches outside your physical body. This is phase two.

"Once you have become comfortable with phase two," Brock said, "you have the option of moving onto phase three. For phase three, you will imagine how it feels to be loved by the divine and then create a facial expression to match it. You hold this facial expression for the full four parts of the breath. This is one of my favorite parts of the process. I feel the effects from head to toe. This is phase three.

"Once you have become comfortable with phase three, you have the option of moving onto phase four. You will need to do phase four in a private setting. You are going to speak the words aloud with your eyes closed. This will give them an extra-strong resonance within you. The words spoken during the breath retention are 'I am,' and when you hold the breath out, you say, 'loved.'

"The meditation goes like this. As you breathe in with your eyes closed, imagine the golden light pouring down through your crown and filling your heart. When you hold the in-breath, say with strength, 'I am.' As you breathe out, see the golden energy expanding your heart. When you hold the out-breath, say the word, 'loved.' As you become familiar with this process, you can adapt it to suit your own creative needs. This one-breath, credit-card meditation is a powerful and easy process. I use it throughout the day."

Brock asked us to make ourselves comfortable so that we could experience the credit-card meditation. He took us through the steps one by one. It was easy to learn. Then we all did phase four together, saying in unison, "I am...loved." It was an incredibly powerful experience and seemed to energize me from head to toe. There seemed to be a great buzz of energy in the group.

Brock asked the elderly gent how it was for him. The man was in tears. Brock allowed him some time, then he asked if the man would share why he was crying.

The elderly gent pulled himself together. "You see, Brock, because I was unable to focus on even three breaths, I was feeling a bit of a failure. This was diminishing how I felt about myself, and I was on a downward spiral. This credit-card meditation is fabulous and has given me a sense of control again. The meditation itself makes me feel wonderful, and I know that I can use this throughout my day in any situation. It is a game changer for me. My tears are out of gratitude for taking the time to teach this to me."

Brock took his seat in the group again, and Tuku suggested we take a fifteen-minute break. I headed outside with Goth Girl.

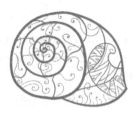

Chapter 63

The Golden Breath Introduction

As soon as we got outside, Goth Girl wanted to know what I thought of the credit-card meditation. I pointed to the sandals I was wearing without socks. I joked that I was wearing big, heavy-wool socks when I arrived, and Brock had blown them off. We had a good laugh.

I told her that he had just redefined meditation for me. Instead of aiming to meditate for thirty, twenty, or even ten minutes, this seemed to take away the subtle pressure to achieve my goal. One breath at a time flipped everything upside down and gave me a whole new freedom. And what I really loved about it was that I could do it anywhere, anytime, with or without my eyes being open. I used to think that I was restricted to certain times and places to meditate. I also liked the facial part. Just creating a warm smile of being loved shifted my emotions in a beautiful way.

Brock popped his head out and invited us back in for the second part of the evening. There was something about the term *golden breath* that resonated with me, and I was really looking forward to Tuku's presentation.

As we took our seats, Tuku was sitting quietly at the front of the group with her eyes lowered to the floor. I could feel the same energy radiating from her that I experienced when she was sitting quietly in the coffee shop booth. I knew she was doing the golden breath.

The group became quiet, and she continued to keep her eyes lowered to the floor. I think she was providing us with an experience of the golden breath before she explained it.

I found myself becoming peaceful, and soon her radiating presence seemed to fill the room. After a few minutes, she slowly raised her head and beamed a loving smile at everybody in the group. *Wow!* I thought. *The whole room is glowing. It seems that this golden breath—whatever it is—is contagious in the best of ways.*

She took a sip of tea and began. "Welcome. It is my pleasure to share with you the golden breath process. The golden breath process leads naturally on from the three oceans meditation, when you arrive at the center of the golden ocean. I was taught the golden breath process by the Shaolin monks over ten years ago.

"It was a process they developed from their many years of deep spiritual practices," she said.

"I would like to share with you my own personal experience of the golden breath process. The golden breath brings me into direct relationship with the Divine Presence. *Divine Presence* is the term I use. Some of the other terms used are God, Divine Mother, The Beloved, Jesus, and Higher Power, to name just a few. It is important that you use a term that speaks to your own belief system. People who are atheists and who do not believe in a higher power, can use *love* or any word that has deep meaning for them.

"There are four stages of the golden breath. Each of the first three stages has a set of words. The fourth state is experienced in silence.

"I will explain the breathing process later, but the three sets of words for the first three stages are *I am loved. You are loved. We are loved.* Then the words dissolve or melt into the experience of love. Another way of saying this is that first you receive love. Then you give love. Then you give and receive love. And then words are not needed, because love is all there is.

"A series of visualizations supports this breathing process. First, I will explain how the process works, and then I will guide you through it. To learn this process, you will be lying down. Once you have fully learned and mastered the process, you will be able to use it in a sitting or standing position too. Today, you will be lying flat on your back and may use small supports under your knees and head. You should make yourself comfortable, so feel free to use a blanket.

"Your ankles will be crossed, creating a circuit of energy through your legs. Your hands will also be connected and placed over your chest with your fingers interlocked. The tips of your thumbs should be touching each other. Once they are in this position, you will slowly lift your thumbs in the direction of your chin, maintaining contact, to create a three-sided triangle. The center of the triangle should be in the center of your chest. The triangle symbolizes ascension, illumination, and manifestation. The middle of the triangle will be the focal point for the golden breath.

"The process begins with your imagination. Use the image of a downward spiral with three turns to take your awareness into the center of your chest. You will begin by gently breathing through your nose. Visualize a small flame like a candle flame in the center of your chest. As you breathe gently in and out, the flame will slowly grow, extending up through the center of the triangle, up through the roof, up through the clouds, and up into the solar system.

"As you gently breathe in and out, you will become aware of a nurturing warmth coming from the flame that makes you feel good all over. Inside the flame is a special chamber that is pitch black. The outer surface of the flame represents a purification process that will burn off all aspects of ego and projections. The aim is to use your imagination to enter the flame with the innocence of a child," Tuku said.

"Inside the flame, you will imagine that there are two chairs. You cannot see them. One chair is for you, and the other is for the Divine Presence. In the empty chair, you will imagine that the Divine Presence is sitting there. Once again, the chamber is pitch black, so you will be gazing through darkness at the Divine Presence. And you know that in the darkness, the Divine Presence is gazing back at you.

"After a couple of breaths to center yourself, you will begin the series of four stages. For the first three stages, you will use the 'ocean breath.' You breathe in and out through the nose. The ocean sound is created by narrowing the throat and air passages, which creates a rushing sound like the ocean. The final stage is silent," she said.

"The first stage consists of three ocean breaths. Breathe in and out slowly, pausing at the end of the inhale and exhale. Imagine that the Divine Presence is sitting across from you, listening to your breath.

"For the second stage, you will continue to use the ocean breath, but you will imagine that the sound is coming from the Divine Presence and that you are listening to the sound of the breath.

"For the third stage, you will use the same ocean breath and imagine that you and the Divine Presence are both breathing at the same time. Together you are creating the sound of the ocean breath.

"For the fourth stage, you will imagine that you are both breathing together in silence without any words. You will breathe in and out in silence, imagining that you and the Divine Presence are breathing together. At this point, you will feel a beautiful union between you and Divine Presence taking place. Although this is a very personal experience, I have heard many reports of it being a transcendental moment. You may continue with the three silent breaths, repeating them for as long as you want. When you are ready, you can thank Divine Presence and imagine yourself moving out of the flame. In your own time, see the big golden flame getting smaller and returning to the size of a candle in the center of your chest," Tuku said.

"When you are ready, the flame becomes smaller and smaller until you can no longer see it. It will wait for your return. When you cannot see the candle flame in the center of your chest, begin the spiral up to the surface, following three turns of the spiral. You will arrive back in the center of the triangle made by your thumbs and fingers. When you are ready, you can begin the outward series of nine spirals to take you out of the golden ocean, through the white ocean, and into the blue ocean.

"When you are ready, you will release the hands and uncross your ankles," she said.

"In your own time, come back to the room and begin to move your fingers and toes as you come back into your body.

"So, the golden breath occurs when you and the Divine Presence merge into one with the silent breath. At this point, words become as garments you release to the floor, and you become naked in order to enter a relationship with the Divine Presence," Tuku said.

"The silence you experience in the golden breath is not simply the absence of sound. This silence is palpable—a kind of subtle substance that you can almost touch. This silence is like a holy place you enter to be with and merge with the Divine Presence. So, when you take these three, silent golden breaths, you are breathing as one with the Divine Presence.

"When you breathe the golden breaths, you have no sense of control or of being in your body. I can only describe it as a luminous experience beyond anything that words can describe. Each person who does the golden breath will have his or her own experience," she said.

"There are two other things I need to mention. First, it will take time and practice to find that place of pure release into the golden breath. It is important that you practice simply for the joy of the practice. If you are doing the practice to gain some result, it means that your ego is involved, and you will negate the opportunity to experience the gifts of the golden breath. The keys here are trust and humility. If ego raises its head, then you will not be able to experience the full luminosity of the golden breath.

"The second thing you must know is that Divine Presence may not always show up. There may be some days when you enter the flame that you do not feel the nearness of Divine Presence. On these days you may still have a deeply relaxing experience. Divine Presence is not your right or something you can ever own. It is a gift that is given, if you are deemed worthy. Your worthiness is based on humility and love. You can't achieve or earn a relationship to the Divine Presence. It can only be given. The fundamental attitude should be one of gratitude. You will live with the understanding that everything in life is given to you, beginning with every breath you breathe."

Tuku went silent, allowing us time to absorb what she had shared. Then she asked for questions.

An attractive middle-aged woman asked how the golden breath relates to everyday life.

"The golden breath brings me to a place of luminosity that permeates and informs the three oceans and every part of my life," Tuku said. "It cleanses the distortions that are in my blue ocean, and I feel that I am living with a sense of higher guidance. It is as if the blue and white oceans become as clear lenses through which the golden light from the golden ocean shines out into the world. When the blue ocean is in harmony, it means that your divine purpose is expressed through every aspect of your life. Your ego and rational mind become instruments of the Divine Presence."

A young guy in a business suit put his hand up. "What is the relationship of the golden breath to birth and death?"

Tuku paused for a few seconds before answering. "Now, that is a lovely question," she said. "The golden breath existed before you were born into this world, and it will continue after you leave this world. The golden breath represents the relationship of your soul to the Divine Presence. When you are born, it is placed inside the blue ocean of your ego and rational mind, which is formed by your parents, teachers, and experiences in life. To reclaim your connection to the Divine Presence, often a person needs to release many early life experiences that served a purpose at the time, but later in life act as constrictions.

"The practice of the golden breath is a way to restore true purpose and meaning to your life. The Shaolin monks created a special metaphor to help the villagers understand birth and death. Imagine that being born is like showing up on the first day of college. There is a chosen curriculum ahead of you for a certain period. The curriculum that you and Divine Presence chose was appropriate for the gifts you brought to this life and what you want to learn during your life.

"There is a basic design or template to your life, but you are also given free will, which means you will be steering your own life. The way to fulfill your destiny is to live in accordance with the call of your soul and Divine Presence. The challenge comes as the blue ocean of ego and intellect is developed: you may choose to follow a different path than the one your higher purpose has for you.

"As with college, there will come a time when your life or curriculum is complete, and you will be called to your home in spirit. You in the West often call this death. The Shaolin monks call it a sacred homecoming. They know that their spirits will someday join again with those they are connected to in this life. They understand that what we call death in this existence is but a birth back into the realm of spirit. Because everybody has a unique curriculum or journey in life, it is important not to compare your life to the lives of others. It is natural to want a carefree life without any major challenges, but this mostly comes from the cultural messages created by Disney and Hallmark.

"When you go to college, the tough task-master teacher often teaches you more than the laid-back, easygoing one does. A more challenging curriculum will teach you more. So, it is with life; the more difficulties and challenges life throws at you, the more lessons you will learn."

I loved her answers. Everything she said made so much sense. I loved the golden breath process and couldn't wait to experience it. Tuku suggested a break, and I headed to the restroom.

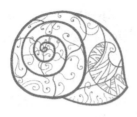

Chapter 64

The Golden Breath Experience

When I returned from the bathroom, I noticed that the chairs had been moved away, and blankets were spread out all over the floor. I joined the other people who were lying down in preparation for the golden breath process.

Goth Girl was helping, and she came along and slipped a bolster under my knees. Then Tuku came along with a lavender eye pillow, which really made me feel nurtured. When everybody had settled down, Tuku asked us to deepen our breathing to get ready for the golden-breath process. She suggested that we allow the process to unfold and not let the mind try to work out what is happening. Next thing we had to do was cross our ankles and cross our hands over our chests with fingers interlocking. Our thumb tips had to touch, and then we moved them upward along the chest until they formed a triangle. The center of the triangle was over the center of our chests. I was feeling very comfortable. Tuku directed our attention to the outer point of our blue ocean and gently guided us along the nine spirals that led us to the center of our chests and the golden ocean.

Next came the downward spiral of three turns, taking my attention to the center of my chest. I had the sense of leaving the outer world and entering deeply into my own internal world. Tuku's voice was soft and warm. With the next few breaths, I imagined a small yellow flame coming out from the center of my chest and moving up through the triangle on my chest. The flame continued to grow and reach upward through the ceiling, the roof, the clouds, and up into the heavenly realms.

After several slow, deep breaths, Tuku invited us to release all expectations as we prepared to enter the flame. I used my imagination to move through the outer flame and enter the inner chamber. I felt an incredible sense of silence. She suggested we imagine taking our seat in the dark chamber within the flame. I imagined a chair in front of me, with the Divine Presence sitting there, gazing at me in the darkness. I imagined that my eyes were open and that I was gazing through the darkness and into the eyes of the Divine Presence. I was surprised at how real it felt.

Tuku invited us to start the ocean breathing by narrowing the backs of our throats and breathing through our noses.

"Bring your awareness to the sound of the ocean breath coming in and going out," she said. "Feel the sound coming from deep within you and listen to the sound of the in and out breath for the next three full breaths."

This felt really good, and I felt a deep peace throughout my body.

"When you are ready," Tuku said, "imagine that the Divine Presence is sitting in front of you in the darkness. Imagine that the ocean breath is coming from the Divine Presence. Listen to the ocean breath coming from the Divine Presence for three full breaths."

I felt a gentle shift and the expansion of my energy. It was an immediate sense of some other presence being with me. It was very comforting.

"When you are ready, imagine that the ocean breath is coming from both you and the Divine Presence. Your breathing is merged into one. Listen to the sound of this beautiful merged breath for three full breaths," Tuku said.

I had the sense of expansion again and an absence of needing to exert any effort. It was as if I was being lifted by some beautiful energy, and all I had to do was surrender.

"When you are ready," Tuku said, "ease into the silent breath and imagine that you and the Divine Presence are breathing together."

The shift from the ocean breath to silence made me feel as if I had released my whole body and had become pure spirit. I wanted to stay there forever. I could not separate the Divine Presence from me. We had become one. The darkness of the chamber seemed to fill with golden light. I had transcended the denser, earthbound energies and had become one with my soul and the Divine Presence. I had the sense that this was who I was before I came into this world and it would be what I return to when my journey in life was complete. I felt that the blue ocean of my ego and rational mind was like a sort of outfit I was wearing for my journey on Earth. Now I understood what I kept feeling in Tuku. It was her soul body merged with the Divine Presence.

Tuku invited us to stay with the silent breath for a few more rounds and then make our way out through the wall of the flame and back into our bodies. I didn't want to leave. I wanted to stay here forever. I sensed that this is what lives on the other side of what we call death. I sensed that what we know as death is simply a shedding of the robe of ego and rational mind. In this place of union with Divine Presence, I had become pure love. I now understood how the blue ocean of ego and rational mind could be used to share this pure love with the world. I also understood how it could be used to trap this love inside, where it would atrophy through lack of use. The feelings of deep loneliness that I used to experience were, in fact, a cry for me to return to this place of deep luminous love that lived inside me. So, this was the incredible golden breath! I knew that my life would never be the same.

Tuku invited us to take our time in returning to the room and our bodies. When we were ready, she guided us to move our fingers and toes and move gently into a seated position.

We put away the blankets and brought the chairs back. As some of the group took a restroom break, I sat quietly, bathing in the glow of luminous love that I was feeling. It was a luscious feeling, like being in a hot tub full of love.

Tuku was sitting very quietly at the front of the room as the group came back.

"Welcome back!" she said beaming a big smile at us. I glanced around the room and noticed that everybody seemed to be emanating peace. There was a sense of radiance in the room that had not been there before. Tuku asked if there were questions. Nobody moved. I had the sense that we all just wanted to stay in this soft and gentle place. She suggested that we drink some water and get some air before the last lesson of the evening: how to do the golden breath in a seated position. Goth Girl handed me a bottle of water, and together, we walked—or rather, floated—outside for some air.

She was keen to hear my thoughts about the golden breath. I ran it through my thoughts but struggled to find words to describe it. I was still feeling the deep inner glow and felt that if I tried to put it into words, I would lose something of the actual experience. My full heart was the true answer. I tapped my heart a couple of times, and Goth Girl knew immediately. We spent a few minutes in silence and then headed back in.

Tuku said that we could also experience the golden breath when we were seated in a chair. It was like the lying-down process. We should sit comfortably and close our eyes as we take some deep, relaxing breaths. Then we should imagine that we were in a dark room and that the Divine Presence was sitting in a chair directly in front of us, gazing lovingly into our eyes. We follow the same breathing process, listening to the ocean breath within us for three breaths. Then we imagine the next three ocean breaths coming from the Divine Presence. After that would come the three shared ocean breaths. The final piece was the three silent breaths shared with the Divine Presence.

I loved the sound of this and was keen to try it out.

Tuku asked if we would like to experience the seated golden breath. Everybody nodded.

We all began the seated golden breath process. I was amazed at how quickly I could feel my energy lighten and shift into a higher vibration. When we arrived at the three silent breaths, I felt the same sense of golden luminosity in and around me. There was the same sense of union with the Divine Presence. It was glorious. When Tuku brought us all back into the room, there was that same sense of radiating peace.

"Any questions?" asked Tuku.

A middle-aged woman in the back row put her hand up. "The golden-breath process is truly remarkable. I have been meditating for many years for long periods at a time, yet I have not experienced the same sense of inner luminosity as I did with the golden breath. And the golden breath is so much quicker and takes me much deeper. Why is this?"

Tuku thanked her for the question. "You raise an important point. The Shaolin monks devote much of their lives to the study of meditation and deep inner work. In the early days, they also spent extensive periods in meditation. As the spiritual vibration of the planet has evolved, the vibrational frequencies available to us have all sped up. Look at technology and how fast computers can process information. As spiritual beings, we have different processing chips than we had many years ago. The golden-breath process was developed by the monks in accordance with the spiritual vibration of the planet. Many of the old systems of meditation were perfect when they were created, but they have not moved forward in harmony with the vibrational evolution of the planet.

"One of the problems is the entrenchment of the old mental formulas that many systems of meditation are based on. The key to the golden breath is using and trusting the imagination to create what we ask it to create. The Shaolin monks know that the imagination is one of the most powerful spiritual tools we have. The problem is that people do not trust their own spiritual creativity and rely on old trusted methods. So yes, the golden-breath process will seem much quicker, and yes, it will take you much further, if you trust and allow it to," she said.

I really loved her answer, and it all made so much sense. Tuku closed the evening with a blessing, and I headed joyfully home.

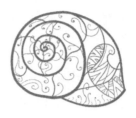

Chapter 65

A Big Surprise

I woke up thinking about Brock. He was like a beautiful presence within my heart, and I was ready to let myself fully love him with all my body and soul. All the touches, the gazes, and the sense of soul connection had brought me to the place of realizing and naming the love I knew we shared.

Ahead of me was a lazy Saturday. Over my morning cup of Joe, I started to put some plans in place for moving Brock and me to the next level. A candlelit dinner here would be the next step. I loved French-style cooking and taking hours and several glasses of wine to prepare a meal. My husband was a picky eater and never appreciated this part of me. But I had a sense that Brock really loved his food and would be seduced by the romance-laced French cuisine I would lavish on him.

The house needed a spring cleaning. Then there was the strong potential that we would end up spending the night together in each other's arms. But those plain, old, worn sheets! It was time for some sensuous new sheets for my bed.

Pink? Red, maybe? Something satin would do the trick. Then I thought about my underwear. Ah, the alarm bells started ringing. Since David left, I had resorted to my old granny underwear. *Who cares?* had been my rational. But the game was changing, and it was time for some new lace flimsies and a tantalizing nightgown. This made me think of the new lingerie shop downtown. The write-up in the paper said that it carried the finest European lingerie.

What better way to spend my Saturday afternoon? I put a second pot of coffee on and sent a text to Brock inviting him to dinner a week from today. Then I pulled out my notebook to write some love poetry. I could see the scene—the candles, the fine wine, the dark-chocolate mousse topped with fresh strawberries. Our eyes on each other's in lingering, teasing, and alluring gazes. The two of us holding back our love as mighty pent-up oceans, waiting to launch our all into each other's tides. I could see him between the sheets, his naked body lying still, his eyes pensive as I perfumed the crevices of my body he would soon be exploring. He would be like a knight errant and I would become his holy grail. I felt a deep, lust-filled desire to inhabit him like breath. I wanted my passion to be as essential as breath to him. I was feeling a sensual pulse of anticipation all over my body, so I took a cold shower.

My route downtown took me past my favorite burger bar. Since my diagnosis, I had cleaned up my diet, but every now and then I allowed myself a burger treat. I had not had any breakfast, so I felt justified in stopping for a greasy burger, fries, and large vanilla milkshake. It was yummy, and I felt nicely full as I continued my journey downtown.

I found on-street parking one block away from the fancy lingerie store. Angels must have been with me. I couldn't remember when I'd felt so good. I heard a text come in and hit the read button. It was from Brock, and I felt a spark of excitement flash through me.

Would love to share dinner with you. May I bring something? he wrote.

I wanted to respond, *Just bring your three beautiful oceans, and we can swim together as one.* But I thought it best to keep it simple.

Just bring yourself, all is good, I wrote.

As I hit the send button, I felt a spark of excitement.

Soon we would be together again. The sharing, the caring, the intimacy of trusting and being trusted. I was also aware of the physical attraction and potential, or I should say, predictability of sexual intimacy. I wanted to be beautiful and sensual for him. My thoughts went back to my lingerie and what would honor our soul, heart, and physical connection.

Black for mystery and allure? White for the virginal purity of the genteel seduction? Red for exciting, steamy-hot passion? Purple for the spiritual connection? My head was full of colorful, spinning thoughts. I arrived at the lingerie store and gazed at the sexy and sultry garments adorning the window. Talk about skimpy! I could feel my temperature rise. A variety of colors were on display. Black seemed to be the sexiest—that dark sense of mystery beckoning. I had a sense that black would hit Brock's bell. Just perusing the sexual delights in the window gave me quite a flush, and I could feel my neck glowing red. I just wanted to throw myself into his arms and lose myself forever.

I walked into the store, and a slim, well-dressed, heavily made-up sales assistant of about thirty spotted me. I could sense her scanning my body, and I had the funny sense of being undressed. It was kind of strange but sensual at the same time. Never, ever in my entire life had I bought lingerie to seduce and be seduced by a man in such a flagrant manner. Perhaps there was hope for me yet.

The young lady was very upbeat and easy to talk to. My lingerie was her job. She asked some leading questions, wanting to get a sense of intended use and the occasion. *This must be one hell of a fun job*, I thought. I gave her a quick outline of the intended scheme of seduction, and she led me to an area where mannequins stood, barely wearing filmy black garments. One good sneeze and I would have lost them. I was definitely getting in the mood.

Soon I was heading to the changing room with an assortment of skimpy garments. I felt very naughty stripping in the pink-velvet walled changing room. And when I pulled the first pair of panties up, I felt like an electric kettle being plugged in. I felt a hot flush go all through my body. This was so much fun! I settled on two sets of black panties and matching bras. Then the saleswoman led me to the negligee section. Talk about hot! One negligee in particular quickened my breath. I asked the saleswoman if it was fire retardant, and we both burst out laughing. Two negligees joined my lingerie.

Next came satin sheets in a deep fuchsia. They would be sensuous for our coursing passion and sublime for lying in stillness with our souls as one. To wrap up my buying expedition, I needed some knock-your-socks-off French perfume—only in my case, it was "knock-Brock's-pants-off" perfume. As I strode out of the store with my bags of sensual delights, I could feel an extra swagger in my hips. Then I flashed to *Pretty Woman*, the movie starring Julia Roberts. Yeah, baby, we could be twin sisters.

It was now midafternoon, and the warm sun felt good on my face.

If only Brock knew the torrent of love and seduction that was headed his way.

Or perhaps he was out doing the same? A grin broke out on my face at the prospect of Brock buying some diamond-studded Y fronts. How about some Italian aftershave? I could feel myself getting hot again. As I turned the corner and headed to my car, I glanced across the intersection and saw what looked like the back of Brock's pickup truck. *It can't be!* I thought. *Why would he be downtown?* I was curious and crossed the road to investigate. As I came within ten yards of the truck, I recognized the plates. I felt excited. *I may get to surprise him*, I thought.

I looked around and didn't see him, so I decided to hang out across the street. I would give him ten minutes. If he didn't show up, then I would head home. If he did appear, I would make a point of showing him the bags I was carrying as a tease. I found a doorway to a jeweler's store that allowed me to loiter out of sight. I could see his truck through the glass as I pretended to look at the jewelry on display.

I had been there for about five minutes when I saw the door to a coffee shop near his truck open, and out he walked. My heart jumped, and I was just about to rush toward him when I saw a petite woman with long blond hair behind him. They stood side by side, talking, for a few moments, and then they turned to walk down the street together.! What I saw next stunned me. He reached out his arm and put it around her waist.

I felt as if a cold knife had just pierced my heart. Together, with his arm around her waist, they walked slowly down the street. I was frozen and in shock. *This is not happening*, I thought. The next minute, I was out of the doorway, discreetly following them down the street. They seemed to be sharing an intimate conversation. My stomach started to feel queasy.

They turned a corner, and I followed. Halfway down the block was a posh hotel called The Gables. When they arrived outside the hotel entrance, Brock gave her a kiss on the cheek, and they walked together into the hotel lobby. It was four o'clock in the afternoon!

My whole body suddenly became like ice. My lungs felt clamped. Then my legs seemed to lock and would not move. I was headed into some form of emotional meltdown. I moved into the entrance of a pawn shop and crouched down before my legs collapsed under me.

It was difficult to breathe. I felt as if my heart had just been cut open and I was bleeding out on the street. The door to the pawn shop opened, and a creepy little man with thick, dark-rimmed glasses peered out at me.

Quick as a flash, I said, "Diabetic! Need some sugar and I'll be fine!" I started to rummage in my bag, pretending to look for something to eat.

He was staring at me with a creepy look. Then he noticed my wristwatch. "Hey, lady," he said, "how about twenty bucks for your watch?"

I felt a flash anger. "How about you give me fifty bucks for my miserable, heartbroken life, and I will throw in the watch!" I shot back.

He pulled back in surprise and retreated into his store.

My car. It was one block away. Could I make it? I wasn't sure my legs would get me there. And what about my bags of lingerie? I pulled myself back up to standing and opened the door of the shop. With one powerful swing of my arm, I launched my bags of lingerie at creepy little guy. "Here! Knock yourself out!"

I eased myself onto the sidewalk and headed to my car. My lungs still felt tight, and I was sucking in air. My legs were wobbly. I kept saying to my legs, "Right, left, right left." I walked like a zombie with my head down, doing everything I could to freeze the impending meltdown. Somehow, I made it to my car and fumbled for my keys. As I thrust the key toward the lock, I missed and scratched the paint. "Shit," I said. I got the door open and threw myself in. Then it came, the flood of icy-cold tears. I felt as if there was a cold knife in the bottom of my stomach, and I was bleeding tears. Then came the stabbing pain in my heart. I collapsed over the steering wheel as wave after wave of pain, anger, and rage poured through me.

For a good ten minutes, I was in emotional meltdown. "No, no, no!" I kept saying. But my eyes did not lie. The arm that had once been around my waist was now around the waist of some blond bitch. "Brock, not Brock!" I lamented through my tears.

Then I noticed outside the car a figure in blue, hovering. I looked up to see a traffic cop writing me a ticket. I tried to deepen my breath to get me through. Then, with no warning, the burger, fries, and vanilla milkshake ejected themselves all over the steering wheel and dashboard. It just flew out of me like a geyser! After several heaves, the wrenching feeling abated. The parking cop stood outside, staring in at me in disbelief.

I thought I should try to explain my problem. I started to wind down my window. The parking cop's head shot backward as the stench of vomit hit him. He put his hand over his nose and mouth and shouted, "You got a real problem, lady!" And he turned and quickly walked away.

The mess was unbelievable. It was all over me and the inside of the car. I pulled out a box of tissues and wiped my face and hands. I was in a bad way. I put the car in drive, and gingerly headed home. To try to drown the messages of betrayal spinning around in my head, I turned on the radio. I screamed when I heard my husband's lousy song. I punched the off button with my fist, and pain shot up my arm.

I made it home and after putting the car in the garage, I threw my clothes into the washer. Naked, I walked upstairs for a shower. Even though the house was warm, I was chilled to the bone. I put on a heavy tracksuit and climbed into bed. There was a constant pain in my heart as I replayed the sight of Brock with his arm around the blonde. Soon, the tears came. They went on and on. It was impossible to stop them. It felt as if I was crying my soul out. This went on for a couple of hours, until I just seemed to run out of tears. I needed strong coffee and headed downstairs. As the coffee brewed, I pulled out a bag of chips and started loading them into my mouth. I was trying to numb the pain I was feeling. With my big cup of joe, I crashed onto the sofa and tried to pull my thoughts together. What to do?

Slowly, Brock's betrayal was becoming reality. And Goth Girl? They were so close that I had to guess that she knew about this. I was done with these cheating assholes! But how to ease myself away from them without poisoning myself with rage?

Should or shouldn't I confront him? He deserved a good slap in the face in public for his lying and cheating, right? I felt I had the right to vengeance.

But this would wreck me emotionally, and with my new treatment beginning soon, I felt it best to slip away silently. The question was how to break away with the smallest amount of angst on my part. Brock did not know what had happened between my husband and me, so I felt justified in telling a few lies. I picked up my phone and started to type a text to him.

> Dear Brock, I need to cancel our dinner date. I have come to realize that I was attracted to you on the rebound from my husband. I am writing to inform you that I have decided to go back to my husband. He is my one and only true love. I have enjoyed our friendship, but that is all it ever was for me. My husband and I will be moving to Denver soon to pursue new career opportunities. I think it best if we have no further contact. Good-bye. Jane.

I read it over a couple of times and then thought about Goth Girl and how I would pull away from her. I did not want to see or speak with either of them again. I needed to deal with my pain before I could deal with her, so I needed a way to keep her away until I was strong again. I picked up my phone again and typed a text to her.

Dear Goth Girl, Just got a wicked good opportunity to attend a conference in Denver for work. Rushing out in a few minutes to catch a plane. Back in five days. I will be in touch when I return. With hugs, Jane.

I sent both texts.

I knew that I was in no state to go to work, so I sent a text to my boss.

Dear Mark, on new chemo, and it is really beating me up. I need to take five days. Thanks, Jane.

I was lost. My heart hurt, and all I could feel inside was despair.

I cried and cried my sadness into a pillow. The sobbing continued until I fell into a light sleep. I woke up about half an hour later with a heart hurting like hell. I went to all the windows and pulled down the shades, so it would look as if nobody was home.

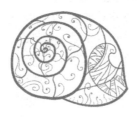

Chapter 66

An Uninvited Visitor

I spent two days in bed, living on salt. The salt came from tears and multiple bags of potato chips. There was a dark grief inside of me that had many faces.

I was grieving Brock. I was grieving Goth Girl, and I was grieving my broken hope of finding true love. I kept playing over and over my interactions with Brock. He had seemed so genuine, so honest. Why had he taken my heart when I offered it? And Goth Girl. She had become like a sister to me. I adored her. Yet, like Brock, she had betrayed me. Would I ever be able to trust my heart again? Was there something flawed in me that everybody else could see, but I could not see? I was a failure. I needed to move away to start a new life. Maybe I needed to buy an Airstream and take to the open road. Or I could go to Italy, find a room above a wine bar, and write poetry as I drank myself to death with cheap wine. I was adrift from everyone and everything. My loneliness woke me in the night screaming, "Failure, failure, failure." I had tried so hard to get everything right, but it had all gone so wrong. My only companion now was my pillow, soaked with bitter tears. I didn't know how to get out of this dark place. I didn't know that I wanted to. The image of Brock's arm around the waist of the blonde haunted me.

On my third day of misery, I was disturbed by a knock on the front door around 10:00 a.m. I thought it might be the mailman with a package. I went to the window and peeked out. I was shocked to see Goth Girl.

She must have used her "psychic seeing" that gave her a way of seeing deeper things. She was tuned into me, and I could not hide. Maybe she didn't get the text saying I was out of town. I would pretend not to be at home. After a couple of knocks, she was sure to give up and leave.

She knocked again, a little louder. I waited in silence behind the curtained windows. She knocked again, even louder. I could sense that she was impatient. I peeked again through a narrow gap in the curtains. Then I saw her turn and walk away. I felt relief. But she did not walk down the path. Instead, she turned right off the front porch and went around the side of the house. My mind flashed to the back door. I knew it was firmly bolted. Then I heard the garage door being lifted. *Oh crap*, I thought. *She's seen my car in the garage*. I heard the garage door slam. Then I saw her walk over to the garden shed. Why the hell was she going in there? I heard some rummaging around, then she appeared carrying my husband's shiny titanium ax! Oh my God, now what? She marched back to the front door and banged on it loudly. I was frozen in fear.

Then she shouted, "Listen up, Wig Girl. I know you're in there. We have two choices for how this frickin' door gets opened: You can open it. Or I can open it. If I open it, you will probably need a new front door!"

I pulled the curtains back urgently and lifted the window. "Give me five minutes," I shouted. My mind was racing now. Perhaps I should call the police. Should I take a photo of this crazed Goth Girl trespassing with an ax in her hand? I pulled on a bathrobe and headed downstairs. Fear turned into anger. Why was I cowering from her? She had been a conspirator in Brock's deceit. She had betrayed me.

I was the one who had the right to be angry. And this was my home! How dare she come banging on my door! By the time my hand touched the doorknob, I was full of anger and rage and ready to blitz this Goth Girl bitch right off my porch.

I flung open the door. I stood with my legs apart, hands on my hips. "And what the frickin' hell do you want?" I barked at her.

She slowly lowered the ax and stood there gazing at me. I could tell she was in her psychic mode. She did that "inner stare" thing. We stood there like gunslingers at the OK Corral, each waiting for the other to make a move.

I scowled at her. After a few minutes, she said softly, "Truth, honey. I have come here for the truth."

Suddenly, I felt my armor and anger being pierced. What was my truth? That I was really angry? That I had been betrayed?

She spoke again. "I have come for the truth."

She hit the release button with that one. "Brock!" I screamed. "That piece-of-crap, no-good bastard! I saw him downtown with his arm around a frickin' blond bimbo! This is the truth, and if you want more truth, I know that you know about this. Don't even begin to tell me that you didn't know, oh almighty spiritual person full of bullshit and light!"

Goth Girl just stood there, quietly gazing at me. "Your truth is beautiful," she said. "Is there more?"

My second wave of rage was brewing, and I let her have it. "I loved you both, and you both betrayed me! I trusted your sorry asses! I did not deserve this! Why? Why? Why? No! I don't want to know why! I only know that I am going to call the police to get your sorry ass off my porch!" Then came the tears. They flooded out of me. Goth Girl was crying as well.

"Is there more truth you need to share?" she asked in a gentle tone.

"No!" I screamed. "Now, piss off!" Then it dawned on me that she showed no surprise that Brock had been with the blond bimbo, which confirmed her guilt. Another torrent of rage poured out of me. "You knew! You knew! All the time, you knew! How could you have done this to me?" I was tired and spent and sobbing uncontrollably.

She stood there in silence. When my sobbing stopped, she said, "May I share my truth?"

"You're wasting your time," I replied. "But sure, knock yourself out." Then my rage rose again, and I shouted, "You've got two minutes!"

She waited for a few seconds, and when she spoke, her voice was relaxed and calm. "The blond hair was a wig."

Ah-ha! She admitted her guilt. "See? I knew it! You are nothing but a dirty cheat too!"

Goth Girl raised an index finger in a powerful gesture that communicated that it was her time to talk.

"Whatever," I said and became silent.

"Brock's little sister was wearing the blond wig when she came to town two weeks ago from Kansas to have a double mastectomy. Brock had been nursing her at the hotel where she was staying. Yes, I knew about her. Brock and I agonized over whether to tell you. We both felt strongly that your breast cancer was healing, and that you would not have to have your breasts removed.

We both felt that if you knew that his sister was having surgery, it would throw your healing into confusion and send you the wrong message. Because she was staying downtown near the hospital, we thought it best to let it unfold with discretion and tell you later."

I collapsed to my knees and started to wail loudly. She knelt by my side and wrapped her arms around me to comfort me. We both kept saying, "Sorry, sorry, sorry." After a few minutes, she helped me to the couch.

"Have you any idea how much Brock loves you? When he received your text saying you were going back to your husband, it almost killed him. He kept saying that he felt that your souls were connected, and the spiral of love would guide you both."

I sprang to my feet and dashed to the kitchen to get my phone. With urgency, I said, "I will call him and make it good. I am ready to get down on bended knee to apologize. He will understand. I just want to look into his eyes and tell him I love him with all my heart and soul."

I dialed his number and waited.

Goth Girl was shaking her head. "It's too late."

The phone kept ringing. Then I heard a phone ringing in Goth Girl's pocket, and she pulled it out. It was Brock's phone! "I'm sorry," she said. "It's too late. He's gone."

"Gone where?" I asked.

"He decided to take a couple of months away and is headed back to the monastery. He doesn't know when he will return."

"No!" I screamed. "I need to look into his eyes and tell him I love him."

Goth Girl looked at her watch, and then she typed something into her iPhone. "Well, he is almost gone," she said. "His flight leaves at noon."

I looked at my watch. It was 11:05 a.m. I had made it to the airport once in thirty minutes, but that was at three o'clock in the morning when there was no traffic. At this time of day, it would take at least ninety minutes.

Goth Girl seemed in a trance. She held her fingers up to her temple as if she were listening. I knew she was tuning into her psychic-seeing. She looked up suddenly and asked if I still had the new phone that could not be traced. "Yes," I said and went to get it from the kitchen.

She grabbed it out of my hand and dialed a number. The she did something very odd. She picked up a napkin and put it over the microphone to disguise her voice. What the hell was she up to?

A male voice answered the call. "Yes?"

"This is Mrs. Jones," she said. "I am calling to report an explosive device on flight 1204 to Hamburg, Germany, scheduled to take off at 12:10 p.m. I can identify who is carrying it. The bomb cannot be detected with scanners. I can ID the person, and I know where the bomb has been planted."

"Okay, ma'am," the man said. "What's your location?"

She gave him my address.

"I will be there in ten minutes. Please be by the curb and ready to go."

"Will do," she said and hung up. She had a wicked grin on her face.

"What are you doing?"

She laughed and explained that her boyfriend, Tony, was not just a regular cop; he was assigned to an antiterrorism squad. He had an operator-monitored emergency phone, and that was what she had called. He would be arriving soon to rush us to the airport.

I was in shock! I could not believe this was happening. Waves of fear and excitement washed though me.

"Clothes!" said Goth Girl, pointing to my bathrobe and pajamas.

I dove into the laundry basket and threw on some jeans and a sweater. Next were a pair of sneakers. I grabbed my handbag, and we were sprinting down the path to meet Tony.

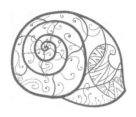

Chapter 67

The Police Cruiser

As we waited at the curb, Goth Girl wore a big grin. She said she'd get me to gate 45 before Brock's flight took off. A couple of minutes later, we heard a police siren. Then a cruiser shot around the corner and screeched to a halt outside my house. The driver's door sprang open, and out jumped Tony. When he saw Goth Girl, he shouted, "What the hell are you doing?"

"Don't ask," she said. "Just shut up and drive."

"Listen," he said. "You don't know me, and I don't know you, right? I am duty-bound to respond to all calls. I don't know what the hell you both are playing at, but get your sorry asses in the cruiser." He pulled open the back door, and we spilled in.

I was in disbelief that this was happening. The cruiser suddenly took off, throwing Goth Girl back against the seat.

I had a sense that what we were doing was really wrong, but my true love, Brock, was at the airport, and all I could think about was looking into his eyes and telling him how much I loved him. I had a funny thought that this would be a great scene in a movie. We screeched through the back streets and soon we were on the highway. What puzzled me was that there were no other cars on the road, yet this was a busy time of day. I glanced at the speedometer; we were doing over seventy miles an hour.

Up ahead, I could see blue flashing lights. Had they put up roadblocks to catch us? As we approached the flashing lights, I could see that instead of blocking us, they were blocking adjoining roads. There was a police car on each side of the road, blocking traffic and keeping our road open. I couldn't believe it.

Then Tony pulled back the glass divider between us. "What the hell are you two playing at?"

Goth Girl slid forward and said, "You just gotta trust me, honey. Brock is at the airport, and we have to stop him from leaving so Wig Girl can look into his eyes and tell that she loves him."

"What?" he shouted in disbelief. "This is your hokey-pokey psychic crap, right? Have you lost your frickin' brain cells?"

Goth Girl seemed really relaxed. "Now, honey, is that any way to speak to your girlfriend?"

Tony suddenly screeched to a halt and spun around in his seat. His face was flushed with anger. "Don't you know that you are breaking a federal antiterrorism law?" he shouted. He pointed his finger menacingly at her and said, "You, Miss Psychic Wonder Woman, will get at least three years for this. With parole, you may get off with two years in a state penitentiary." Then he pointed at me. "And *you* are an accomplice. You'll be up for at least two years. With parole, you may get it down to one year in a state pen. All because of this woo-woo stuff! Remember, I don't know you, and you don't know me. Got it?" Then he turned, and we accelerated away.

Goth Girl did not seem at all fazed by Tony's angry pronouncement that we would both end up in jail. She very casually glanced at her watch and said, "We're on track. We're going to catch him! Love rocks, baby!" And she let out a big laugh.

We were still hurtling along at ninety miles an hour. Every now and then, I saw Tony's angry eyes in the mirror. I could tell he was seething.

Then I realized that she had not reported a bomb on Brock's flight, but on another flight. I asked her, "Why didn't you report Brock's flight?"

"My guides," she said as she tapped her temple.

I was incredulous. "What, those spiritual beings you talk about?"

"Yeah!" she said. "I was going to report Brock's flight, but when I ran my finger over the flights that came up on my iPhone, I picked up a strong energy reading for the flight to Hamburg that's leaving from gate 54."

"So, what does this mean?" I asked.

"Don't know," she said. "Spirit does not send emails. It sends guidance, and I listen, trust, and respond. That's all I know how to do."

I looked at her in amazement. "But you're going to lose your dream of becoming a famous psychic," I said. "You'll be going to jail for two years. We'll *both* go to jail! This is one hell of a mess we are in! We really screwed up this time, didn't we?"

Goth Girl turned to me and smiled. "Listen up, honey. We set our intention right. Now we must sit back and let the Universe do what it has to do. I don't know how this is going to turn out. I just know that we're in good hands. Remember the white horse story? Focus on Brock and those gorgeous blue eyes of his."

As we approached the airport, I could see more blue flashing lights outside the departure terminal. We stopped near two burly cops, who were standing next to a dark-blue police vehicle I'd seen in the airport on other occasions. One of them reached out and pulled the door of the cruiser open. I noticed that Tony had turned to look at us. He was in shock. Goth Girl reached up and gently stroked his cheek, saying, "Just trust me, honey. That's all I ask of you!"

He angrily pulled his head back.

We both climbed out of the cruiser and hopped onto the waiting police vehicle. The two cops jumped on the front seat, and we shot forward. This must have been a turbo cart, and we zoomed into the terminal building with the blue light flashing.

Goth Girl looked at her watch and said that Brock's flight was due to depart at noon. The gate would close at 11:55; I would get there at 11:46, with nine minutes to spare. She used her iPhone to confirm the flight and gate number. Then she moved her finger slowly over the other flights and looked up at me, concerned. "We have to drop you off at gate 45 for Brock's flight, then I need to go to gate 54. Can't explain why. I just have this sense I have to do this."

We both clung to the seats of the car as it sped through the terminal.

"You have just given up two years of your life for me and the person I love. How can I ever repay you?" I said.

She beamed a big smile at me. "Sometimes for love, you just gotta set that intention and let it all hang out, baby!" We both roared with laughter. One of the cops turned to look at us. "All is good! Gate 45!" shouted Goth Girl.

As we approached gate 45, she shouted at the cops to stop before heading down the corridor to the gate. The driver braked, and both cops spun around to see what was going on. Goth Girl pointed down the corridor and told me, "Run like the wind. He will be waiting for you!"

I gave her a quick kiss on the cheek, realizing that this may be the last time I would see her for two years. Goth Girl barked at the cops to get her to gate 54, and they took off.

As I sprinted down the corridor to the departure lounge, people jumped out of the way. I was three minutes from being in the arms of the man I loved! I knew he would be standing by the gate waiting for me. I knew he would know that I was coming for him. I glanced at my watch; I was three minutes ahead of schedule. I was four minutes away, then three minutes away, then two minutes away, and then one minute away. I sprinted into the departure lounge.

What I saw shocked me: the departure lounge was deserted but for a petite airline representative typing on a computer at the desk near the locked boarding door. As I ran to her desk, I could see through the window behind her an airplane pulling back from the loading ramp. I pointed to the clock. "It's 11:50!" I shouted. "What's going on?"

She looked a little taken aback, and I thought she was considering calling security. I was breathing heavily, and my eyes were now full of tears. Without saying anything, she pointed to a TV screen showing a weather channel. Then in a Southern accent, she said, "The plane was boarded early and because of thunderstorms, it left ten minutes early."

"No, no!" I cried out. "My true love is on that plane!"

She looked quizzically at me. I walked to the large window and pressed my face up against it, saying his name. "Brock, Brock, Brock!" As the plane slowly taxied toward the runway, tears gushed down my cheeks. My chest felt tight, as if something had just been ripped from it. I was sobbing into the cold sheet of glass. Then I heard a polite little cough, and I turned to see the airline representative standing next to me, holding a box of tissues. She gestured toward a row of chairs and said the departure lounge would not be used for an hour or so, and I could take some personal time without being disturbed. She very gently took my arm and guided me to a chair. She gestured for me to sit down. I was feeling dazed. It was as if a bomb had just gone off in my heart.

There was a deep sense of sadness in my stomach. A little voice in my head shouted, "Five frickin' minutes!" That was all. I had lost my true love by five minutes! I slowly lowered myself onto the chair.

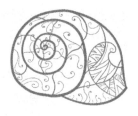

Chapter 68

The Universe Delivers

As I sat there sobbing, I realized that I had reverted to my old pattern of cause-and-effect behavior in responding to a crisis. I took a deep breath and brought myself back into the moment. I brought my awareness to the blue ocean and started to follow the spiral of love through the deep peace of my soul and into my golden center and place of Divine Presence. I immediately felt inner peace and calm wash over me. Even though I knew that the police would soon be coming to arrest me, the idea that I was loved gave me a warm golden feeling. This was the spiral of love in action. I was aware that I was an accomplice to a federal crime, yet the thought of one whole year of my life in jail did not cause me panic or regret. The reality I faced was that I would have to resign my position, and my career would be over. After all, who would want to employ a felon? I wondered how they would arrest me. Would they use cuffs? The prospect of walking out of the airport in handcuffs was something I would just flow with. And would I see Goth Girl again? The woman whose dream I had just stolen because of love? I knew that life would unfold as it needed to, and ultimately, I would use this experience *for* my growth and not remain a victim. The sense of inner peace was still in my golden center.

I heard footsteps approaching. It sounded as if just one cop had come for me. The other was probably taking Goth Girl into custody. I felt a gentle touch on my shoulder. At least the cop wasn't aggressive.

Then I heard a cough. I turned slowly and opened my eyes, expecting to see a cop. Much to my shock and amazement, Brock was standing over me.

I screamed and leaped from the chair, throwing myself into his arms.

"You came," he said. "You came. You came for me!"

Our lips hungrily found each other's, and they writhed together as we wrapped our arms around each other, clamping our bodies together tightly. Then I pulled back and explained the mistaken text I'd sent and how I had been confused when I saw him with his sister.

"I knew there had to be something else going on," he said. "I just knew our love was real. I should have told you about her. I'm sorry."

"No!" I said. "I'm sorry. I should have asked you to explain." Then I brought my hands up to cup his face and looked into his deep-blue eyes. I took a big breath and said, "Brock, I love you, I love you, I love you."

He kissed me again, and the sweetness and softness of his lips felt like heaven. This was the moment I had waited for all my life. It was glorious. I was lost and consumed in his passion and love for me, and I felt our souls merge into the golden ocean as one, luminous being.

Then we pulled back, and I asked him why he was not on the plane. He explained that security personnel had identified him as suspicious because he did not have a cell phone or any checked bags, and he had purchased a one-way ticket. The TSA officer thought he might be on the run from the law, so he was pulled off the flight for screening.

The thought that I was going to be arrested any minute popped into my mind. I told Brock the story and said the police would soon be coming for me.

"But we have the rest of our lives together, Jane," he said. "We'll get through this."

It was so comforting to hear him say "we." Then, over his shoulder, I saw Goth Girl walking toward us with the cops behind her. She was expressionless. The officers looked very serious. I was relieved to see that they had not handcuffed her. But now I would have to say good-bye to the love of my life. A year apart! What a price to pay.

I could have lost him forever, though. I knew that a year would go quickly. I turned to Brock and gave him one last kiss.

As Goth Girl approached, her expression suddenly shifted, and a big grin broke out on her face. "You'll never guess what shit just went down," she said. "So, they stopped the Hamburg flight from taking off, as per my report of an explosive device. They unloaded all the passengers and put them through security again. They searched the whole plane and found nothing. Then, as a matter of security protocol, they brought in a sniffer dog, and he found plastic explosives molded like orthotic devices inside the shoes of a passenger. They haven't found the detonator yet, but he could have triggered it with his phone. There were 410 passengers on board and eight cabin crew. Depending on where the plane went down, more lives could have been lost. So, I, with my psychic powers, have just saved hundreds of lives! These guys are taking me to a press conference. The airport wants me to be a part of their security team. Can you believe it? No jail for me or you, babe."

She pulled out her psychic business card and held it up as if offering it to heaven. "Thank you, guides! Thank you, Universe!" she said, looking up and smiling.

I was in complete and utter shock. So was Brock. I turned to him and said, "Seems I am a free bird, honey!"

Then I heard the footsteps of somebody running, and around the corner came Tony. He ran up to Goth Girl and took both her hands in his. "I am oh so sorry," he said. "I just heard what you did and all those lives you saved. I was wrong to call it woo-woo stuff. I am so sorry to have misjudged you and your spiritual gifts. Can you ever forgive me for acting like an asshole?"

Goth Girl stood on tiptoes and planted a kiss on his forehead. "Honey, I knew it was going to come out well. I just didn't know *how* it was going to come out well."

What he did next absolutely blew me away. He lowered himself onto one knee and reached out to take her hand. He looked up into her eyes and said, "Dar, will you marry me?"

She let out a scream that startled even the two burly cops. "Yes!"

Tony stood and swept her up in his arms, and they kissed as we all looked on. Then Goth Girl said, "Honey, I got this fame thing to do with the press. How about we continue with this tonight?"

"Sure thing," he said, and he put her down.

She turned to the two cops. "Okay, guys. Time to take Cinderella to the ball." And they all started laughing. Goth Girl gave me a kiss on the forehead and said, "Don't ever doubt your intentions, honey. Remember: be patient; the Universe has your back." Then they all walked off together.

I turned to Brock, and we fell into each other's arms again. Then I heard the airline representative cough to get our attention. We both turned to look at her. "Please excuse me, Mr. Williams, but on behalf of the airline, I would like to apologize for the inconvenience we caused you in missing your flight. We have booked you on the next flight to Myanmar, departing in sixty minutes, with a free upgrade to first class. Would that be okay with you?"

Without thinking about it, I reached into my bag, pulled out my credit card, and handed it to her. "Any chance the seat next to his might be available?"

She took my credit card and said to give her a few moments to see what she could do.

Brock and I were in another clingy hug when she coughed again, and we turned to look at her. She said that a seat had been reserved next to Brock's. I yelped with joy. Then she handed back my credit card and said, "Thank you, but this will not be necessary. This flight is on us."

I yelped again turned back to Brock. Our lips were hungry for each other's, and we were lost in a long and intense kiss when the airline rep cleared her throat. "Please excuse me," she said, "but while I have reservations on the line, they asked about your return flight. When would you like to come back?"

We looked at each other. Sparks flew between us, and we both spun to face the airline rep. Together, at the tops of our voices, we sang the refrain to that country song, "We ain't never coming back!"

The Author—My Cancer Story

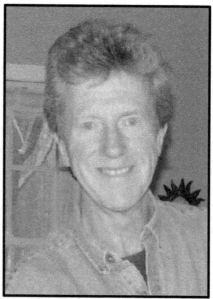

Fifteen years ago, I went for a routine annual physical examination. I had been exercising regularly, ate a healthy diet, and my life was full of color. I was feeling in excellent health and expected a good report.

I walked into my primary care doctor's office at 2:30 p.m. I walked out of his office at 3:25 p.m. with a dual diagnosis of colon cancer and prostate cancer. My life of color turned to black and white. I went home to bed, where I stayed for 24 hours. I was frightened, angry, depressed, and felt as if my life was about to end, soon!

I have had many low points in my life, and I can honestly say that this was the lowest. After 24 hours in bed, I went to the bathroom and looked in the mirror. The man looking back was unknown to me. I felt lost, adrift, empty, sad, and clueless as to how to move forward.

Cancer, like a strong wind, had just blown into my life, and I was like a ship that had just capsized. My mast and rudder were both gone, and the maps for my life were lost at sea. I felt very isolated and could not see beyond the dark, stormy clouds of the dual diagnosis of colon and prostate cancer.

I knew that I had to make a very important decision that would affect the rest of my life. Was this game over, or game on? Even though I felt as if I was about to lose everything, there was a voice deep within me that wanted me to live. I listened to the voice and chose game on, which began my journey back to health, hope, and happiness. I chose to live, to love, to create, and to claim what I wanted from my life.

And so it was, I restored my broken mast, fixed the rudder, and made new maps for where I wanted my life to go. The cancer that had blown me over and capsized my life had now become the wind in my sails.

I am pleased to say that I am now cancer free.

Author with his
own wood sculpture

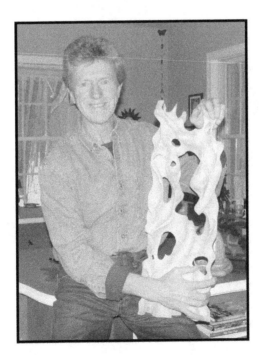

 From chapter...43

Experiencing the Wood Sculpture

THE SURGEON GENERAL'S

Certificate of
Appreciation

Presented to

Robert W. H. Wilkins (Woody)

In recognition of your extraordinary efforts on behalf of the children of this Nation. God bless your hard work and creativity on their behalf.

_____
Surgeon General

Anthonia C. Novello

Books and Programs by Woody

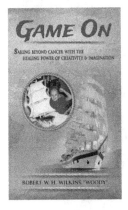

It was my own journey with cancer that inspired me to write my first book about childhood cancer, *Game On* in 2015.

GAME ON is an inspirational book about overcoming the emotional and psychological challenges of cancer. It is a fictionalized account of the true story of an eight-year-old boy called Jack, who spends ten weeks in hospital undergoing chemotherapy treatment for leukemia. Jack learns to use his creativity and imagination to partner with his medical team by fighting cancer's two assassins: fear and anxiety.

It is a fun and educational read - one that has the potential to redefine one's relationship to cancer and teach one about the power of the human spirit to overcome and rise above life-debilitating circumstances. Parents and teachers will find insights for helping children to engage and apply their own inner creative will force in the fight against cancer.

"Robert "Woody" Wilkins is one of the best I have seen working with children who have cancer and other life-threatening diseases. Woody uses his experience and keen insight to write *Game On*. It is a worthwhile book for not only families whose children are ill but also all who are in contact with them."

Howard A. Pearson MD
Past President American Academy of Pediatrics
Professor of Pediatrics Yale University Department of Pediatrics

Game On – Love it! This book is filled with truth and healing and should be read by everyone caring for and about children with cancer or other health problems. It can coach us all and help us to find peace and healing.

Bernie Siegel MD
Author of The Art of Healing and Love, Medicine & Miracles

Available at online vendors and www.DancesWithWood.org.

The Butterfly Ship Adventure Program ™

A Wellness and Empowerment Tool for Women with Cancer

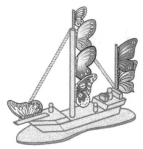

The Butterfly Ship Adventure empowers and inspires women with cancer to reclaim the direction of their lives and rekindle purpose and passion for life.

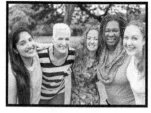

The program provides women with a series of specifically designed processes and tools, including a journaling workbook that builds self-esteem and belief in their ability to heal and overcome cancer.

The Butterfly Ship Adventure is designed to create happy and posi-tive emotions. It boosts self-confidence and self-esteem. Healthy emotions strengthen the immune system, and a strong immune system helps heal and prevent cancer.

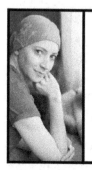

The program is designed to be used in a variety of settings.

HOSPITAL-BASED PROGRAMS
CLINIC-BASED PROGRAMS
HOME-BASED FAMILY PROGRAMS
DAY AND EVENING WORKSHOPS
PRIVATE COACHING SESSIONS

The Butterfly Ship Adventure Program *is provided by Dances With Wood.*

For more information or to make a donation, please contact:

Robert W. H. Wilkins "Woody" *Executive Director*

Email: Woody@butterflyshipadventure.org

www.danceswithwood.org

Dances With Wood is a 501(c)(3) Nonprofit Organization

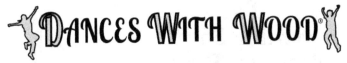

DANCES WITH WOOD

Empowering and inspiring children and adults with cancer and other serious illnesses for 20 years.

More than 40,000 people served in 40 states!

Dances With Wood is a creative arts program that serves children in hospitals who have cancer and other serious illnesses.

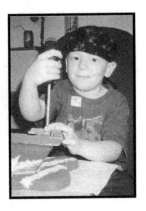

The program provides children with the opportunity to experience the transforming power of their own imagination and creativity through woodworking projects that can be undertaken while a child is sitting or lying in a hospital bed.

Provides a distraction from fear and negative thoughts.

Promotes emotional and psychological growth.

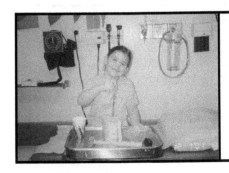

Empowered Creativity:
Heals the spirit,
provides hope,
and strengthens
the will to live.

For more information or to make a donation, please contact:

Robert W. H. Wilkins "Woody" *Executive Director*

Email: Woody@danceswithwood.org

www.danceswithwood.org

Dances With Wood is a 501(c)(3) Nonprofit Organization

The Sailing Ship Adventure Program™

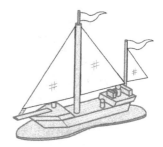

A Wellness and Empowerment Tool for Men with Cancer

The Sailing Ship Ship Adventure empowers and inspires men with cancer to reclaim the direction of their lives and rekindle purpose and passion for life.

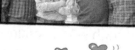

The program provides women with a series of specifically designed processes and tools, including a journaling work- book that builds self-esteem and belief in their ability to heal and overcome cancer.

The Butterfly Ship Adventure is designed to create happy and posi-tive emotions. It boosts self-confidence and self-esteem. Healthy emotions strengthen the immune system, and a strong immune system helps heal and prevent cancer.

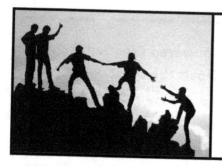

The program is designed to be used in a variety of settings.

HOSPITAL-BASED PROGRAMS
CLINIC-BASED PROGRAMS
HOME-BASED FAMILY PROGRAMS
DAY AND EVENING WORKSHOPS
PRIVATE COACHING SESSIONS

The Sailing Ship Adventure Program *is provided by Dances With Wood.*

For more information or to make a donation, please contact:

Robert W. H. Wilkins "Woody" *Executive Director*
Email: Woody@sailingshipadventure.org
www.danceswithwood.org

Dances With Wood is a 501(c)(3) Nonprofit Organization

Heart to Heart™

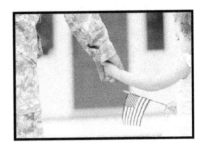

A Program to Help Heal Veterans with PTSD

Heart to Heart is a program for disabled active-military service personnel and disabled veterans. It provides an opportunity for veterans to work in community, building and painting wooden toys for hospitalized children battling cancer and other serious illnesses.

The program offers creative opportunity to "grow" the healthy, functioning aspects of the veteran, diminishing the effects of

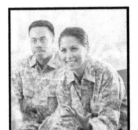

psychological dysfunction caused by post-traumatic stress disorder.

The Heart to Heart program gives these men and women a sense of purpose and meaning, which is essential to healing and living a meaningful life.

Working together with other veterans creates a sense of belonging and camaraderie that helps to promote caring, friendships, and feelings of well-being. It also encourages a sense of belonging that reduces isolation and strengthens self-esteem.

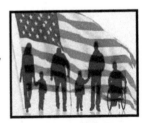

The Heart to Heart Program *is provided by Dances With Wood.*

For more information or to make a donation, please contact:

Robert W. H. Wilkins "Woody" Executive Director

Email: Woody@danceswithwood.org

www.danceswithwood.org

Dances With Wood is a 501(c)(3) Nonprofit Organization